Healthcare in the United States

Navigating the Basics of a Complex System

Deanna L. Howe | Andrea L. Dozier | Sheree O. Dickenson

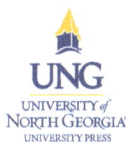

UNG
UNIVERSITY *of*
NORTH GEORGIA™
UNIVERSITY PRESS

Blue Ridge | Cumming | Dahlonega | Gainesville | Oconee

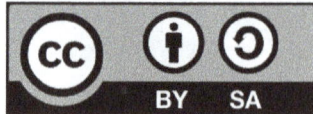

ISBN: 978-1-940771-91-5

Produced by:
University System of Georgia

Published by:
University of North Georgia Press
Dahlonega, Georgia

Cover Design and Layout Design:
Corey Parson

For more information, please visit http://ung.edu/university-press
Or email ungpress@ung.edu
Instructor Resources available upon request.

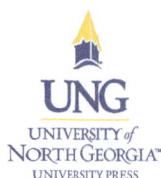

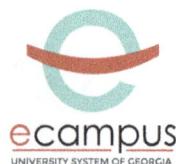

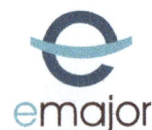

TABLE OF CONTENTS

HEALTHCARE SETTINGS ## 80

FEDERAL AND STATE FUNDED HEALTHCARE ## 104

PRIVATE INSURANCE   124

SPECIAL POPULATIONS   138

ACCESS ISSUES IN HEALTHCARE   160

COST OF HEALTHCARE   180

Acknowledgements

Contributors

Thanks goes to the individuals who provided a first-person perspective on specific topics throughout the book: Dr. Joan Darden, Dr. Michael Daugherty, Misty A. Spanberger, Deb Hairr, James Brooks, Sheila Graddy-Bennett, Brandy Bass, Samantha Wells, Terri M. Mitchell, Nicholas K. Johnson, Cynthia Chaney, Sarah Schrader and Josh Lipkowitz.

Thanks to our administrators for supporting us throughout this writing process: Dr. Sarah Brinson, Dean, Darton College of Health Professions; Dr. Cathy Williams, Department Chair, Nursing.

Thanks to the administrators from Affordable Learning Georgia, in particular Mr. Jeff Gallant, for initiating this project which serves students through no cost textbooks.

Our Team

We wish to extend a special thanks to eCampus Administrative Services, especially Dr. Sarah Kuck and Ms. Christy Talley Smith, for providing faculty authors, guidance, and support throughout the development process. We also want to acknowledge Ms. Yinning Zhang, the project manager, who guided us from the beginning to the end, and Kristy Gamble, the graphic designer, who promoted the aesthetics of this book. The peer reviewers who took the time to read all of the chapters and provide us with constructive feedback. To all the UNG Press staff, in particular Dr. Bonnie Robinson and Ms. Corey Parson, who worked diligently to ensure this book is published and in the hands of students.

Dr. Howe would like to personally thank: *my supportive and thoughtful husband for being a sounding board, reading content, and giving feedback; for supporting me through the many long nights and long months of the researching and writing process; to my children Courtney and Bailey (and their partners) for being such great people who I can call my own! You both inspire me! To my mother who has and probably always will brag about my accomplishments.*

Everyone needs a cheerleader and you have always been that for me. To my colleagues Andrea and Sheree for agreeing to work on this project with me! What a great team we are!

Dr. Dozier would like to personally thank: *God, for allowing me the opportunity to be involved in this endeavor. To my sons William, Christian, and Isaiah, thanks for your patience and sacrifices while I worked on this project. Thank you to my mom, Elizabeth Lovett, and my brother Dr. Andrew Lovett for their unwavering support and encouragement. I could never have done this without you all.*

Dr. Dickenson would like to personally thank: *my friends and colleagues Dr. Howe and Dr. Dozier for inviting me on this exciting journey. Much love and appreciation is given to my incredible husband and family who, once again, had to adapt to many nights and weekends without me. And, most importantly, I thank the Lord God Almighty, Maker of heaven and earth who makes all things possible for those who believe in Him.*

Preface

Authors Note

This text provides an overview of the basic structure of the U.S. healthcare system. Each chapter contains content describing and explaining our current healthcare system's complexities. Easy to understand terminology explains the components of the U.S. healthcare system. In an effort to create foundational knowledge, readers and students are able to focus on the basics of our healthcare system by reading this textbook.

About this Book

This book is a collaborative effort among three faculty members from the Darton College of Health Professions, Nursing Department, at Albany State University, a Historically Black College and University (HBCU), and part of the University System of Georgia. The book idea originated from a grant-funded program to create open education resources (OER) for students learning in University System of Georgia's eMajor courses. The cost of education in the United States is remarkably expensive, and the added burden of purchasing textbooks for each course can be prohibitive. The opportunity to create free educational materials has been a rewarding experience. A free pdf form of this text is available for download.

The authors of this book are registered nurses who have each worked 25 or more years in various roles and specialties within our healthcare system. There have been many changes throughout the years. The authors' experience and knowledge are from a nursing perspective not found in other texts of similar content.

The healthcare system has advanced tremendously since the very beginning of our formalized system. The most significant growth has been in technology use to support, diagnose, increase patient safety, and document patient outcomes. However, more can be done to ensure a system that meets all our citizens' healthcare needs.

Readers of this text will learn a brief history of our healthcare system and explore the current state of health in the U.S. In the next 12 chapters, readers will:

- consider health as defined using determinants of health
- discover the many types of healthcare providers seen throughout the system
- differentiate between the different types of healthcare settings
- explore state and federal programs that provide oversight
- examine private insurance and managed care plans
- survey access issues and the cost of healthcare
- review how state and federal government provides support to special populations
- discover the quick expansion of technology use in healthcare
- assess quality determinants and accreditation standards
- compare national healthcare systems presently used to the present U.S. healthcare system
- identify advantages of a national healthcare system for the United States

This book will describe and explain our current healthcare system's complexities by providing the basics of many components in easy to understand terminology. Each chapter includes essential features to assist the student in learning and understanding

- Learning outcomes, noting what the student can expect to learn by the end of each chapter.
- Key terms for each chapter content, explained and defined within the chapter and in a glossary.
- Tables, figures, pictures, and weblinks to enhance learning.
- Pause and Reflect scenarios with questions to stimulate thought about the topic.
- First person perspectives which bring richness and depth to the topic.
- Review questions to challenge the reader's comprehension.
- The current state of the U.S. healthcare system in the year 2020, including the impact of COVID-19.

The authors have written this book using APA writing format, consistent for social science and education majors, with in-text citations. This should make it easier for readers to locate the many resources used to develop each chapter. Included as companion materials are supplemental/instructor resources.
Each chapter includes:

- A course map that ensures alignment between the course learning objectives, chapter learning objectives, learning activities, and assessments.
- Student learning assessment assignment suggestions, including discussion forums, individual learning activities, and group learning activities.
- Chapter Powerpoint presentations.

General grading rubrics are also included to assess discussion forum activity and assignments. Instructors will need to update the grading rubrics to meet specific assignment criteria..

The authors hope you enjoy this book and are inspired to enter the healthcare system with newfound knowledge and a better understanding of how to navigate through the U.S. healthcare system.

Deanna Howe, Andrea Dozier, and Sheree Dickenson

1   Introduction

1.1 LEARNING OBJECTIVES

By the end of this chapter, the student will be able to:

- Define "system" in relation to the U.S. healthcare system

- Discuss the evolution of healthcare coverage in America

- Explain various government-sponsored healthcare programs

- Discuss factors influential to the development of the U.S. healthcare system

- State the goals of the American Association of Labor Legislation (AALL)

- Recall the original purposes of the American Medical Association

- State at least three historical events that influenced U.S. healthcare

1.2 KEY TERMS

- Children's Health Insurance Program

- Flexner report

- Health Insurance Marketplace

- Health Insurance Portability and Accountability Act

- Medicaid

- Medicare

- Patient Protection and Affordable Care Act

- Social Security Act of 1935

- system (U.S. healthcare)

1.3 HEALTHCARE SYSTEM DEFINED

Have you ever had to define something that was incredibly complicated? The idea can get jumbled in the head, and trying to express it coherently might be difficult. Rather than come up with one broad definition, it might be best to break the idea into smaller parts. The "idea" here is the healthcare system, which is broad, bold, and full of complexities. The "parts" are the many components of the healthcare system. The challenges are to describe the broad concept so as to make this complicated system understandable and bring a deeper meaning to the topic.

Let's start with the question: What is a system? Defining the term system is necessary to better understand its context within U.S. healthcare. Merriam-Webster (2020) defines the term system as "a regularly interacting or interdependent group of items forming a unified whole" (para. 1). For the purposes of this book, the authors have defined the U.S. healthcare **system** as being made up of an interconnecting network which provides multi-layers of components to manage the health of U.S. citizens. As noted in Figure 1.1, each colored circle signifies a component within our nation's healthcare system. The noted components are not exhaustive but represent many of the "parts" which this book will cover when describing the "idea" of our U.S. healthcare system. Each noted component contains many subcomponents which you will learn more about throughout this book. Here's an example that illustrates only a few of the many possible subcomponents within this concept: healthcare settings include hospitals, clinics, and surgical centers; federal and state funded programs include Medicare, Medicaid, and Indian Health Services; and healthcare workers include physicians, nurses, and other health professionals.

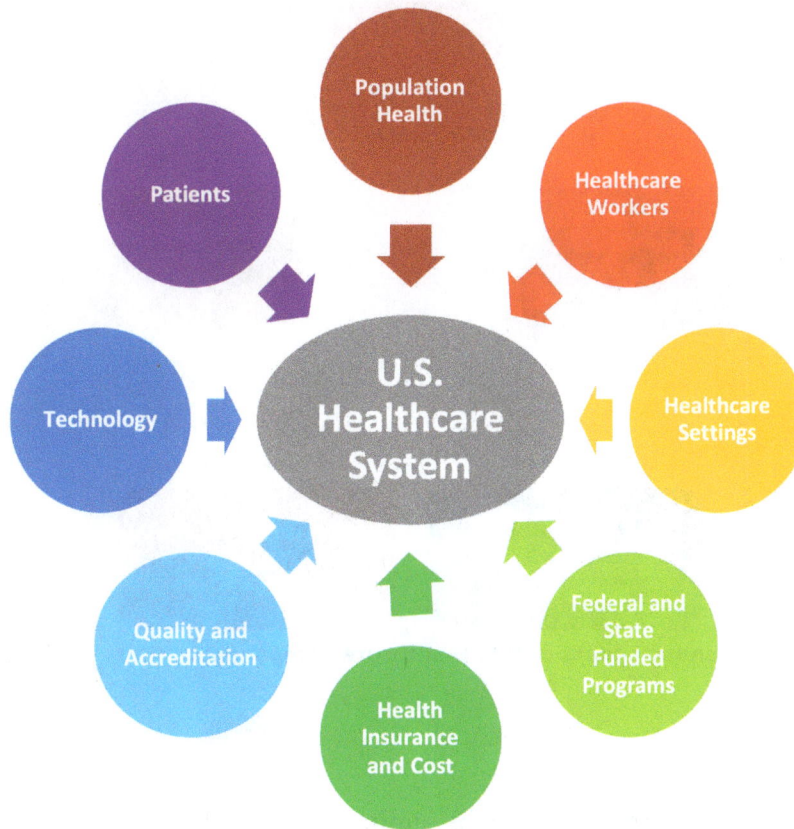

Figure 1.1: Components that make up the U.S. Healthcare System

Source: Original Work
Attribution: Deanna Howe
License: CC BY-SA 4.0

Organizations—such as The Joint Commission, Centers for Disease Control and Prevention (CDC), American Medical Association (AMA), and hospital systems—work *independently* (alone) to meet the goals and objectives of the organization and the needs of its stakeholders. Yet, each also work *interdependently* (reliant on one another) to meet goals and objectives regarding the health of U.S. citizens. This scenario exemplifies this interconnectedness: the CDC publishes a guideline for hospitals regarding hand hygiene (washing hands with soap and water) before and after patient contact to decrease the incidence of healthcare acquired infections (HAI). The hospitals then create an employee policy requiring all health workers to wash their hands prior to and after each patient interaction. Healthcare workers then implement the new hand washing policy, which may or may not reduce HAIs in patients. Hospitals will begin tracking and recording the incidence of HAIs through use of patient medical records (data collection) and will report findings to HAI surveillance systems, such as the National Healthcare Safety Network (NHSN). The CDC will collect this data and adjust or create new goals or guidelines for HAI as needed (Figure 1.2). In effect, components within the system have to work together (*interdependently*) to meet the needs of health, safety, and quality in patient care.

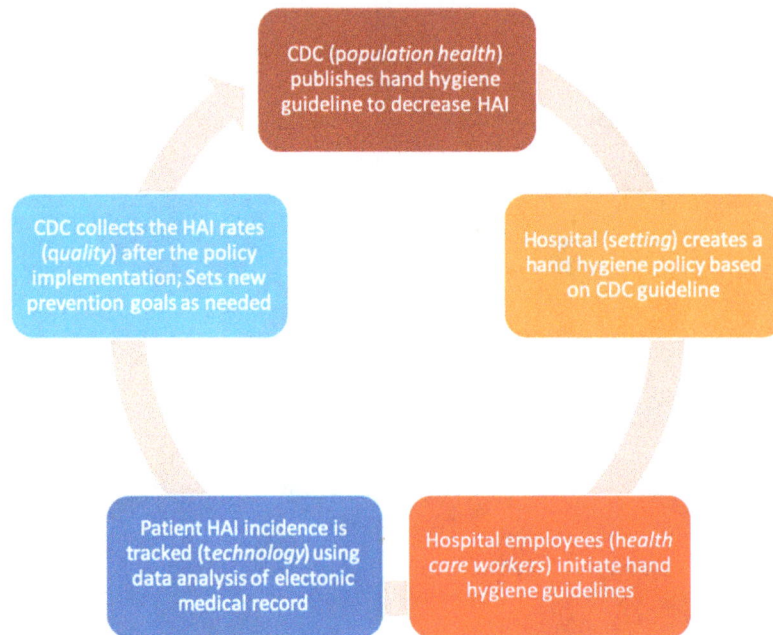

Figure 1.2: Interconnectedness of U.S. Healthcare Components

Source: Original Work
Attribution: Deanna Howe
License: CC BY-SA 4.0

The U.S. healthcare system is influenced by legislation, government organizations, employers, private organizations, and self-interest groups. These different influencers create laws, policies, and regulations which can expand or restrict access to healthcare. As a result, some U.S. citizens can rely on quick access to care and positive outcomes. However, other citizens have difficulty accessing healthcare, and many millions are without healthcare insurance. Consider the impact of COVID-19 on the U.S. economy and the millions of people forced out of work and, thus, the millions more who have lost their health insurance coverage. We will discuss the idea of a national health system in Chapter 12. This chapter will focus on the history of the U.S. health system. Looking to the past gives a better understanding of where our nation started in terms of providing healthcare.

Pause and Reflect

Have you ever had to work within a team? What was your experience? What about a sporting team? For example, consider you are on a football, basketball, or baseball team. What if only half or three-quarters of the team members were playing? How would this affect the overall structure of your team? What is the likelihood your team could win?

Now consider the healthcare system. What if only some of the components were to work together? How would this impact the overall health of the U.S. healthcare system? How could this affect an individual's healthcare?

1.4 HISTORY OF THE U.S. HEALTHCARE SYSTEM

The healthcare system in the U.S. originated in the seventeenth century (Health Entrepreneur, 2015). Historical healthcare developments during the First Industrial Revolution, Progressive Era, and the Great Depression are the foundations of the U.S. healthcare system. The advent of public hospitals as well as the evolution of nurse and physician education allowed our health system to rapidly develop. Government programs that have influenced U.S. healthcare have allowed expansion of healthcare nationwide.

1.4.1 Healthcare Workers Evolution: Women, Physicians, and Nurses

The role of women

According to Health Entrepreneur (2015), before the eighteenth century, women played a significant role in providing health to those within their household using domestic medicine. At that time, women were expected to be responsible for the healthcare needs of the home. For example, women conducted the birthing process during this time. Doctors were involved only when serious illnesses occurred (Health Entrepreneur, 2015).

Physicians

In the seventeenth century, healthcare was home-based, with traveling doctors providing basic care, such as surgery, to those in need. As the profession grew and the practice advanced, the first college for physicians was started at the University of Pennsylvania in 1765. No formal educational schools for doctors existed before this time. This college offered two educational options for attendees: Bachelor of Medicine and a Doctor of Medicine degree (Fee, 2015).

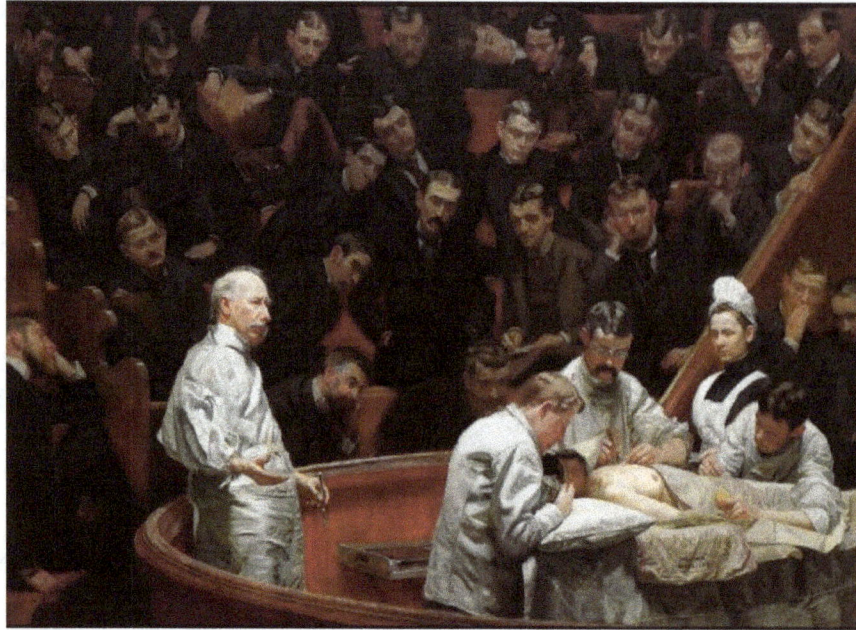

Figure 1.3: The Agnew Clinic

Source: Wikimedia Commons
Attribution: Thomas Eakins
License: Public Domain

In 1847, the **American Medical Association (AMA)** was formed to help set standards for medical training, ethics, and the improvement of public health. The AMA symbolized the beginning of organized medicine in the U.S. (American Medical Association, 2020). In 1910, Abraham Flexner published the **Flexner Report**, which was extremely instrumental in the educational preparation of physicians. This report helped with organizing medical school curricula and licensing. For example, this report suggested admission requirements for medical school and an educational emphasis on science from colleges or universities, followed by additional years of medical training (Stahnisch & Verhoef, 2012).

Nursing

Florence Nightingale (1820–1910), known as the "Lady with the Lamp," is credited with establishing the first formal care practices of the nursing profession. During the Crimean War, she reduced hospital death rates by two-thirds after initiating sanitation and hygiene standards, clean water, nutritious food, and compassionate care (*History*, 2020).

In the U.S., formal nursing education began at the New England Hospital for Women and Children in 1872 (Petiprin, 2016). The first American-trained nurse was Linda Richards. The profession of nursing evolved tremendously. While early nursing training was conducted in hospital settings, nursing education migrated into more collegiate environments with standardized examinations. The profession progressed with national standards created and state licensure to practice.

- -
First Person Perspective

Dr. D. has worked for fifty-three years as a registered nurse and forty years as a nurse educator and administrator. She is Professor Emeritus and is active in national nursing education organizations.

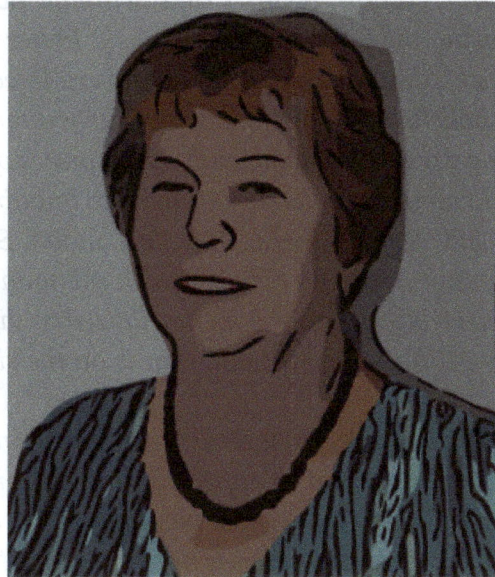

Figure 1.4: First Person Perspective

Source: Original Work
Attribution: Deanna Howe
License: CC BY-SA 4.0

In spite of the fact that my nursing career spans over fifty years, I continue to practice in our profession. Aside from laboring on days and nights in the NICU and on the Pediatric unit, I have taught over 3,000 nurses in ASN through Ph.D. programs at a variety of institutions. One of the many wonderful things about the nursing profession is that members are offered a wide range of practice options. Early on, I incorporated my love of travel with some professional opportunities. So far, I have travelled to every state in the U.S. and twenty-eight countries where I have had the privilege of meeting nurses in far flung places like China, Japan, England, Turkey and Russia, just to name a few.

One of the highlights of my adventures was to actually spend three nights in the Georgian mansion that was Florence Nightingale's home at Embley Park in Hampshire, England. What a thrill to tour her home, see her parlor and her bedroom. Then, to be able to sit in chairs that she actually used and to hear the tapes of her voice that were housed there. The grounds around the home are impressive including the tree that she used to sit under. Not too far from Embley Park is the quaint town of East Wellow where we travelled down a dirt path lined with sheep to St.

Margaret's Church yard to Miss Nightingale's grave site. Her grave is marked with an obelisk with only her initials, FN, engraved on one side. Known for her humility, she requested that her grave be marked with her initials only, as not to draw too much attention to herself.

The trip continued to Istanbul and onto Scutari, where Nightingale developed life-saving nursing practices for the British troops fighting the Crimean War. Today, Scutari and Selimiye Barracks is an active army base housing the First Army of Turkey. In her day, the floors were dirt where cots holding wounded soldiers were lined up. Now, Selimiye Barracks has polished marble floors and large windows. Nightingale's small office is on the second floor, with many pieces of handwritten Notes on Nursing adorning the walls. It was hard to imagine the difficulties she encountered while serving there. Back in London, St. Thomas' Hospital and the Nightingale Training School which she founded in 1860 actively still exist. Florence Nightingale is memorialized in the hospital lobby and in the Florence Nightingale Museum that is on the site of the original St. Thomas' Hospital.

In order to understand where we are in nursing today and where we are going, it is important to appreciate our history or where we have been. Stepping back into the 1850s, heightened my appreciation for the talents, skills and compassion nurses have exhibited for over one hundred and fifty years.

First person perspective vignette collected and created by D. Howe, 2020.

For your consideration: Dr. D. shares her travels and experience of visiting Florence Nightingale's home and other important landmarks. Centuries of health discoveries and practices have been adopted by the U.S.

Consider how the U.S. could improve from the past and create a healthcare system that meets the needs of all citizens. What aspects should be included? Based on your knowledge right now, what is good about the U.S. healthcare system? What needs improvement? After reading the content within this book, return here and answer these questions again. How do your answers differ?

1.4.2 Historical Events and Healthcare

Public hospitals

The first public hospitals in the U.S. were founded in 1736 (America's Essential Hospitals, n.d.). Bellevue Hospital, located in New York City, is known as the first public U.S. hospital. Bellevue, which started as a six-bed ward, later became home to the first U.S. hospital maternity ward. Charity Hospital, located in New Orleans, also opened in 1736. Later, in 1751, Dr. Thomas Bond and Benjamin Franklin founded Pennsylvania Hospital.

The development of hospitals symbolized an upward shift in the healthcare available to U.S. citizens. The care that was once given at home would now be offered at hospitals under the supervision of physicians and nurses. Many more cities recognized the need for hospitalization and followed suit. Between 1860 and 1930, there was an insurgence of public hospitals (America's Essential Hospitals, n.d.).

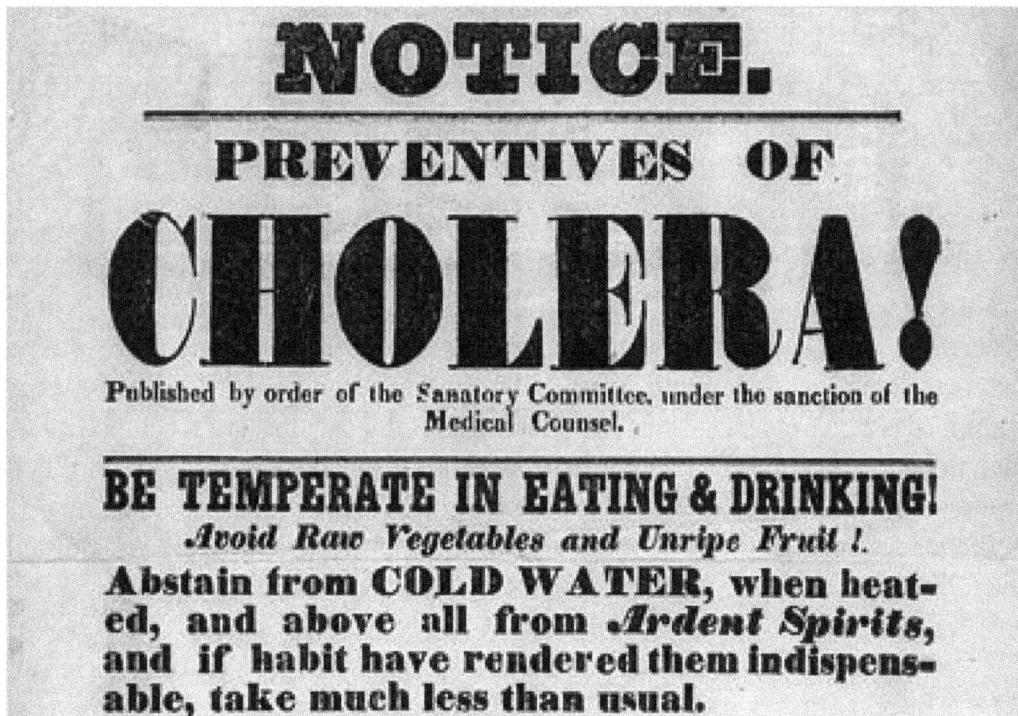

NOTICE.

PREVENTIVES OF

CHOLERA!

Published by order of the Sanatory Committee, under the sanction of the Medical Counsel.

BE TEMPERATE IN EATING & DRINKING!

Avoid Raw Vegetables and Unripe Fruit !.

Abstain from **COLD WATER**, when heated, and above all from *Ardent Spirits*, and if habit have rendered them indispensable, take much less than usual.

Figure 1.5: A poster warning about cholera

Source: Wikimedia Commons
Attribution: Sanatory Committee, New York City
License: Public Domain

The First Industrial Revolution, 1760s–1840s

The First Industrial Revolution began in Great Britain around 1706 and spread to other countries. During this time, an increase in migration from rural areas into cities occurred. Although the Industrial Revolution provided an economic boom to many towns, it held a plethora of disadvantages as well. Hazardous working conditions exposed workers to unsafe working practices within industries and to harmful substances, such as toxic dust, solvents, and heavy metals (Office of Teaching & Digital Learning, 2015). Factory workers worked around dangerous equipment and were forced to work long hours, which made them more susceptible to injury. Poor sanitation, overcrowded housing, and air pollution made matters worse.

Unsurprisingly, working and living conditions during the Industrial Revolution created new problems in healthcare in Europe and the U.S. (Office of Teaching

& Digital Learning, 2015; Grayson, 2011). Cholera, tuberculosis, and typhus were among the most prevalent diseases (Wilde, 2019). Additionally, other diseases such as measles and smallpox were problematic as well (Grayson, 2011). The impact of the Industrial Revolution—and these diseases—would have a devastating impact on the U.S. and its citizens. For example, families were not able to receive needed medical treatment due to the high cost of healthcare, which led to many deaths, particularly among children (Grayson, 2011). These issues became a concern for many. Although there were adverse effects on the nation's health, some noteworthy changes occurred due to this era's rapid urbanization, changes such as increased jobs, trade, and demand for goods (Office of Teaching & Digital Learning, 2015). A positive outcome during this time frame was the invention of the smallpox vaccine by Edward Jenner in 1796.

Progressive Era, 1890s–1920s

In the U.S., the years between the 1890s and 1920s are known as the Progressive Era. During this time, many social, political, and health reforms took place. There occurred a great deal of fervor in addressing some of the problems that resulted from the Industrial Revolution (World History Education Resources, 2017). Many committees and reform groups were created. Some of this era's achievements include women's reproductive and suffrage rights, alcohol prohibition, and food and drug acts. These acts, along with many others, helped to improve the quality of life for Americans. In his first inaugural address in 1913, Woodrow Wilson said the following:

> We have been proud of our industrial achievements, but we have not hitherto stopped thoughtfully enough to count the human cost, the cost of lives snuffed out, of energies overtaxed and broken, the fearful physical and spiritual cost to the men and women and children upon whom the dead weight and burden of it all has fallen pitilessly the years through. The groans and agony of it all had not yet reached our ears, the solemn, moving undertone of our life, coming up out of the mines and factories, and out of every home where the struggle had its intimate and familiar seat. (Wilson, 1913)

Committee on the Cost of Medical Care. Numerous healthcare advances occurred during the Progressive Era. Unfortunately, as medical advances took place, the cost of healthcare increased (Hoffman, 2003). As a result, the Committee on the Cost of Medical Care (CCMC) was formed in 1927 to help discover ways to make healthcare more affordable. The CCMC became an enormously influential reform group.

Compulsory health insurance. During the Progressive Era, reformers pushed for compulsory health insurance for laborers. These reformers maintained that with compulsory health insurance, workers who experienced illnesses (which

HEALTHCARE IN THE UNITED STATES

were very prevalent during this time) and concomitant loss of income would be able to benefit from this health insurance, if it were approved. However, compulsory health insurance was met with opposition for several reasons. One reason was a low demand for health insurance during the time, as prior to 1920, people regarded health insurance as unnecessary (Economic History Services, n.d.). Another reason was that pharmacists and physicians opposed compensatory insurance out of fear that this type of insurance would limit the payments they would receive.

American Association of Labor Legislation. Around 1906, the Progressive Era American Association of Labor Legislation (AALL) reform group began. Its goals were to establish safer working conditions, ensure unemployment pay, and create benefits for workers no longer able to work (Chasse, 1994). This assembly was met with much opposition. The AALL assembly created a model bill stipulating three essential requirements: comprehensive and required benefits for low-income employees; insurance organization and oversight by the worker and employer representatives; and health insurance contributions by employers, workers, and states. One problem associated with the proposed bill was it lacked input from the working constituents it intended to benefit (Hoffman, 2003). Instead, the AALL spent its efforts on garnering support from physicians. Although the AALL push for an obligatory health insurance bill was short-lived, the bill's ideologies helped form health policies in the U.S. for future decades (Chasse, 1994).

The Great Depression, 1929–1939

The Great Depression began in 1929 and continued for 10 years, until 1939. The impact of this time caused devastation to U.S. industries such as agriculture, mining, construction, automobiles, and many more. Before the Great Depression, workers often received healthcare from their employers. As the Great Depression deepened, many workers could no longer afford healthcare coverage because of its cost (Emanuel, 2016). Consequently, workers previously covered were left without any reasonable means of healthcare.

Starting in the 1930s, the U.S. began to recover from the Great Depression, and the quality of life began improving. This time saw advances in medicine through discoveries and experiments. Doctors discovered ways to treat patients and, in some cases, alleviate illnesses that once were deemed fatal (Gordon, 2018). Awareness of disease transmissions lead to initiatives for providing clean water and new vaccinations. Additionally, people became more knowledgeable regarding food preparation and safety.

When the Great Depression began, the U.S. was the only industrialized country that did not offer some type of unemployment insurance or social security (A&E Television Networks, 2020). This would change in 1935 with the help of Congress. The **Social Security Act of 1935** provided coverage for underprivileged, jobless, or aging Americans. Social Security provided public support and helped to improve the quality of life for Americans.

Historical Events

Vaccines. As mentioned above, the smallpox vaccination was developed in 1796 by Edward Jenner. It took nearly 200 years for the disease to be eradicated in 1975 (CDC, 2016). Although initially met with hesitation and resistance, vaccines would eventually become widely accepted in the U.S. Figure 1.6 shows a brief history of vaccine accomplishments. Pharmaceutical companies have developed several vaccines to protect against the COVID-19 virus. Clinical trials were fast tracked and three vaccines received emergency FDA approval. These three are being distributed nationwide. Most companies developed a two-shot vaccine while another has developed a one-shot vaccine. These vaccinations have shown early promise of providing acceptable levels of immunity and/or a decrease in life-threatening symptoms against current virus mutations. However, our overall health as a country and arguably across the world relies on a majority of persons to become immunized against COVID-19.

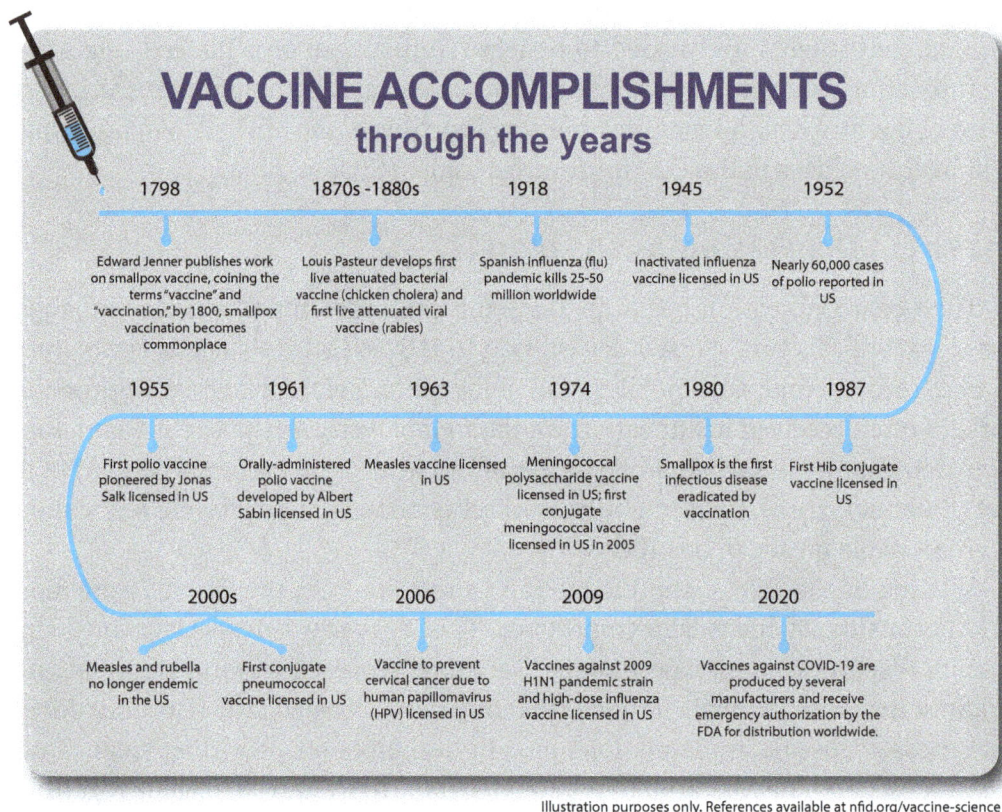

Figure 1.6: Vaccine Accomplishments Through the Years

Source: Original Work
Attribution: Kristy Michelle Gamble
License: CC BY-SA 4.0

Healthcare coverage. Historically, an unfortunate characteristic of the U.S. healthcare system was and is the vast number of citizens without healthcare coverage (Black, 2020). Over the years, government-sponsored programs were created for individuals who may not be able to afford the financial strain of quality healthcare. It is reported that the idea of healthcare for all Americans spans back to Teddy Roosevelt's presidency (1901—1909) (Anderson, 2019). While numerous presidents attempted to formulate affordable healthcare for Americans, most of their efforts were unsuccessful or short-lived. This would change in 1965 with the foundation of Medicare and Medicaid during the first presidential term of Lyndon B. Johnson.

Medicare. The first individuals to obtain Medicare were President Harry Truman and his wife (Anderson, 2019). The U.S. **Medicare** program (1965) provides healthcare coverage to those individuals 65 or older, diagnosed with end-stage renal disease, or under 65 years old receiving Social Security Disability Insurance for a period (Medicare Interactive, 2020).

Medicaid. Created in 1965, Medicaid is a government-sponsored healthcare program that offers coverage to lower-income individuals (Medicare Interactive, 2020). Although the federal government provides guidelines for every state, the actual implementation and management of the Medicaid program varies for each state (Centers for Medicare & Medicaid Services, 2019). After Lyndon B. Johnson's presidential terms, other healthcare initiatives would follow those of Medicare and Medicaid.

Social Security Amendment of 1972. President Richard Nixon signed into action the Social Security Amendment of 1972. Much discussion and debate surrounded this amendment that would eventually become law (Social Security, n.d.). The Social Security Amendment had several parts and provided provisions, such as increased benefits for widows and widowers, an established minimum benefit for workers who earned low income and had worked in employment for many years, disability insurance protection improvements and improvements on the Medicare program, just to name a few.

Health Maintenance Organization Act of 1973. In 1973, President Richard Nixon enacted the Health Maintenance Organization (HMO) Act of 1973. The goal of this act was to control consumer healthcare cost and ensure delivery of quality healthcare for Americans (Muller, 1974). HMOs were considered an alternative to fee-for-service healthcare.

Emergency Medical Treatment Act (EMTALA) of 1986. The EMTALA allowed patients to be able to receive emergency medical treatment regardless of their ability to provide payment for services (Findlaw, 2018). This is also known as the "anti-dumping" law. The law ensures patients receive appropriate examination and stabilization regardless of ability to pay for services.

The Consolidated Omnibus Budget Reconciliation Act (COBRA). COBRA was signed into action in 1986 by President Ronald Reagan. COBRA provides individuals the opportunity to continue health insurance coverage for a temporary extension once the qualified member has left employment (Griffin, 2020). Employees with a spouse and dependents would also be able to remain covered with COBRA. These guidelines help individuals obtain healthcare coverage more easily while changing jobs.

Health Insurance Portability and Accountability Act (HIPAA) of 1996. HIPAA was created to help secure the privacy of patient information. It also helped decrease waste and fraud in health insurance organizations. HIPAA was the first federal regulation of its kind (Potter & Perry, 2018). Under HIPAA guidelines, patient information is only shared with others on an as-needed basis. HIPAA also requires patients to receive a notice of their privacy rights when receiving services. Because of HIPAA, patients are required to acknowledge receipt of these privacy rights notices. See Figure 1.7 for a summary of information protected by HIPAA.

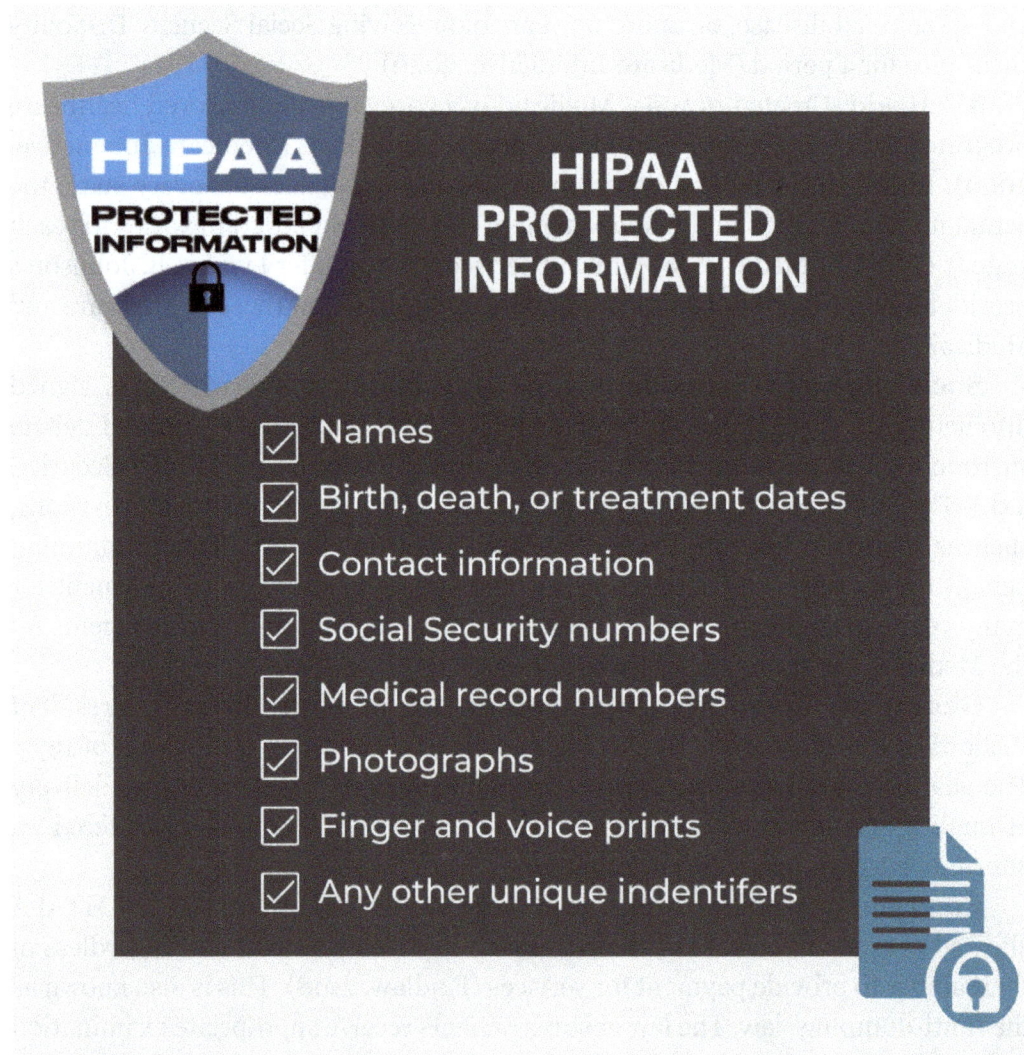

Figure 1.7: HIPAA Protected Information

Source: Original Work
Attribution: Kristy Michelle Gamble
License: CC BY-SA 4.0

Children's Health Insurance Program (CHIP) (1997). CHIP was created to provide healthcare to children whose family income exceeds the guidelines set forth by Medicaid yet who are not able to purchase private coverage (Centers for Medicare & Medicaid Services, 2019). CHIP was a part of the Balanced Budget Act of 1977 and became an achievement of President Bill Clinton (Griffin, 2020). This program provided coverage for children 19 years old or younger.

Medicare Prescription Drug, Improvement and Modernization Act (2003). In 2003, President George W. Bush signed the Medicare Prescription Drug, Improvement and Modernization Act. This act helped senior citizens obtain payment for prescription drugs through private insurance plans. The Medicare Part D Plan was created as a result of this law. The amount of prescription coverage an individual may receive varies. However, the Center for Medicare and Medicaid Services outlines the minimum payment amount with which all Medicare Part D plans must comply.

The Patient Protection and Affordable Care Act (2010). The Patient Protection and Affordable Care Act, also known as the **Affordable Care Act (ACA)** or Obamacare, was created to help resolve the issue of uninsured Americans. Individuals who may not otherwise receive healthcare coverage for reasons such as pre-existing conditions and gender-related issues were now able to receive coverage with the ACA (ObamaCare Facts, 2020). The ACA of 2010 provided Americans with increased affordability, access, and quality healthcare (Burwell, 2018). Because of the ACA, the number of individuals with healthcare coverage because has drastically increased (Broaddus & Park, 2016). Although it has made available many more healthcare provisions, the ACA has met with some disapproval and remains a topic of much debate and upheaval.

Table 1.1: ACA at a Glance
• Creates healthcare exchanges where uninsured can buy coverage and the poor can apply for subsidies.
• Prohibits denials for pre-existing conditions
• Expands Medicaid to everyone within 133% of federal poverty level

Source: New York Daily News
Attribution: New York Daily News
License: Fair Use

There are many provisions within the ACA. For example, individuals who are employed yet do not have healthcare coverage with their employer have the option of obtaining coverage under the ACA's **Health Insurance Marketplace.** While some states oversee their marketplace, the federal government oversees states that choose not to provide oversight. Employers may opt to use this marketplace to offer healthcare coverage for their employees (Savel & Munro, 2018).

Another component created as a part of the ACA is the Basic Health Program (BHP) (2015). Each state can decide if they wish to participate in the BHP or not. The BHP allows low-income individuals whose income ranges between 133–200%

of the federal poverty level to obtain healthcare coverage (Centers for Medicare and Medicaid Services, 2019). These individuals have incomes that are above and below the threshold for Medicaid and Children's Health Insurance Program guidelines (Centers for Medicare & Medicaid Services, 2019). This program also allows lawfully present non-citizens the option to enroll.

1.5 TIMELINE OF IMPORTANT HEALTHCARE EVENTS

1736—First public hospital founded
1796—Smallpox vaccine developed
1847—American Medical Association (AMA) formed
1935—Social Security Act passed
1965—Medicare and Medicaid established
1973—Health Maintenance Organization Act (HMO) passed
1986—Consolidated Omnibus Budget Reconciliation Act (COBRA) created
1986—Emergency Medical Treatment Act (EMTALA) created
1996—Health Insurance Portability and Accountability Act (HIPAA) began
1997—Children's Health Insurance Program (CHIP) started
2003—Medicare Prescription Drug, Improvement and Modernization Act
2010—Patient Protection and Affordable Care Act (ACA) began

> **Pause and Reflect**
>
> In your opinion, which historical development has had the most impact on U.S. healthcare? Explain your answer.

1.6 SUMMARY

This chapter has defined the term *system* and provided a description of the U.S. healthcare system to be used within the context of this book. Healthcare transformations have been occurring since the early 1700s. The First Industrial Revolution, the Progressive Era, and the Great Depression all had impacts on healthcare in the U.S. The American Medical Association helped establish better training, education, and standards for physicians. The evolution of healthcare workers and their formal education has led to an upward shift in the quality of care now offered to those in need. The historical events of U.S. healthcare have helped to provide a framework through which healthcare has continued to thrive.

1.7 REVIEW QUESTIONS

1. Describe how the components which make up the "system" of U.S. healthcare are interrelated.

2. What impact did the American Medical Association have on the training of physicians in the U.S.?

3. Identify an example of government-sponsored healthcare programs.

4. What were the goals of the American Association of Labor Legislation?

5. List two factors influential in the development of the U.S. healthcare system.

REFERENCES

A&E Televisions Networks. (2020). Great Depression history. Retrieved June 11, 2020, from https://www.history.com/topics/great-depression/great-depression-history

America's Essential Hospitals. (n.d.). History of public hospitals in the United States. American's Essential Hospitals. Retrieved October 1, 2019, from https://essentialhospitals.org/about-americas-essential-hospitals/history-of-public-hospitals-in-the-united-states/

American Medical Association. (2020). AMA history. Retrieved October 12, 2019, from https://www.ama-assn.org/about/ama-history/ama-history

Anderson, S. (2019). A brief history of Medicare in America. Retrieved October 10, 2019, from https://www.medicareresources.org/basic-medicare-information/brief-history-of-medicare/

Black, B. (2020). Healthcare in the United States. In B. Black (ed.), Professional Nursing, Concepts & Challenges. 9th ed. Elsevier, pp.311–340.

Burwell, S. M. (2018). The simple reality of our complex system: The future of healthcare. The Journal of Law, Medicine & Ethics, 46(4), 825–828. https://doi.org/10.1177/1073110518821973

Centers for Disease Control and Prevention (CDC). (2016, August 30). History of smallpox. Retrieved from https://www.cdc.gov/smallpox/history/history.html#:~:text=The%20basis%20for%20vaccination%20began,symptoms%20of%20smallpox%20after%20variolation

Centers for Medicare & Medicaid Services. (2019). Basic health program. Retrieved October 9, 2019, from https://www.medicaid.gov/basic-health-program/index.html

Centers for Medicare & Medicaid Services. (2019). CMS' program history. Retrieved October 9, 2019, from https://www.cms.gov/About-CMS/Agency-Information/History/index.html

Chasse, J.D. (1994). The American Association for Labor Legislation and the Institutionalist Tradition in National Health Insurance. Journal of Economic Issues, 28(4), 1063–1090. Retrieved from www.jstor.org/stable/4226887

Economic History Services. (n.d.). Health insurance in the United States. Retrieved June 12, 2020, from https://eh.net/encyclopedia/health-insurance-in-the-united-states/

Ezekiel, E. (2016, December 13). The American healthcare system with Ezekiel J.

Emanuel, MD, Ph.D. [YouTube Video]. University of Pennsylvania. Retrieved from https://www.youtube.com/watch?v=i0bHLTGuK8U&t=54s:

Fee, E. (2015). The first American medical school: The formative years. Lancet, 1940–1941. DOI: https://doi.org/10.1016/S0140-6736(15)60950-3

Findlaw. (2018, July 31). What is the Emergency Medical Treatment and Labor Act (EMTALA)? Retrieved June 12, 2020, from https://healthcare.findlaw.com/patient-rights/what-is-the-emergency-medical-treatment-and-labor-act-emtala.html

Gordon, J. S. (2018). Is there hope in the healthcare-cost crisis? USA Today Magazine, 147(2882), 2832

Grayson, R. (2011). The U.S. Industrial Revolution. Abdo Publishing.

Griffin, J. (2020, March 27). The history of healthcare in America. Retrieved October 12, 2019, from https://www.griffinbenefits.com/blog/history-of-healthcare

Health Entrepreneur. (2015, June 6). US healthcare system-The origin. Retrieved October 12, 2019, from https://www.healthentrepreneur.com/resources/USHealthcareSystem-TheOrigin.aspx

History. (2020, April 17). Florence Nightingale. Retrieved from https://www.history.com/topics/womens-history/florence-nightingale-1

Hoffman, B. (2003). Healthcare reform and the social movements in the United States. American Journal of Public Health. 93(1). Retrieved from https://www.ncbi.nlm.nih.gov/pmc/articles/PMC1447696/pdf/0930075.pdf

Medicare Interactive. (2020). Introduction to Medicare. Retrieved October 8, 2019, from https://www.medicareinteractive.org/get-answers/medicare-basics/medicare-overview/introduction-to-medicare

Merriam-Webster. (2020). System, noun. Retrieved from https://www.merriam-webster.com/dictionary/system

Muller, M. (1974). Health maintenance organization act of 1973. Retrieved from https://www.ssa.gov/policy/docs/ssb/v37n3/v37n3p35.pdf

ObamaCareFacts.com. (2020, January 27). What is ObamaCare? Retrieved May 21, 2020, from https://obamacarefacts.com/whatis-obamacare/

Office of Teaching & Digital Learning. (2015). Boston University School of Public Health. The Industrial Revolution. Retrieved October 1, 2019, from http://sphweb.bumc.bu.edu/otlt/MPH-Modules/PH/PublicHealthHistory/publichealthhistory4.html

Potter, P., Perry, A., Stockert, P. & Hall, A. (2018). Nursing Assessment. In: Fundamentals of Nursing, 9th ed. St. Louis: Elsevier, p.215.

Savel, R. & Munro, C. (2018). The health of our health care system. American Journal of Critical Care 27, 258-260. DOI: 10.4037/ajcc2018521

Social Security. (n.d.). Legislative History. Retrieved from Retrieved from https://www.ssa.gov/history/1972amend.html

Stahnisch, F. & Verhoef, M. (2012). The Flexner Report of 1910 and its impact on complementary and alternative medicine and psychiatry in North America in the 20th century. Evidence-Based Complementary and Alternative Medicine. Retrieved from https://www.ncbi.nlm.nih.gov/pmc/articles/PMC3543812/

U.S. Department of Health & Human Services. (2019). Healthy People. Retrieved October 10, 2019, from https://www.cdc.gov/nchs/healthy_people/index.htm

Vogenberg, F. R. (2019). US Healthcare trends and contradictions in 2019. American Health & Drug Benefits, 12(1), 40–47. Retrieved from https://www.ncbi.nlm.nih.gov/pmc/articles/PMC6404804/

Wilde, R. "Public health during the industrial revolution." ThoughtCo, Retrieved August 31, 2019, from www.thoughtco.com/public-health-in-the-industrial-revolution-1221641

Wilson, W. (1913). First Inaugural Address, Inaugural Addresses of the Presidents of the United States from George Washington 1789 to George Bush 1989: Bicentennial Edition (Washington, D.C.: U.S. Government Printing Office, 1989), in Original Sources. Retrieved from http://originalsources.com/Document.aspx?DocID=WI48J53FWS6M9WH

World History Education Resources. (2017). Progressive era (United States, from the 1880s to the 1920s). Retrieved from http://www.world-history-education-resources.com/articles/progressive-era-united.html

2 Overview of Health

2.1 LEARNING OBJECTIVES

By the end of this chapter, the student will be able to:
- Define health
- Describe health determinants that affect the health of a person and a population
- Discuss measures used to assess the health status of the U.S.
- Define chronic disease and list behaviors contributing to the cause of a chronic condition
- Identify personal behaviors and local or national initiatives to improve the health of Americans

2.2 KEY TERMS

- acute
- chronic disease
- disability
- epidemiology
- health
- health determinant
- health status
- incidence
- infant mortality
- life expectancy
- morbidity
- prevalence

2.3 INTRODUCTION

This chapter provides an overview of health in the United States and explores questions such as the following: What is health? How do we measure health status? What are health determinants? What is the health of the U.S. population? What are chronic diseases? What are suggestions to improve health in the U.S.?

2.4 HOW IS HEALTH DEFINED?

The World Health Organization (WHO, 2020), the global agency for advising and supervising health throughout the world since the formation of the United Nations in 1945, reaffirmed its definition of **health** in 1998 as "a state of complete physical, social and mental well-being, and not merely the absence of disease or infirmity" (WHO, 1998, p. 1). Figure 2.1 illustrates the multidimensional concept of health from the WHO.

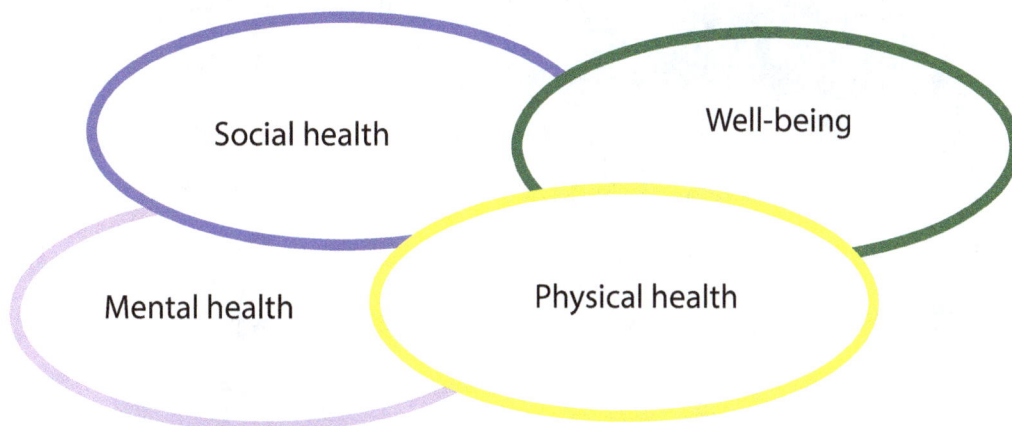

Figure 2.1: The Definition of Health by the World Health Organization (WHO)

Source: Original Work
Attribution: Kristy Michelle Gamble
License: CC BY-SA 4.0

Although the WHO's definition was originally developed in 1948 and many believe it is outdated (Fallon & Karlawish, 2019; Leonardi, 2018; Badash et al., 2017), the main constructs of health are still applicable—physical health, mental health, social health, and a feeling of well-being. These main constructs of health may be viewed differently now as society has evolved. Today, people are living longer and enduring greater challenges to physical health (Fallon & Karlawish, 2019). There is greater awareness of how social issues of poverty, educational levels, and cultural differences affect our health (Ashcroft & Van Katwyk, 2017). Mental illness is no longer a taboo subject for many (Jutras, 2017). Feelings of well-being are explored more in healthcare settings than they were in the past. These factors, plus others, and their relationship to each other affect the health of an individual and a population. These variables are called **health determinants**.

Many agencies and organizations such as the WHO, the U.S. Office of Disease Prevention and Health Promotion (ODPHP), the Centers for Disease

Control and Prevention (CDC), and the Federal Interagency Forum on Child and Family Statistics (FIFCF), have proffered health determinants that cover various biological, socioeconomic, environmental, and health access factors. These health determinants are interrelated and involve all aspects of a person's life, health and well-being, as well as where they "live, learn, work, and play" (CDC, 2018a). See Figure 2.2 for the WHO's 2008 pictorial of health determinants and their interrelationship. Figure 2.2 depicts early thinking concerning social determinants of health. Figure 2.2 represents our society's evolving view of health determinants.

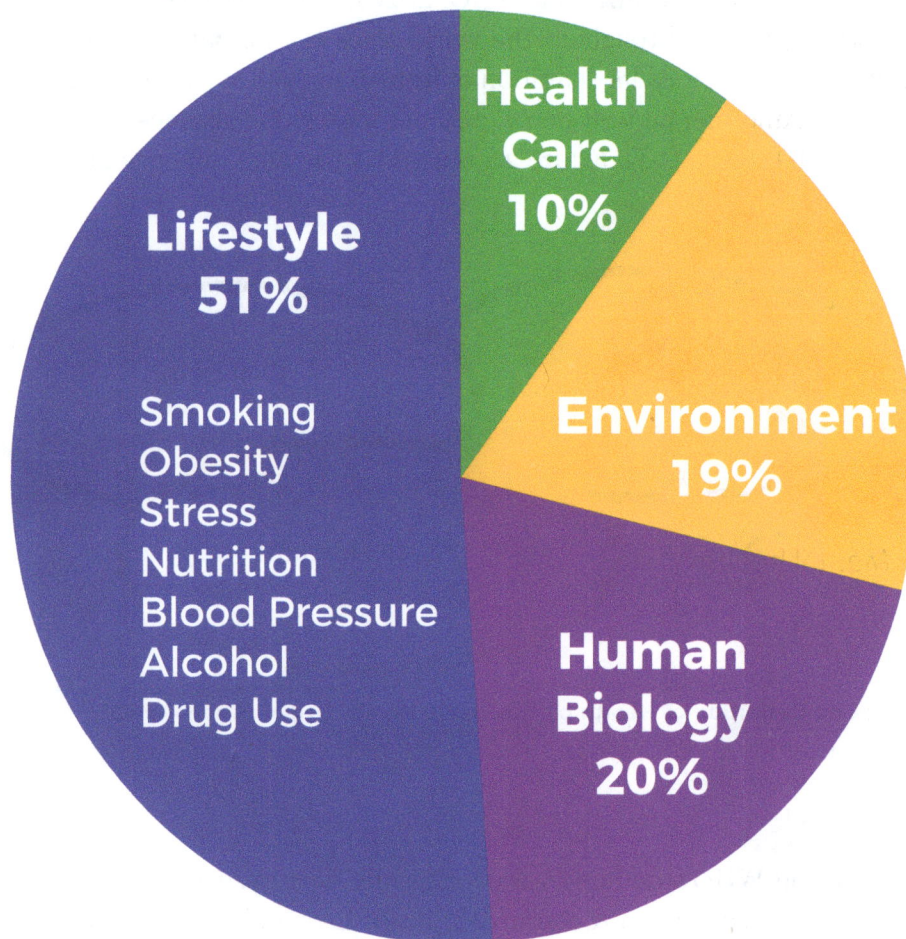

Figure 2.2: 2008 Social Determinants of Health from the WHO (Early Thinking)

Source: Original Work
Attribution: Kristy Michelle Gamble
License: CC BY-SA 4.0

Pause and Reflect

What comes to your mind when you think of health? Is there anyone whom you would consider healthy? Unhealthy? What characteristics separate them? Which characteristics would you use to define good health and poor health?

In 2008, the WHO's report indicated that 51% of a person's health was determined by lifestyle choices of smoking, obesity, stress, nutrition, blood pressure, alcohol use, and drug use. Twenty percent was thought to relate to a person's biological or genetic makeup. Nineteen percent was thought to be related to the person's environment, where they lived and worked. Finally, 10% was determined to be related to the access or quality of healthcare a person received. As society has evolved, more recent descriptions and images of social determinants, although varied, emphasize socioeconomic factors (Figure 2.3). The biological, socioeconomic, behavioral, environmental, and access-to-healthcare determinants are discussed further.

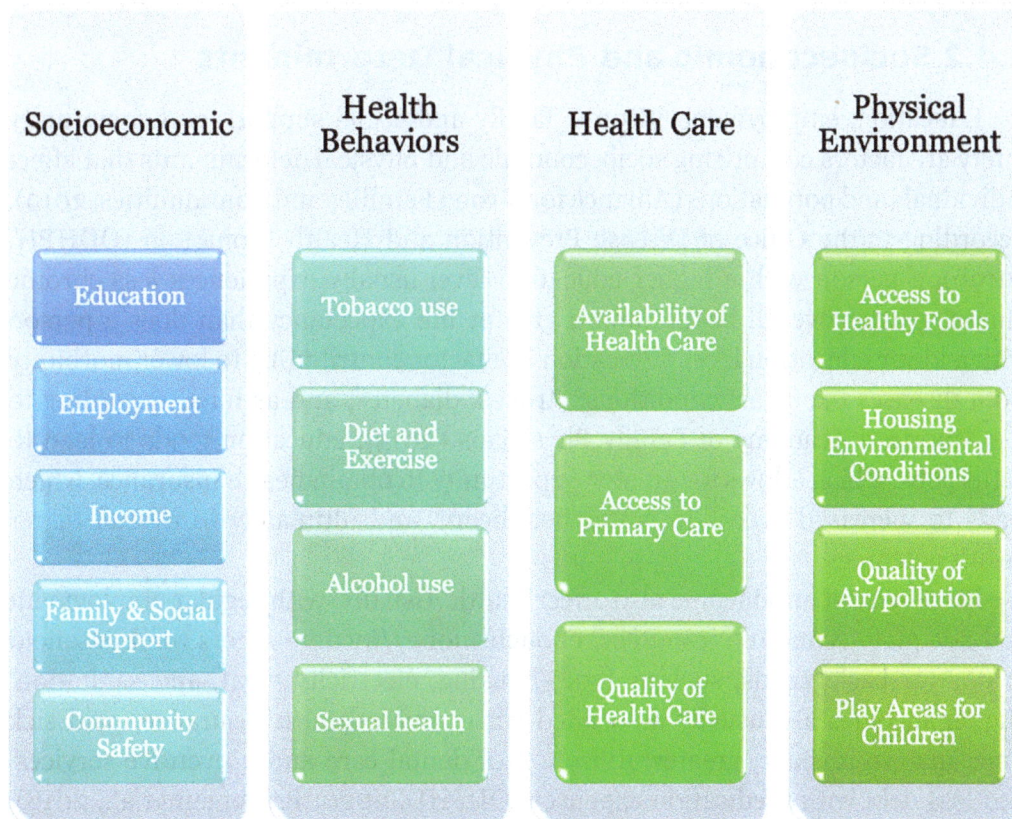

Figure 2.3: Updated Social Determinants of Health (from various models)

Source: Original Work
Attribution: Deanna Howe
License: CC BY-SA 4.0

2.4.1 Biological Determinants

Biological determinants of health include such factors as age, gender, inherited conditions, and genetics. According to the Office of Disease Prevention and Health Promotion (ODPHP, 2019a), the chief causes of death in the U.S. have a hereditary component. These include heart disease, cancer, diabetes, stroke, and Alzheimer's disease. In fact, greater than half of the population is at an increased risk of cancer, diabetes, or heart disease due to having living or deceased blood relatives with at least one of these debilitating disease processes.

Some diseases are more typical of certain races or ethnic groups (National Institute of Health [NIH], 2020). For example, sickle cell anemia occurs mostly in Blacks or African Americans or those of Mediterranean descent (NIH, 2020). Diabetes occurs more often in the Black, Hispanic, and Native American populations (NIH, 2020). Cystic fibrosis and multiple sclerosis are examples of conditions that mainly affect the white or Caucasian race (NIH). Gender also affects prevalence of a disease. According to the National Institute of Health (2018), osteoporosis is more common in females, while muscular dystrophy is more common in males (NIH, 2020).

2.4.2 Socioeconomic and Physical Determinants

Education, employment, income, family and social support, and community safety are factors comprising socioeconomic and physical determinants that affect individuals and populations (Alliance for Strong Families and Communities, 2019). According to the Office of Disease Prevention and Health Promotion (ODHPH, 2019b), a person with a higher education level usually experiences less chronic illness, greater overall health, and a greater life expectancy than does a person with a lower education level. Education is a factor contributing to lower morbidity from diseases like heart conditions, strokes, diabetes, and asthma. According to the American Academy of Family Physicians (2015), education tends to lead to better jobs, which allows for greater opportunity to obtain health insurance, which leads to increased access to better healthcare, and ultimately to overall better health outcomes.

Employment and income also affect health. Usually, with regular employment and adequate economic resources, enough money/income enters the household to pay for basic needs, such as food, housing, electricity, heat, and sanitation. Higher incomes are usually associated with private health insurance, paid sick time, maternity leave, greater utilization of dental care and preventive services, and less debt with medication expenses (ODPHD, 2020; Braveman et al., 2018). Those employed and with higher incomes are usually able to live in homes free of environmental concerns, such as lead contamination, and live in healthier neighborhoods with grocery stores and parks within close distance (Braveman et al., 2018). Job security promotes positive mental health with decreased reports of depression and anxiety (ODPHD, 2020). Prolonged psychosocial stress from not having adequate finances or being impoverished can cause harmful bodily effects to those with low economic resources, thereby also increasing an individual's chance of developing a stress-related or chronic illness (ODPHD, 2020; Braveman et al., 2018).

Family and support systems also affect health. Familial and support system factors that may affect children and adolescents' health resulting in unsafe conditions and emotional harm include mistreatment of children, exposing children to risky behaviors, and incarceration of a parent. Rejection and bullying from family members and/or the community can also impact health and lead to mental health problems, depression, suicide, and other harmful activities, especially in the adolescent years (Federal Interagency Forum on Child and Family Statistics [FIFCF], 2019).

Community safety can also influence health (FIFCF, 2019). Poor outdoor air quality, with such pollutants as ozone, cigarette smoke, carbon monoxide, sulfur dioxide, and others, can be especially harmful to vulnerable children, possibly causing long term respiratory complications (FIFCF, 2019). Contaminants in drinking water can affect the health of the community, causing long- or short-term gastrointestinal problems or diseases (FIFCF, 2019). Crowded housing, inadequate housing, or homelessness exposes individuals to greater opportunities for infection or disease (FIFCF, 2019). Lead exposure, although declining, is still a concern in some neighborhoods (FIFCF, 2019). Crime and violence in the neighborhood may result in physical harm or mental health illnesses (FIFCF, 2019).

2.4.3 Health Behavior Determinants

Unhealthy behaviors—such as cigarette smoking, poor diet, lack of exercise, and alcohol consumption—are commonly cited as conditions that perpetuate an unhealthy lifestyle (CDC, 2019a). Along with those four, the Alliance for Strong Families and Communities (2019) includes sexual health. Unsafe sexual behaviors, as well as exposure to or participation in violence and criminal activity, also promote risky and unhealthy behaviors (Office of Disease Prevention and Health Promotion [ODPHD], 2019b).

Of all the known health behavior determinants, cigarette smoking continues to be the number one factor causing health problems in the U.S. (CDC, 2019a). According to the CDC, "tobacco use is the leading cause of preventable disease, disability, and death in the United States" (2019a, para. 1). Cigarette smoke—either through direct inhalation, second-hand smoke, or maternal smoke while pregnant (causing sudden infant death syndrome [SIDS], prematurity, low birth weight, or other conditions)—has contributed to more than 20 million deaths in the last 50 years, according to the 2014 Surgeon General's report (CDC, 2014). Currently, the U.S. has the lowest-ever prevalence of cigarette smoking at 14% of the population (U.S Department of Health & Human Services [HHS], 2020a). However, 16 million Americans are presently suffering from some form of illness related to smoking, such as asthma, cancer, chronic obstructive pulmonary disease (COPD), and heart disease and stroke (HHS, 2020a).

Inadequate nutrition and lack of physical activity are two additional known health behavior determinants that can impact every stage of the lifespan. Adequate nutrition is essential for growth and development, maintenance of bodily functions, and prevention of illnesses and diseases (Ohlhorst et al., 2013). Many Americans do not eat the recommended amounts of fruits, dairy products, oils, vegetables, and whole-grains but, instead, are consuming approximately 600 more calories per day than needed in the form of sugars, refined grains, and unhealthy fats (U.S Department of Health and Human Services [HHS], 2017). Rates of obesity are dramatically increasing, with close to half of those children who live in poverty being overweight compared to around a fifth of those children who live in households with four times the poverty level income (HHS, 2017). Obesity is related to greater illness, disease, disability, and mortality. Obesity is also associated with higher healthcare costs (HHS, 2017). Other nutritional considerations are that many households live in areas where supermarkets with fresh foods and produce are miles away while some Americans live in food-insecure households where food is limited.

According to the U.S Department of Health and Human Services (2017), only a third of American children are physically active each day. Over 80% of adolescents and over 80% of adults do not perform the amount of aerobic or muscle strengthening physical activity recommended for their age group (HHS, 2017). The HHS also reports that "children now spend more than seven and a half hours a day in front of a screen" (TV, video games, tablets, and computers) and that approximately one third of high school students are involved in video or computer games for three or more hours per average school day. Health benefits of exercise include controlling weight, reducing risks of heart disease, managing diabetes, improving moods, improving cognitive functioning, strengthening bones and muscles, reducing risk of falls, and improving sleep (National Institutes of Health [NIH], 2019). Regular exercise may also reduce the risk of some cancers, improve sexual health, and increase the chance of a longer life (NIH, 2019). The NIH cites a 2011 meta-analysis, performed by Gontved and Hue, where viewing TV, rather than exercising, was found to have a linear relationship to the development of type 2 diabetes, cardiovascular disease, and all-cause mortality.

The next significant health behavior is the use of alcohol. According to the National Institute on Alcohol Abuse and Alcoholism (NIAAA), alcohol is considered "the third leading preventable cause of death in the United States" (behind tobacco and diet and exercise), with a reported estimated 88,000 deaths per year(NIAAA, 2019). Over half of persons eighteen years of age and older report drinking within the previous month and over one-fourth of those have admitted to binge drinking in the previous month (NIAAA, 2019). White et al. (2020) report almost a million alcohol-related deaths between 1999 and 2017. However, the U.S. Department of Transportation (2019) reports a 3.6 percent decrease in alcohol-impaired-driving deaths for 2018.

The most known alcohol-related illnesses and diseases are abuse or dependence, cirrhosis, and cancer (NIAAA, 2019). White et al. (2020) found 31% of alcohol-related deaths in 2017 were from liver disease, while 18% were from overdoses of alcohol imbibed independently or in combination with other drugs. Females and young adults aged 25–34 experienced the greatest increase in alcohol-related deaths (White et al., 2020). According to the American Academy of Child and Adolescent Psychiatry (2019), 20% of adults in the U.S. lived in a home with an alcoholic relative during their childhood. Alcohol abuse effects are far reaching and include mental health and physical health of self and others, but recovery from alcoholism is possible (National Institutes on Alcohol Abuse and Alcoholism [NIAAA], 2019).

Risky sexual behaviors can also affect health and are considered another significant health determinant. Early sexual activity among youth increases the risk of sexually transmitted diseases (STDs), as that behavior generally increases the number of sexual partners in a lifetime (FIFCF, 2019). From 2014 to 2018, there have been dramatic increases in STDs including the following: chlamydia (increase of 19%); gonorrhea (increase of 63%); primary and secondary syphilis (increase of 71%); and congenital syphilis (increase of 185%), with a 22% increase in infant deaths from 2017 to 2018 (CDC, 2019b). The CDC reports that the age group between 15 and 24 are responsible for half of the STDs in the U.S. STDs can cause miscarriages and pelvic inflammatory disease leading to infertility. The economic impact of STDs is in the billions annually (CDC, 2019b). In addition to the physical consequences of early sexual activity, the FIFCF (2019) notes there can also be emotional consequences for those involved.

Stress is another factor that affects health and is listed as a social determinant of health in some models. Everyone is affected by stress at some time. However, continued, long-term stress from overwork, discrimination, or job insecurity may increase the risk of heart disease and other conditions (ODPHP, 2019b). Stress increases a person's blood pressure and heart rate and may cause mental disturbances (ODPHP, 2019b). Stress is manageable, and there are treatments to help reduce stress, such as physical exercise, meditation, and some medications. The National Institute of Mental Health has a 24-hour, seven-days-a-week hotline available for anyone who feels overwhelmed and is having thoughts of suicide, which sometimes may also be attributed to stress (National Institute of Mental Health [NIMH], 2020).

Pause and Reflect

Individual stress levels are at an all-time high in the U.S. as a result of financial instability, burn out from putting others first, social isolation, and technology use. While some temporary stress can be good—like preparing for an important college exam—excess stress can lead to severe health problems. Many common symptoms which can be visible include anxiety or nervousness, excessive alcohol consumption, overeating, or lack of sleep. Other symptoms which may not be visible include increased breathing, higher heart rate, high blood pressure, and muscle tightening.

Have you ever noticed a high stress level in someone? What symptoms did you see? Conduct a literature review regarding reduction of stress and describe which types of activities could help reduce high stress levels.

2.4.4 Physical Environmental Determinants

The physical environment is another major category of determinants of health, and many variables that fall in this category also fall under community safety. Home and neighborhood environmental determinants are factors that affect a person's health and well-being throughout the age spectrum. The growth, development and overall health of young children may especially be impaired due to secondhand smoke, lead-based paints, poor quality of drinking water, and pests in the home. Outdoor pollution or poor air quality may also affect all ages. For example, asthma, a respiratory condition, is more common in poor neighborhoods (FIFCF, 2019).

Other factors affecting the health of all ages in a neighborhood are a lack of amenities. Safe neighborhood parks are important for children to have places to play in. As touched on above, local grocery stores with healthy and affordable foods are needed without individuals having to travel far distances. Over 23 million people live in what the Office of Disease Prevention and Health Promotion (2019b) call "food deserts," where individuals are unable to easily purchase healthy, affordable food. A lack of adequate transportation can also lead to unhealthy lifestyles where individuals have long distances to travel, making it difficult to prepare and cook meals, be at home with family, and get adequate rest (ODPHP, 2019). One model of social determinants cites the overall quality of the physical environment as accounting for approximately 10% of a person's health (FIFCF,2019).

2.4.5 Healthcare Availability, Access, and Quality

The availability of healthcare resources nearby, including easy accessibility of competent and caring primary care providers have an impact on an individual's health (FIFCF, 2019; ODPHP, 2019c). Having access to quality primary care healthcare providers affords individuals opportunities to receive preventative services, have illnesses and diseases detected and treated early, thus reducing complications and heavy financial burdens. Therefore, access to quality primary healthcare providers leads to better health and well-being (ODPHP, 2019c).

Conversely, those without access to quality primary healthcare obtain fewer preventative services, experience illnesses and diseases that may not be detected and treated early, and may have poorer health outcomes. Compared to those without health insurance coverage, those individuals with health insurance coverage generally not only have easier access to healthcare resources but also utilize them more frequently. Thus, not having health insurance, along with the high cost of healthcare, are two factors making healthcare access more difficult for some individuals. Not having needed healthcare services available and not having culturally competent healthcare providers of choice are also barriers to obtaining healthcare services (ODPHP, 2019c). See Chapter 8 for an in-depth analysis of access issues and concerns in healthcare.

2.5 HOW IS HEALTH STATUS MEASURED?

The general health status of a population is most commonly measured by life expectancy. **Health status** is "a description and/or measurement of the health of an individual or population at a particular point in time against identifiable standards, usually by reference to health indicators" (WHO, 1998, p. 12). Arias and Xu (2019) explain **life expectancy** as the "average number of years of life remaining for persons who have attained a given age (x)" (p. 2). The ODPHP (2019d) has established the 2020 Healthy People initiative, a 10-year comprehensive plan—developed using evidence-based research and historical data—to improve each American's health. In the 2020 Healthy People initiative, the two life expectancy measures evaluated are life expectancy at birth and life expectancy at age 65. According to the Office of Economic Cooperation and Development (OECD, 2019), "Life expectancy at birth is defined as how long, on average, a newborn can expect to live, if current death rates do not change" (para. 1). Infant mortality is universally accepted as a reliable criterion for general health of a population (Murphy et al., 2018). **Infant mortality** is "the ratio of infant deaths to live births in a given year" (Murphy et al., 2018, p. 5). Current life expectations at birth, life expectancy at age 65, and infant mortality rates will be discussed in the following sections.

2.5.1 Analyze the Health Status of the U.S. and the Increase of Chronic Diseases

Identifying the causes of mortality in population groups are important in evaluating the health of a population and charting a course for improved health. **Morbidity** is the term used to describe illness within a population (National Cancer Institute, [NCI], n.d.) and may refer to short-term or **acute** episodes of symptoms or illness or to **chronic illness,** disease, or disability. According to the CDC (2019c), "chronic diseases are defined broadly as conditions that last one year or more and require ongoing medical attention or limit activities of daily living or both" (para. 1). A **disability** may be an impairment of a body part or function, an activity limitation, or a restriction preventing participation in life situations (WHO, n.d.). The **incidence** (or rate of individuals developing chronic illness, disease, and disability) and the **prevalence** (or the number of actual cases) is increasing as our population ages. The study of diseases and illnesses and the factors that determine their presence in a population is **epidemiology** (NIH, 2020).

Life expectancy at birth and life expectancy at age 65

The 2017 statistics reveal that life expectancy at birth is 78.6 years for all the U.S. population; 76.1 years for males and 81.1 years for females (Murphy et al., 2018). This is a slight decrease from 2016. Life expectancy at age 65 in 2017 has essentially not changed compared to 2016, with females living 20.6 years past age 65 compared to 18.1 years for males (Murphy et al., 2018). (Life expectancy in the U.S. compared to other countries is discussed in Chapter 12.)

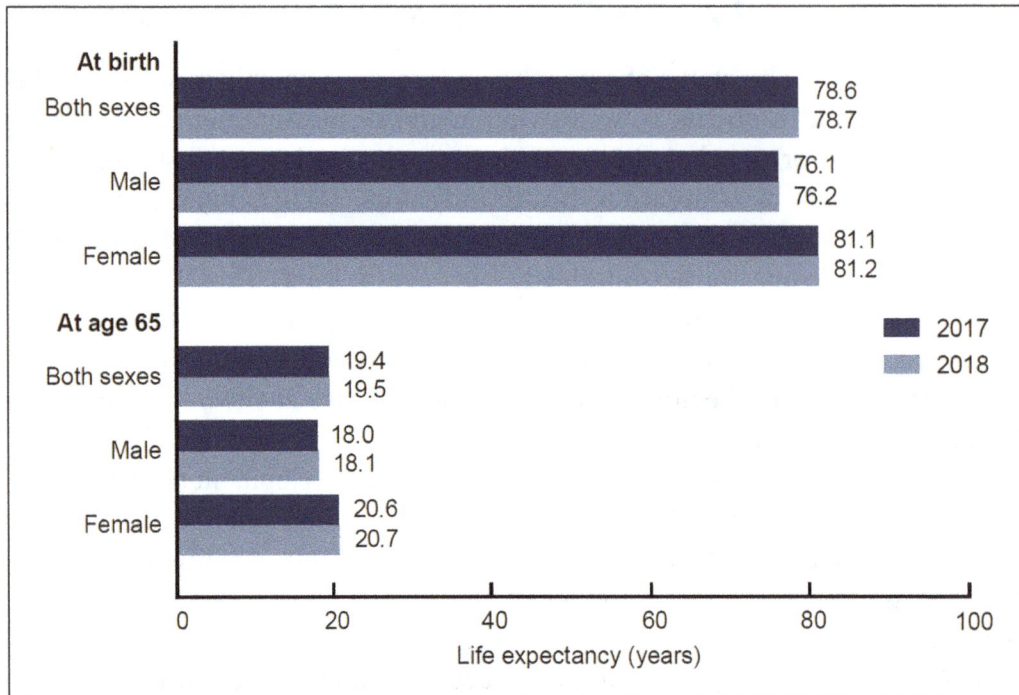

NOTE: Access data table for Figure 1 at: https://www.cdc.gov/nchs/data/databriefs/db355_tables-508.pdf#1.
SOURCE: NCHS, National Vital Statistics System, Mortality.

Figure 2.4: Life Expectancy at Selected Ages, by Sex: United States, 2016 and 2017. Note: Life expectancies for 2016 were revised using updated Medicare data; therefore, figures may differ from those previously published.

Source: US Department of Health and Human Services
Attribution: Centers for Disease Control and Prevention
License: Public Domain

Death rates in the U.S. by race, ethnicity, and gender

The non-Hispanic black male population have the highest death rates in the U.S. Non-Hispanic white males have the second highest death rates in the U.S. Hispanic females have the lowest number of deaths in the U.S. (Figure 2.5).

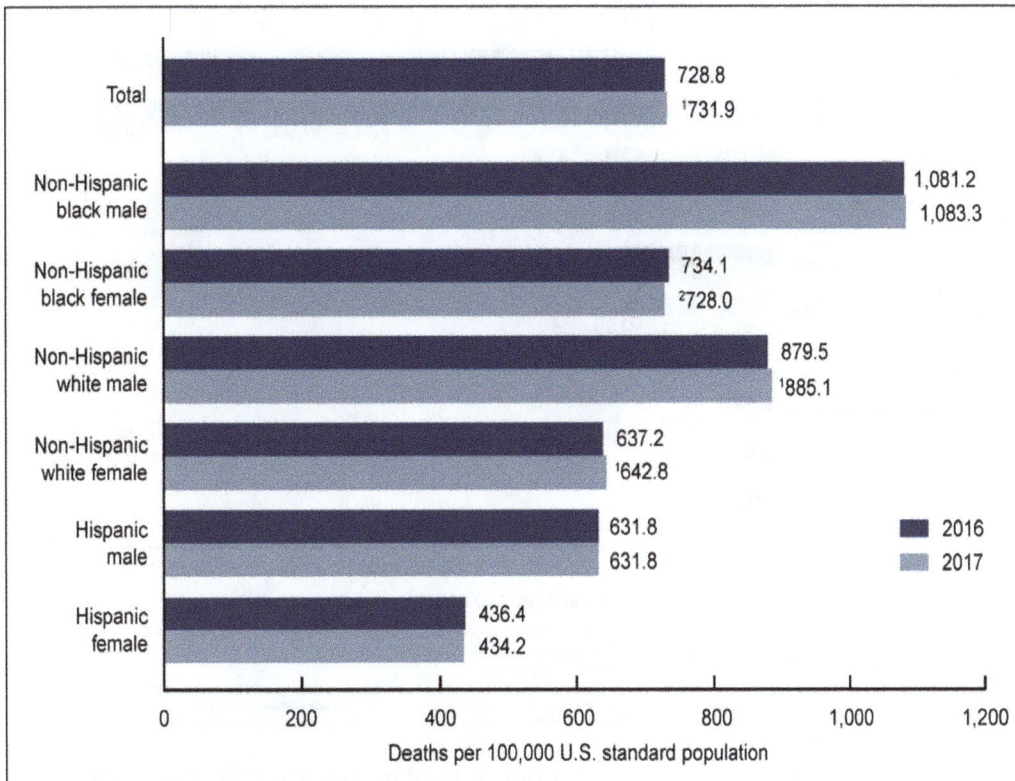

¹Statistically significant increase in age-adjusted death rate from 2016 to 2017 (*p* < 0.05).
²Statistically significant decrease in age-adjusted death rate from 2016 to 2017 (*p* < 0.05).
NOTE: Access data table for Figure 2 at: https://www.cdc.gov/nchs/data/databriefs/db328_tables-508.pdf#2.
SOURCE: NCHS, National Vital Statistics System, Mortality.

Figure 2.5: Age-Adjusted Death Rates, by Race and Ethnicity and Sex: United States, 2016 and 2017

Source: US Department of Health and Human Services
Attribution: Centers for Disease Control and Prevention
License: Public Domain

Chief causes of death in the U.S.

The top ten causes of deaths in the U.S. in 2017 continue to be the same as in 2016. Interestingly, nine of the ten top causes of death are the same as in 1998. The top two—heart disease and cancer—are the same top two in 1998 and in 2017. Only Alzheimer's disease has replaced chronic liver disease in the top ten causes of death (Murphy et al., 2018).

In 2017, ranked in order of numbers of deaths caused, are heart disease as number one and suicide tenth. It is noteworthy that the ten highest causes of death are responsible for 74% of the total deaths in 2017 in the U.S. (Figure 2.6).

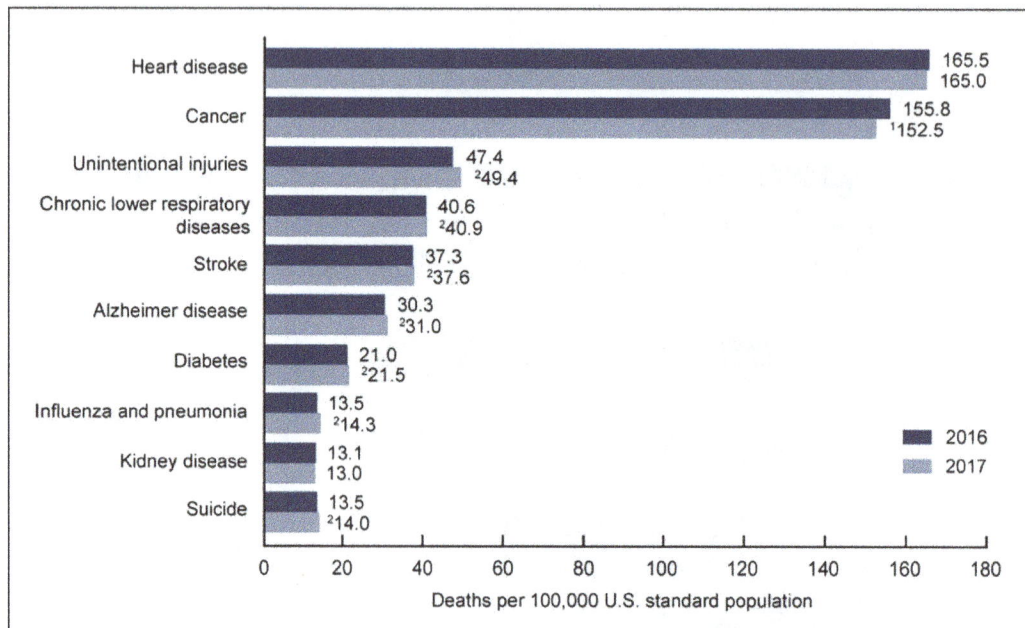

¹Statistically significant decrease in age-adjusted death rate from 2016 to 2017 ($p < 0.05$).
²Statistically significant increase in age-adjusted death rate from 2016 to 2017 ($p < 0.05$).
NOTES: A total of 2,813,503 resident deaths were registered in the United States in 2017. The 10 leading causes accounted for 74.0% of all deaths in the United States in 2017. Causes of death are ranked according to number of deaths. Rankings for 2016 data are not shown. Data table for Figure 4 includes the number of deaths for leading causes. Access data table for Figure 4 at: https://www.cdc.gov/nchs/data/databriefs/db328_tables-508.pdf#4.
SOURCE: NCHS, National Vital Statistics System, Mortality.

Figure 2.6: Age-Adjusted Death Rates for the 10 Leading Causes of Death: United States, 2016 and 2017

Source: US Department of Health and Human Services
Attribution: Centers for Disease Control and Prevention
License: Public Domain

Infant mortality

Any infant death before the first birthday is considered in **infant mortality rates (IMR)** (CDC, 2019d). The IMR decreased some but was not statistically significant from 2016 to 2017, with 5 to 5.7 infant deaths per 1,000 live births, respectively (CDC). Worldwide, the U.S. ranks 174 out of 228 countries and territories in IMRs (Central Intelligence Agency [CIA], n.d.). Comparatively, Slovenia has the lowest IMR ranking at number 228 with 1.7 deaths per 1,000, and Afghanistan has the highest IMR and ranks first at 104.3 deaths per 1,000 live births (CIA, n.d.). The 2016 Infant Mortality Rate by race and ethnicity indicate that the majority of infant deaths were in the Black population (11.4), followed by American Indian/Alaska Natives (9.4), Hawaiian/Pacific Islanders (7.4), Hispanics (5.0), Whites (4.9), and Asians (3.6). In 2017, seven southern states (Alabama, Arkansas, Georgia, Mississippi, North Carolina, Oklahoma, and Tennessee) and six midwest or east coast states (Indiana, Ohoio, South Dakota, Delaware, Maryland, and Rhode Island) had the highest IMRs with 7.1-8.6 deaths per 1,000 live births (CDC). The top ten causes of deaths for U.S. infants in 2017 and ranked in order are congenital malformations, low birth weight, maternal complications, sudden infant death syndrome, unintentional injuries, cord and placental complications, bacterial sepsis of the newborn, diseases of the circulatory system, respiratory distress of the newborn, and neonatal hemorrhage (Figure 2.7).

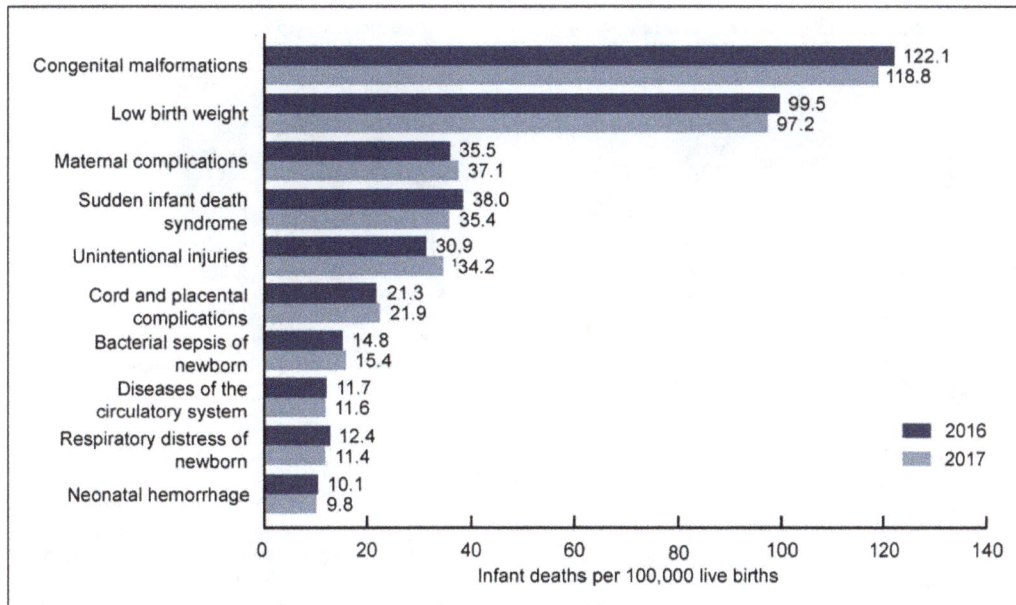

Figure 2.7: Infant Mortality Rates for the 10 Leading Causes of Infant Death in 2017: United States, 2016 and 2017

Source: US Department of Health and Human Services
Attribution: Centers for Disease Control and Prevention
License: Public Domain

Chronic disease

Chronic disease is described as conditions which last one year or more and may progress or get worse over time (National Center for Chronic Disease Prevention and Health Promotion [NCCDPHP], 2020). According to the NCCDPHP (2020), the seven most common chronic diseases in the U.S. are heart disease, cancer, stroke, chronic obstructive pulmonary disease, diabetes, chronic kidney disease, and Alzheimer's disease. 60% of adults in the U.S. have at least one of the above, and 40% of adults are living with at least two of these chronic conditions (NCCDPHP, 2020). Moreover, 90% of the total annual U.S. healthcare dollars are utilized for people with chronic physical and mental health disorders (CDC, 2019e).

The leading cause of death in the U.S. is heart disease. Heart disease, stroke, and other cardiovascular diseases combined cause one third of all deaths in the U.S. The economic toll on the nation is heavy in terms in cost of disease management and lost productivity (CDC, 2019g). High blood pressure, high low-density lipoproteins (LDL), cholesterol blood levels, lack of exercise, poor dietary habits, obesity, and type 2 diabetes are other risk factors for heart disease and stroke (CDC, 2019g) (Figure 2.8).

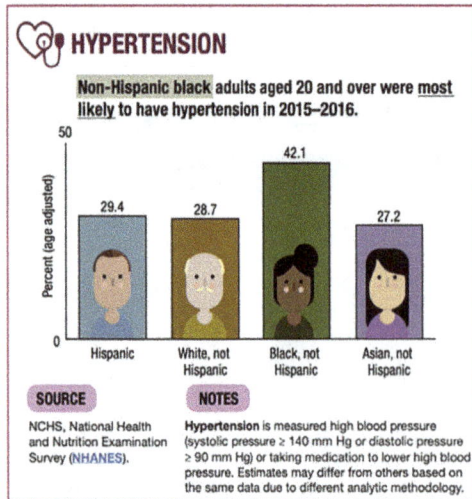

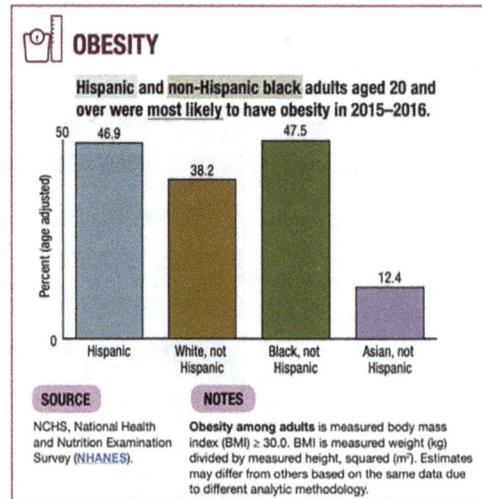

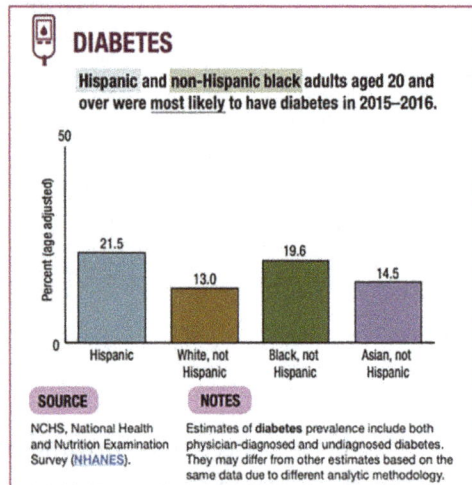

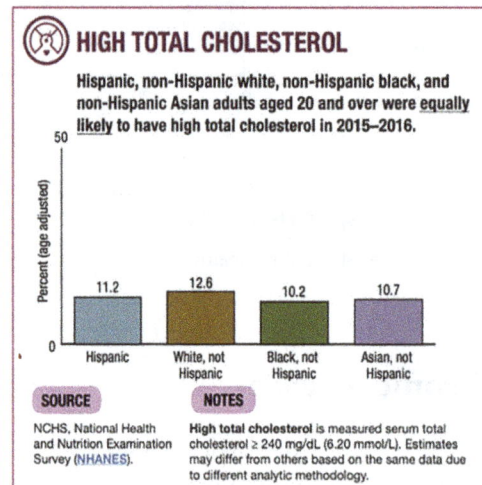

Figure 2.8: Risk Factors for Heart Disease

Source: Centers for Disease Control and Prevention
Attribution: Centers for Disease Control and Prevention
License: Public Domain

Cancer is the second leading cause of death, with 1.6 million people diagnosed with this disease each year. According to the CDC (2019h), there are "600,000 deaths from cancer each year with one in three people developing cancer in their lifetime and $174 billion in cancer care costs projected in 2020" (p. 2). Moreover, research indicates that with appropriate healthy food choices, various cancer screenings, and appropriate vaccinations, greater than half of deaths from cancer could be prevented.

Diabetes is a condition that has more than doubled in the U. S. in the last 20 years. This growth is mainly due to an aging and an overweight population. The latest CDC (2018b) statistics indicate that "more than 30 million Americans have diabetes and another 84.1 million have prediabetes" (p. 2). Diabetes can be a very debilitating disease with long-term complications, such as amputation of a leg, foot, or toe; blindness; and kidney failure. According to the CDC (2018b), $237 billion are spent annually in medical costs, and there is a loss of productivity equaling $90 billion because of this disease.

Pause and Reflect

Obesity is a contributing factor to the development of diabetes. While many factors are associated with obesity, a lack of exercise is a significant one. What is the recommended amount of exercise suggested to maintain weight? How much exercise should a person do for weight reduction. Which exercises provide the best heart-healthy but low-impact? If you were to design a campaign to share with a group of young middle schoolers about exercise for a healthy body, what would you include?

The CDC (2019i) notes that 5.7 million people in the U.S. are living with another chronic condition: Alzheimer's disease—the nation's sixth leading cause of death. Alzheimer's disease is currently incurable and mostly affects those age 65 and older. Research continues to determine the cause. Possible genetic links have been found, but more probably there is a mix of genetic, environmental, and lifestyle factors (CDC, 2019i).

Other chronic conditions seen in the U.S. include arthritis, a debilitating disease affecting 54.4 million people and resulting in inability to work for some or causing ill-health. Epilepsy is another debilitating and chronic condition that affects about 3.4 million people, often beginning in childhood. Lastly, as touched on above, one in ten deaths in working-age individuals between the ages of 20 and 64 are caused by excessive alcohol use, costing $249 billion annually.

Risk factors

The NCCDPHP (2019) identified four main risk factors responsible for most of the chronic conditions people are living with today: tobacco, poor nutrition, lack of exercise, and excessive alcohol use (Figure 2.8). Since tobacco use is the leading risk factor for "preventable diseases, disability, and death" (CDC, 2019f, p. 1) the U.S. must do more to discourage young people from smoking. According to the CDC (2019f), "every day, about 2,000 young people under the age of 18 smoke their first cigarette, and more than 300 become daily cigarette smokers" (para. 2).

--- --- --- --- --- --- --- --- --- --- --- --- --- --- --- --- --- --- --- ---

First Person Perspective

Ms. B. is an African American female with a family history of high blood pressure and stroke. She provides service and outreach in her community.

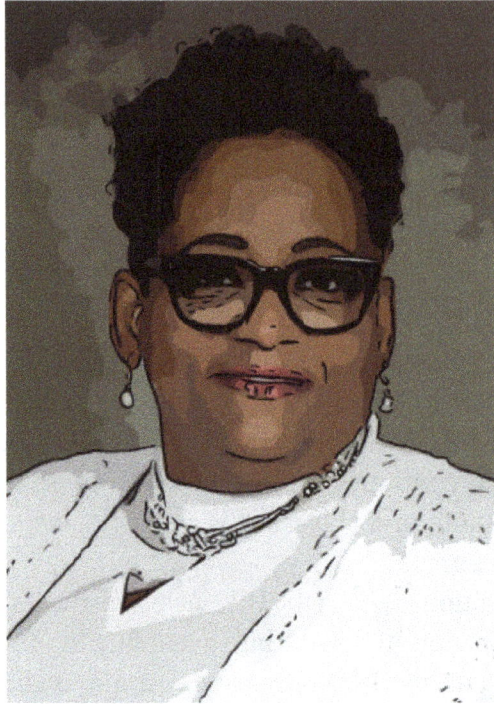

Figure 2.9: First Person Perspective

Source: Original Work
Attribution: Deanna Howe
License: CC BY-SA 4.0

When I began to have persistent headaches in 2002, I went to a local medical care center. At the time I did not have health insurance and was put on a sliding scale payment plan. The doctor diagnosed me with high blood pressure and had me take a diuretic pill. After two weeks on the medicine, I quit taking the pills because they made me have to go to the bathroom too much and made functioning at work difficult. After a few months off the medicine, I started having heart palpitations and could no longer perform my job. Eventually I quit working and had to go back to the doctor. Tests showed I had out of control blood pressure again. After this episode I decided to take my health seriously and started taking blood pressure medications and began feeling better right away.

It wasn't until this initial diagnosis that I began understanding how much high blood pressure affected my family. I come from generations of family members who have had blood pressure problems. My grandmother died from a massive stroke and my granddaddy had a massive stroke that left him paralyzed and unable to walk. He died ten years later.

My uncle also had high blood pressure but did not take his medications because of the side-effects. He also had a massive stroke which left him paralyzed and unable to speak clearly. So far none of my children have high blood pressure, but my grandson had an episode at age ten when the pediatrician discovered a higher-than-normal blood pressure. He was sent to a specialist and after six months released because no more issues were found. The situation has resolved but we continue to monitor his blood pressure often to make sure he is okay.

Today, I am able to work, and I walk daily for exercise and to keep the weight off. My blood pressure has been under control and I continue to take my medications. My life depends on me taking the medications and taking care of myself.

First person perspective vignette collected and created by D. Howe, 2020.

For your consideration: High blood pressure and stroke disproportionately affect African American women (American Heart Association, 2020). Ms. B. states the side effects from blood pressure medications affected her and her uncle. Initially, both quit taking their medications and began having high blood pressure symptoms again.

Ms. B.'s adult children do not have high blood pressure now. Should her children let their doctor know they have a strong family history of high blood pressure and stroke? Should U.S. health experts prioritize gender or culturally specific health campaigns to minimize risk and poor health outcomes of certain diseases? For example, online ads to discourage teens from smoking or the need to report cyberbullying.

2.5.2 Other Concerns for the Nation's Health

Mental health

According to the CDC (2018c), there were approximately 43.4 million adults, or 20% of the adult population, with a mental illness in 2014. Suicide "is the 10th leading cause of death in the U.S. and the 2nd leading cause of death among people aged 15–34" (CDC, 2018c, p. 1). In 2015, approximately one in twenty-five adults had a serious mental illness. Serious illness prevents or limits normal functioning in one or more of life's activities (CDC, 2018c). Mental illness affects all persons, regardless of gender, age, socioeconomic status, or physical health.

Homelessness

Homelessness, an increasing problem, is a public health concern. Some argue that a multidisciplinary approach is needed for this population with programs or laws to address decriminalization of homelessness, public health issues, and laws which support access to healthcare, affordable housing, and mental health services (CDC, 2017). Homeless persons are exposed more frequently to conditions which lead to tuberculosis, respiratory illness, flu, hepatitis, alcohol and drug abuse, HIV infection, and mental illness. Inadequate nutrition, violence, injuries, and poor sleeping conditions, in addition to sanitation and toileting, are concerns for the homeless (Figure 2.10).

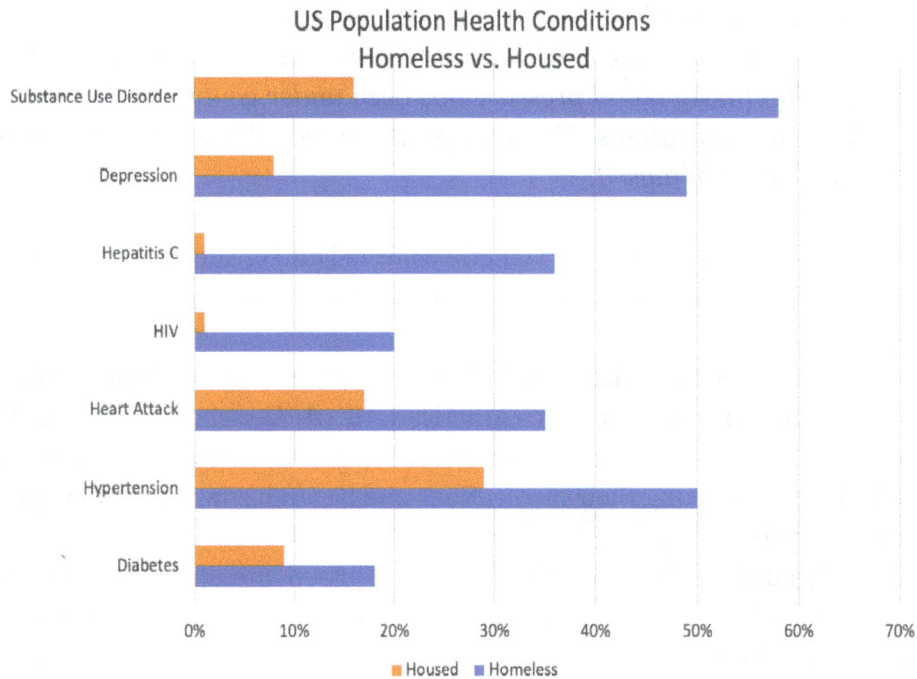

US Population Health Conditions
Homeless vs. Housed

Figure 2.10: Comparison of Health Conditions in Homeless and General U.S. Population

Source: Original Work
Attribution: Kristy Michelle Gamble
License: CC BY-SA 4.0

COVID-19 virus pandemic

The U.S. is facing a grave challenge and adversity as the entire world is affected by the COVID-19 pandemic. COVID-19 is an acronym for coronavirus disease 2019 and is part of a group of viruses that cause respiratory illnesses (Mayo Foundation for Medical Education and Research [MFMER], 2020). The updated name for the virus is severe acute respiratory syndrome coronavirus 2 (SARS-CoV-2) (MFMER). This virus originated around December 2019 in China, and a global pandemic was declared in March 2020 by the WHO (MFMER). As of July 2021, there are nearly 200 million confirmed cases with over 4 million deaths globally, in more than 188 countries, areas, or territories (WHO, 2021). In the U.S., over 34 million cases and 600,000 deaths have been attributed to COVID-19 as of late July, 2021 (WHO, 2021). As variants of the virus emerge and spread throughout the world, more infections and deaths are expected. Persons living in nursing homes or long-term care facilities, and any person of any age with underlying conditions of hypertension, cardiovascular disease, diabetes, chronic respiratory disease, cancer, renal disease, and obesity continue to be at greater risk of severe symptoms or fatality (CDC, 2020). The largest number of deaths thus far have been in the 85+ age population.

2.6 HOW CAN WE IMPROVE HEALTH IN THE U.S.?

Other than the pandemic we are currently facing, and from a standpoint of causes of deaths in the U.S. and preventable chronic disease, the CDC (2019c) clearly points to tobacco use as the number one risk factor. The other three risk factors are poor nutrition, lack of physical activity, and excessive alcohol use. Since most risk factors are related to a person's choice, continued education is the answer to improving health in the U.S. The CDC has many initiatives to educate the population about tobacco use, healthy food choices, cancer screenings and vaccinations, physical activity programs, identifying risk factors for heart disease and diabetes, among others. The ODPHP (2019f) has begun the 2020 Healthy People initiative, utilizing experts to evaluate the biological, economic, environmental, and social health determinants discussed in this chapter and their interrelationships throughout a person's lifespan using twenty-six leading health indicators (LHIs), with twelve main topic areas (see healthypeople.gov). This data will provide additional information about health indicators and the health status of Americans and should serve to motivate all sectors of the U.S. population.

Other ideas for improvement of health include the following:

1. Develop new and utilize existing genetic testing and family health history tools; record information in electronic health records (ODPHP, 2019).

2. "Mobilize community partnerships" and "link people to needed personal health services" (CDC, 2018d, Public Health Professionals Gateway, p. 2). Provide "community-based resources and transportation options for older adults," as research indicates these social support activities can positively affect health status by lowering the risk for physical and mental illnesses and death (ODPHP, 2019).

3. Design programs to facilitate adolescents' positive development by teaching healthy behaviors and encouraging social connections. According to the FIFCF, "The formation of close attachments to family, peers, school, and community have been linked to healthy youth development" (FIFCF, 2019, p. 63).

4. Improve access to healthcare services. Screenings and monitoring of weight, blood pressure, and cholesterol can reduce the risks of heart disease, diabetes, and other physical and mental conditions in adults, adolescents, and young children. Perform cancer screenings for early and treatable signs of cancer in the breast, colo-rectal area, and skin. Educate young people and screen for and treat sexually transmitted

diseases to reduce the risk of serious and long-term health conditions. Education and screening for the older population concerning visual and hearing disorders also are needed.

5. Most states have some type of health insurance, such as Medicaid, for children. Provide education for parents on the importance of reading to children, healthy eating habits, physical activity with limited screen time, oral care, screenings, vaccinations, and other checkups for children and adolescents to ensure they are keeping pace with developmental milestones and staying healthy; also, identify early signs of problems such as obesity and risk factors for chronic health conditions later in life (ODPHP, 2019).

6. Facilitate reading and mathematics achievements in children and youth as well as after school programs to assist youth to complete high school. Additional school counselors are needed to work with youth to find employment or continue education after graduation with college or technical school.

2.6.1 Lack of Use of Evidence-Based Preventive Services

A proposal by the Office of Disease Prevention and Health Promotion (2019) is that the U.S. should initiate preventive services based on statistical evidence. The proposal states the following:

> Prevent illness by promoting healthy behaviors in people without risk factors (diet and exercise counseling), prevent illness by providing protection to those at risk (e.g. childhood vaccinations); identify and treat people with no symptoms, but who have risk factors, before the clinical illness develops (e.g. screening for hypertension or colorectal cancer) (ODPHP, 2019, para 11).

We must continue to research healthcare variables and disseminate the information to improve healthcare for all. Research provided by the various surveys mentioned in this chapter will help us reach these and other objectives.

2.7 SUMMARY

This chapter has included an overview of definitions of health and health determinants that affect the health of individuals and a population. It has also described measures to assess the health status of the U.S. It has discussed chronic conditions and risk factors for chronic illness and disability and has provided measures to improve health in the U.S.

2.8 REVIEW QUESTIONS

1. How is health defined?
2. What are health determinants and how do they affect a person and a population?
3. What measures are used to assess the health status of the U.S.?
4. How is chronic disease defined? What behaviors contribute to an individual's developing a chronic disease?
5. Explain two ways to improve health in the U.S. and support your answers.

2.9 REFERENCES

Alliance for Strong Families and Communities. (2019). Social determinants of health. Social Determinants of Health Issue Brief. Retrieved from https://alliance1.org/web/resources/pubs/social-determinants-health-issue-brief.aspx

American Academy of Child and Adolescent Psychiatry (No. 17, May 2019). Alcohol use in Families. Retrieved from https://www.aacap.org/AACAP/Families_and_Youth/Facts_for_Families/FFF-Guide/Children-Of-Alcoholics-017.aspx

American Academy of Family Physicians. (2015). Learning matters: How education affects health. Leader Voices Blog. Retrieved from https://www.aafp.org/news/blogs/leadervoices/entry/learning_matters_how_education_affects.html

American Heart Association. (2020). Heart disease in African-American women. Retrieved November 16, 2020, from https://www.goredforwomen.org/en/about-heart-disease-in-women/facts/heart-disease-in-african-american-women

Arias, E. & Xu, J. (2019). United States life tables, 2017. National Vital Statistics Reports, 68(7). National Center for Health Statistics. Retrieved from https://www.cdc.gov/nchs/data/nvsr/nvsr68/nvsr68_07-508.pdf.\

Artiga, S., & Hinton, E. (2018). Beyond health care: The role of social determinants in promoting health and health equity. Kaiser Family Foundation. Retrieved from https://www.kff.org/racial-equity-and-health-policy/issue-brief/beyond-health-care-the-role-of-social-determinants-in-promoting-health-and-health-equity/

Ashcroft, R. & Van Katwyk, T. (2017). Joining the global conversation: Social workers define health using a participatory action research approach. British Journal of Social Work, 47, 579–596.

Badash, I., Kleinman, N. P., Barr, S., Jang, J., Rahman, S., & Wu, B. W. Redefining health: The evolution of health ideas from antiquity to the era of value-based care. Cureus 9(2): e1018. DOI 10.7759/cureus.1018

Braveman, P., Acer, J., Arkin, E., Proctor, D., Gillman, A., McGeary, K. A., & Mallya, G. (2018). Wealth matters for health equity. Robert Wood Johnson Foundation.

Centers for Disease Control and Prevention. (2020, September 29). Coronavirus disease

2019 (COVID-19): CDC COVID Data Tracker: United States COVIC-10 Cases and
Deaths by States.

Centers for Disease Control and Prevention. (2019a). Tobacco use. Retrieved from
https://www.cdc.gov/chronicdisease/resources/publications/factsheets/tobacco.htm

Centers for Disease Control and Prevention. (2019b). Sexually transmitted disease
surveillance 2018. DOI:10.15620/cdc.79370

Centers for Disease Control and Prevention. (2019c). About chronic diseases. Retrieved
from https://www.cdc.gov/chronicdisease/about/index.htm

Centers for Disease Control and Prevention. (2019d). Reproductive health:
Infant mortality. Retrieved from https://www.cdc.gov/reproductivehealth/
maternalinfanthealth/infantmortality.htm

Centers for Disease Control and Prevention. (2019e). Health and economic costs of
chronic disease. Retrieved from https://www.cdc.gov/chronicdisease/about/costs/
index.htm

Centers for Disease Control and Prevention. (2019f). Office on smoking and health: At a
glance. Retrieved from https://www.cdc.gov/chronicdisease/pdf/aag/osh-H.pdf

Centers for Disease Control and Prevention. (2019g). Division for heart disease and
stroke prevention. Retrieved from https://www.cdc.gov/chronicdisease/resources/
publications/aag/heart-disease

Centers for Disease Control and Prevention. (2019h). Division of cancer prevention and
control: At a glance. Retrieved from https://www.cdc.gov/chronicdisease/resources/
publications/aag/dcpc.htmstroke.htm

Centers for Disease Control and Prevention. (2019i). Division of population health: At a
glance. Retrieved from https://www.cdc.gov/chronicdisease/pdf/aag/dph-H.pdf

Centers for Disease Control and Prevention. (2019j). Health literacy. Retrieved from
https://www.cdc.gov/healthliteracy/learn/index.html

Centers for Disease Control and Prevention. (2018a). Social determinants of health:
Know what affects health. Retrieved from https://www.cdc.gov/socialdeterminants/
research/index.htm

Centers for Disease Control and Prevention. (2018b). Division of diabetes translation: At
a glance. Retrieved from https://www.cdc.gov/chronicdisease/pdf/aag/ddt-H.pdf

Centers for Disease Control and Prevention. (2018c). Mental health: Learn about mental
health. Retrieved from https://www.cdc.gov/mentalhealth/learn/index.htm

Centers for Disease Control and Prevention. (2018d). Public health professionals
gateway: The public health system and the 10 essential public health services.
Retrieved from https://www.cdc.gov/publichealthgateway/publichealthservices/
essentialhealthservices.html

Centers for Disease Control and Prevention. (2017). Homelessness as a public health law
issue: Selected resources. Retrieved from https://www.cdc.gov/phlp/publications/
topic/resources/resources-homelessness.html

Centers for Disease Control and Prevention. (2014). The health consequences of smoking – 50 years of progress: A report of the surgeon general. Retrieved from https://www. hhs.gov/sites/default/files/consequences-smoking-exec-summary.pdf.

Central Intelligence Agency. (2020). The world factbook. Retrieved from https://www. cia.gov/library/Publications/the-world-factbook/fields/354rank.html. Retrieved May 28, 2020.

Fallon, C. K. & Karlawish, J. (2019). Is the WHO definition of health aging well? Frameworks for "Health" after three score and ten. American Journal of Public Health, 109(8), 1104–1105.

Federal Interagency Forum on Child and Family Statistics. (2019). America's Children: Key National Indicators of Well-Being, 2019. Washington, D.C.: U.S. Government Printing Office.

Jutras, M. (2017). A walk through the drastic transformation of attitudes toward mental illness throughout history. British Columbia Medical Journal, 59(2), 86–88. Retrieved from https://www.bcmj.org/print/mds-be/historical-perspectives-theories-diagnosis-and-treatment-mental-illness

Leonardi, F. (2018). The definition of health: Towards new perspectives. International Journal of Health Services, 48(4), 735–748.

LoRe, D. Ladner, P., & Suskind, D. (2018). Talk, read, sing: Early language exposure as an overlooked social determinant of health. Pediatrics, 142(3). DOI: https://doi. org/10.1542/peds.2018-2007

Mayo Foundation for Medication Education and Research. (2020, May 19). Coronavirus disease 2019 (COVID-19). Retrieved from https://www.mayoclinic.org/diseases-conditions/coronavirus/symptoms-causes/syc-20479963?p=1

Murphy, S.L., Xu, Jiaquan, Kochanek, K.D., & Arias, E. (2018). Mortality in the United States, 2017. NCHS Data Brief, 328. Hyattsville, MD: National Center for Health Statistics.

National Cancer Institute. (n.d.). NCI dictionary of cancer terms. Retrieved from https:// www.cancer.gov/publications/dictionaries/cancer-terms/def/morbidity

National Center for Chronic Disease Prevention and Health Promotion (NCCDPHP). (2020). About Chronic Diseases. https://www.cdc.gov/chronicdisease/about/index. htm

National Health Care for the Homeless Council. (2019, February). Homelessness & Health: What's the connection? Retrieved from https://nhchc.org/wp-content/ uploads/2019/08/homelessness-and-health.pdf

National Institutes of Health. (2020a, May 19). Epidemiology. Retrieved from https://search.nih.gov/ search?utf8=%E2%9C%93&affiliate=nih&query=epidemiology&commit=Search

National Institutes of Health. (2020b). US National Library of Medicine: Genetics Home Reference (2020). Help me understand genetics: Inheriting genetic conditions.

Retrieved from https://ghr.nlm.nih.gov/primer/inheritance/ethnicgroup

National Institutes of Health. (2019). Benefits of exercise. U.S. National Library of Medicine: MedlinePlus. Retrieved from https://medlineplus.gov/benefitsofexercise.html

National Institutes of Health. (2018). Osteoporosis overview. NIH Osteoporosis and Related Bone Diseases National Resource Center. Retrieved from https://www.bones.nih.gov/health-info/bone/osteoporosis/overview

National Institutes on Alcohol Abuse and Alcoholism (NIAAA). (2019). Alcohol facts and statistics. Retrieved from https://www.niaaa.nih.gov/sites/default/files/AlcoholFactsandStats.pdf

Office of Disease Prevention and Health Promotion. (2020). Social determinants – Interventions and resources - Employment. Retrieved from https://www.healthypeople.gov/2020/topics-objectives/topic/social-determinants-health/interventions-resources/employment

Office of Disease Prevention and Health Promotion. (2019a). Genomics. Healthypeople2020.gov. Retrieved from https://www.healthypeople.gov/2020/topics-objectives/topic/genomics

Office of Disease Prevention and Health Promotion. (2019b). Social determinants. Healthypeople2020.gov. Retrieved from https://www.healthypeople.gov/2020/leading-health-indicators/2020-lhi-topics/Social-Determinants

Office of Disease Prevention and Health Promotion. (2019c) Access to health services. Retrieved from https://www.healthypeople.gov/2020/leading-health-indicators/2020-lhi-topics/access-to-health-services

Office of Disease Prevention and Health Promotion. (2019d). Leading health indicators: Injury and violence. Retrieved from https://www.healthypeople.gov/2020/leading-health-indicators/2020-lhi-topics/Injury-and-Violence/determinants

Office of Disease Prevention and Health Promotion. (2019e). Social determinants – Objectives. Retrieved from https://www.healthypeople.gov/2020/topics-objectives/topic/social-determinants-of-health/objectives

Office of Disease Prevention and Health Promotion. (2019f). Leading health indicators. Retrieved from https://www.healthypeople.gov/2020/Leading-Health-Indicators

Office of Economic Cooperation and Development. (2019). Life expectancy at birth (indicator). Retrieved from https://data.oecd.org/healthstat/life-expectancy-at-birth.htm#indicator-chart

Ohlhorst, S. D., Russell, R. R., Bier, D., Klurfeld, D. M., Li, Z., Mein, J. R., Milner, J., Ross, A. C., Stover, P., & Konopka, E. (2013). Nutrition research to affect food and a healthy lifespan. Advances in Nutrition, 4(5), 579–584. https://doi.org/10.3945/an.113.004176

Proctor, B. D., Semega, J. L., & Kollar, M. (2016). U.S. Census Bureau Current Population Reports, P60-256 (RV), Income and poverty in the United States: 2015. U.S.

Government Printing Office, Washington, D.C.

Semega, J., Kollar, M., Creamer, J., & Mohanty, A. (2019). U.S. Census Bureau Current Population Reports, P60-266, Income and Poverty in the United States: 2018. U.S. Government Printing Office, Washington, D.C.

U.S. Department of Commerce. (2020). Poverty thresholds for 2019 by size of family and number of related children under 18 years. U.S. Census Bureau. Retrieved from https://www.census.gov/data/tables/time-series/demo/income-poverty/historical-poverty-thresholds.html

U.S. Department of Health and Human Services (HHS). (2020a). Smoking cessation. A report of the surgeon general. Atlanta, GA: U.S. Department of Health and Human Services, Centers for Disease Control and Prevention, National Center for Chronic Disease Prevention and Health Promotion, Office on Smoking and Health.

U.S. Department of Health and Human Services (HHS). (2020b). Health literacy. Retrieved from https://www.healthypeople.gov/2020/topics-objectives/topic/social-determinants-health/interventions-resources/health-literacy

U.S. Department of Health and Human Services. (2017). President's council on sports, fitness and nutrition. Retrieved from https://www.hhs.gov/fitness/resource-center/facts-and-statistics/index.html

White, A., Castle, I.P., Hingson, R., & Powell, P. (2020). Using death certificates to explore changes in alcohol-related mortality in the United States, 1999-2017. Alcoholism: Clinical and Experimental Research, 44(1), 178-187. https://doi.org/10.1111/acer.14239

World Health Organization (WHO). (2020, Sept 29). World Health Organization: Who we are. Retrieved from https://www.who.int/about

World Health Organization (WHO). (2021). Coronavirus statistics. Retrieved from https://covid19.who.int/table

World Health Organization. (1998). Health promotion glossary. Retrieved from https://www.who.int/healthpromotion/about/HPR%20Glossary%201998.pdf?ua=1

World Health Organization. (n.d.). Disability. Retrieved from https://www.who.int/health-topics/disability#tab=tab_1

Zong, J., Batalova, J., & Burrows, M. (2019). Frequently requested statistics on immigrants and immigration in the United States. Migration Policy Institute, 1-30. Retrieved from https://www.migrationpolicy.org/article/frequently-rquested-statistics-immigrants-and-immigration-united-states

3

Healthcare Workforce

3.1 LEARNING OBJECTIVES

By the end of this chapter, the student will be able to:

- Contrast the many types of healthcare workers in the U.S.
- Differentiate between two types of Advanced Practice Providers
- Identify the work setting for each type of healthcare provider
- Discuss the projections for future employment in healthcare professions
- Explain how the rising numbers of seniors will impact the U.S. healthcare workforce
- Describe the meaning of gender pay inequality

3.2 KEY TERMS

- advanced practice provider (APP)
- allied health provider
- complementary and alternative medicine (CAM) provider
- dentist
- gender pay inequality
- optometrist
- pharmacist
- physician
- psychologist
- registered nurse

3.3 INTRODUCTION

Every individual in the U.S. will likely come into contact with some type of healthcare provider during their lifetime. Whether through birth, a trip to the emergency room, immunizations, filling a prescription, getting teeth cleaned, or moving into a long-term care home, citizens will meet providers in a variety of settings. The healthcare workforce is the backbone of the healthcare system—which is considered the largest employer in the U.S. (Thompson, 2018). According to the Bureau of Labor Statistics (BLS) (2020a), healthcare employment opportunities are expected to grow 14% from 2018 to 2028. This increase is largely attributed to the growing elderly population and to the numbers of healthcare providers entering retirement age. The impact on the workforce will be significant.

This chapter will identify many different U.S. healthcare professions. Definitions of each profession type, roles and responsibilities, and educational requirements will be presented. This chapter will also include the most up-to-date data for health professions in the workforce and projections for the future. According to the U.S. News & World Report (2019), in a 2019 U.S. News Best Jobs Rankings, physician's assistant, dentist, orthodontist, and nurse anesthetist were health professions listed among the top five professions noted.

3.4 PHYSICIANS

Physicians are made up of two types of educated professionals: Doctor of Medicine (MD) and Doctor of Osteopathic Medicine (DO). The major difference between the two is a practice philosophy. Medical doctors practice allopathic medicine, which focuses on diagnosing and treating disease (BLS, 2020a). Doctors of osteopathic medicine view practice more holistically, diagnosing patients by using osteopathic manipulative medicine and emphasizing wellness and health promotion (AACOM, 2019). However, each has the same licensing requirements and prescriptive abilities and practitioners can pursue the same specialties.

- - - - - - - - - - - - - - - - - - -
Most Common Types of Physician Specialties

Specialties A to Z

Allergists/Immunologist; Anesthesiologist; Cardiologist; Colon and Rectal Surgeon; Critical Care Medicine Specialist; Dermatologist, Endocrinologist; Emergency Medicine Specialist; Family Physician; Gastroenterologist; General Surgeon; Geriatric Medicine Specialist; Hematologist; Hospice and Palliative Medicine Specialists; Infectious Disease Specialists; Internist; Medical Geneticist; Nephrologist; Neurologist; Obstetrician and Gynecologist; Oncologist; Ophthalmologist; Osteopath; Otolaryngologist; Pathologist; Pediatrician; Physiatrist; Plastic Surgeon; Podiatrist; Preventative Medicine Specialist;

Psychiatrist; Pulmonologist; Radiologist; Rheumatologist; Sleep Medicine Specialist; Sports Medicine Specialist; Urologist

3.4.1 Specialty

Physicians may choose from a variety of specialties in which to practice medicine. Of the best paying jobs listed in the 2019 U.S. News Best Jobs Rankings report, all five were specialty physicians: anesthesiologist, surgeon, oral and maxillofacial surgeon, obstetrician and gynecologist, and orthodontist (ranked in order) (U.S. News & World Report, 2019). There are hundreds of specialties and subspecialties, which can make finding the right doctor confusing for the average American (Table 3.1). Most citizens have seen a pediatrician as a child for well-baby or sick visits. While pregnant, many women have been followed by an obstetrician-gynecologist (OB-GYN). A broken bone is generally treated by an orthopedist. Depending on the medical issue, a doctor exists who specializes in it. However, general practitioner doctors can diagnose and treat the body as a whole. Most people see a private practice physician or multi-provider clinic for medical concerns or unusual symptoms. If further care or diagnostics are needed, the patient may then be referred to a specialty provider.

Table 3.1: Number of Physicians by Specialty in 2019	
Physicians and surgeons, all other	433,700
Family and general practitioners	126,600
Internists, general	42,800
Surgeons	38,200
Anesthesiologists	34,500
Pediatricians, general	31,700
Psychiatrists	28,600
Obstetricians and gynecologists	20,700

Source: US Bureau of Labor Statistics
Attribution: US Bureau of Labor Statistics
License: Public Domain

3.4.2 Work Settings

Physicians work in a variety of settings, including private or multi-provider clinics, hospitals, surgical centers, public health departments, prisons, elderly care centers, academia, or government. In 2018, there were approximately 756,800 physician jobs in the U.S. (BLS, 2020a). More physicians now work for someone else rather than independently in private practice (Henry, 2019).

3.4.3 Education

The education required to become a physician includes a four-year bachelor's degree, satisfactory medical college admission test (MCAT), four years of medical school, and a three-to-seven year residency program. In addition, upon completion of medical training, a standardized national licensure exam must be passed. MDs take the U.S. Medical Licensing Examination (USMLE), and DOs take the Comprehensive Osteopathic Medical Licensing Examination (COMLEX-USA). All physicians, regardless of degree type, must also apply for a license to the Medical Board of the state in which they wish to practice medicine.

3.4.4 Projections for the Future

According to the Association of American Medical Colleges (AAMC) (2019), physician shortages are expected to reach approximately 122,000 by the year 2032. A major contribution to this shortage is an increase in persons 65 and older, projected at 48% over the next twelve years. This shortage is complicated by physicians' reaching retirement age. Employment is expected to grow 7% from 2018 to 2028 (BLS, 2020a). Prospects are good for employment because of the expected physician shortages but are especially good for physicians willing to work in rural or low-income areas (BLS, 2020a).

Activity 3.1: Match each specialty doctor to the type of symptoms they treat	
1. Pulmonologist	a. increased appetite, increased thirst, and frequent urination
2. Urologist	b. a brown, irregular shaped mole on the leg
3. Neurologist	c. a urinary tract infection that will not go away
4. Endocrinologist	d. difficulty breathing during exercise
5. Dermatologist	e. frequent headaches

Key: 1.d; 2.c; 3.e; 4.a; 5.b

3.5 ADVANCED PRACTICE PROVIDERS

Advanced practice providers (APPs) are significant to the healthcare workforce, providing much needed relief as an extension of the doctor or, in some cases, as independent providers. APPs are a group of "non-physician" providers who can examine, diagnose, and treat patients independently in some states or in collaboration with a physician in other states. APPs include physician assistants (PAs) and advanced practice registered nurses (APRNs), such as nurse practitioners (NPs), Nurse Anesthetists (CRNAs), Clinical Nurse Specialists (CNS), and Nurse Midwives (CNMs). CRNAs and CNMs are generally specific in their work environment—the operating room, surgical centers, and obstetric-gynecological practices—while the CNS's focus is defined by population or setting. In the 2019 U.S. News & World Report Best Healthcare Jobs rankings, physician assistant ranked number one, nurse anesthetist ranked number four, and nurse practitioner ranked number five (U.S. News & World Report, 2019). This chapter will focus on NPs and PAs who serve a primary care role in healthcare.

3.5.1 Nurse Practitioner

Nurse practitioner (NP) training began in 1965 to answer the need for more providers to give care to children and families. The profession has grown in the last fifty-five years, with NPs serving a critical role in today's healthcare system. NPs are registered nurses with an advanced degree. NPs follow a patient-centered model of care and must meet national standards of care. Below lists the responsibilities of nurse practitioners.

The Role and Responsibilities of Nurse Practitioners

- Take and record patients' medical histories and symptoms
- Perform physical exams and observe patients
- Create patient care plans or contribute to existing plans
- Perform and order diagnostic tests
- Operate and monitor medical equipment
- Diagnose various health problems
- Analyze test results or changes in a patient's condition
- Give patients medicines and treatments

The scope of practice for NPs depends on the state where licensure is obtained. NPs practice in these three environments: full practice, reduced practice, and restricted practice. States with *full practice* licensure laws permit NPs to work independently in a primary care role—including prescription rights—under the authority of the state board of nursing. *Reduced practice* licensure laws affect NPs working in specific states and reduce the ability of NPs to engage in at least one element of practice. The states with reduced practice laws require a regulated collaborative agreement with another health provider or limit the setting of NP practice. The *restricted practice* licensure laws also restrict the ability of NPs to engage in at least one element of practice. The states with restricted practice laws also require a career-long supervision for the NP to provide patient care (The American Association of Nurse Practitioners [AANP], 2018).

Specialty

In a 2018 Health Resources & Services Administration (HRSA) (2018) U.S. Health Workforce survey, nurse practitioners numbered 122,858. NPs may choose from several specialties to provide direct patient care, including the following: family, adult, adult-gerontology primary care, acute care, pediatrics-primary care, adult-gerontology acute care, women's health, psychiatric/mental health-family, psychiatric/mental health, and gerontology. NPs work in a variety of settings, such as private practice, hospital outpatient clinics, inpatient hospital units, emergency rooms, urgent care, and community health centers.

Education

Educational requirements for the nurse practitioner include licensure as a registered nurse (RN) and an earned master's degree in a nurse practitioner program with clinical competency from an accredited program. Master's degree programs offer advanced nursing education in areas of clinical nurse specialist, certified nurse midwife, nurse anesthetist, and nurse practitioner (family, pediatric, psychiatric). Passing a national certification examination and licensure in a specific state is required to assume the full NP role. Additional requirements may be cardiopulmonary resuscitation (CPR), basic life support (BLS), or advanced cardiac life support (ACLS) certifications. Individual states may require continuing education credits annually or biannually. NPs may choose to earn a Doctorate of Nursing Practice (DNP) or another doctoral level of education. According to AANP (2019a), approximately 95.2% of NPs hold a master's degree. The National Organization of Nurse Practitioner Faculties (NONPF) are "committed to move all entry-level nurse practitioner (NP) education to the DNP degree by 2025" (p. 1).

3.5.2 Physician Assistants

Physician assistant (PA) training began in 1967 to improve and expand healthcare in response to a shortage in primary care physicians. PA education is modeled after general medicine and trains candidates to practice medicine (American Academy of PAs [AAPA], 2019). PAs have a similar role and responsibilities to NPs. The scope of practice, specific duties, and level of physician supervision differs by state. Below lists the responsibilities of the PA. In the 2019 U.S. News Best Jobs Rankings, physician assistant ranked at number three in the top 100 best jobs and number one in the best healthcare jobs.

- -

Typical Duties of the Physician Assistant

- Take or review patients' medical histories
- Examine patients
- Order and interpret diagnostic tests, such as x rays or blood tests
- Diagnose a patient's injuries or illness
- Give treatment, such as setting broken bones and immunizing patients
- Educate and counsel patients and their families

- Prescribe medicine
- Assess and record a patient's progress
- Research the latest treatments to ensure the quality of patient care
- Conduct or participate in outreach programs

Physician assistants practice in many settings and in several different specialties. The profession has grown 37.2% over the last five years, with a current PA workforce of 131,152 certified in 2018 (NCCPA, 2018). The PA workforce is young. In a 2018 survey of recent physician assistant graduates, 72.5% were under the age of 30 and another 23.4% between the ages of 30 and 39. Women dominate the field and make up approximately 70% of the PA workforce (2018 Statistical Profile of Certified Physician Assistants, 2019).

Education

Educational requirements for physician assistants include a master's degree from an accredited program lasting approximately two years of full-time study. Many educational programs have admission requirements of a bachelor's degree in a science field and patient care experience. Once education is complete, candidates must pass the Physician Assistant National Certifying Examination (PANCE) from the National Commission on Certification of Physician Assistants (NCCPA). In addition, licensure through a state application to practice must be granted. Certification is maintained by earning 100 hours of continuing education credits every two years and passing the Physician Assistant National Recertifying Exam (PANRE) every ten years. PAs may also take an additional examination to earn a specialty certification (PhysicanAssistantEDU.org, 2019).

3.5.3 Future Projections for Advanced Practice Providers

Demand for advanced practice providers is expected to increase, with a continued focus on preventative and primary care. In the Medscape Physician Compensation Report 2019, physicians were asked, "Do you use NPs or PAs in your practice?" (Kane, 2019). The responses noted nurse practitioners are most often employed in outpatient clinics, academic (nonhospital) settings, and in healthcare organizations. Physician assistants are most often employed in healthcare organizations, office-based multispecialty groups, and in hospitals. Significantly, physicians in this same survey said profits increased with the use of NPs and PAs. Nurse practitioner employment in the next ten years is expected to grow 28% (BLS, 2020b). Physician assistant employment is expected to grow 31% in the next ten years (BLS, 2020c).

- -- -- -- -- -- -- -- -- -- -- -- -- -- -- -- -- --

First Person Perspective

Dr. D., DO, FACOS, specializes in urology.

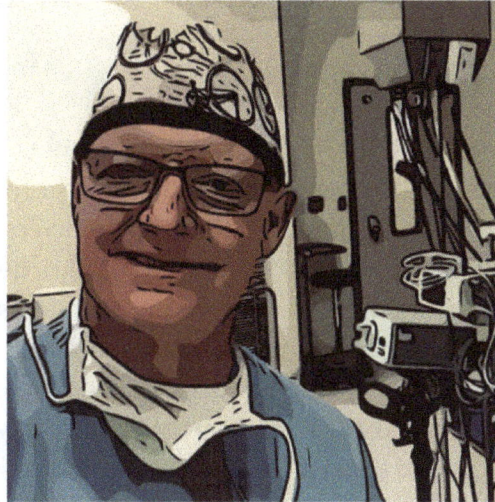

Figure 3.1: First Person Perspective

Source: Original Work
Attribution: Deanna Howe
License: CC BY-SA 4.0

I am a practicing urologist in a rural area in the southwest region of the U.S. We are a private practice and have been in this area for over forty years. When I joined the group in 2002, we had seven full time urologists in a town of 100,000 people that serviced an area of over 300,000. Over the years, due to retirements and loss of personnel, we now have four urologists that cover this same area. My state ranks 45th in the country in need of urologists per population. It had become apparent that due to the lack of urologists in the U.S., we needed to increase our workforce.

Our practice had never had APPs until hiring our first physician assistant three years ago. Our first experience with a PA was so successful that we have since hired two nurse practitioners to work in our clinic and surgery center full time. The APPs see patients in the office and make rounds in the hospital, as well as assisting in complex surgical procedures. Our practice is reliant on these APPs every day; they do remarkable work in caring for our patients.

First person perspective vignette collected and created by D. Howe, 2020.

For your consideration: Dr. D. states physicians in his private practice are decreasing due to retirements and there is a need to increase the workforce available to serve his community. Advanced practice professionals, such as NPs and PAs, are increasing in numbers and able to contribute as primary care providers by helping meet patient needs.

Have you ever had an NP or PA as a primary care provider? What was your overall impression? Do you feel that advance practice providers will help stabilize the workforce as the physician population is declining?

- -

3.6 REGISTERED NURSES

Registered nurses (RNs) are without a doubt the most abundant professionals in the U.S. healthcare system, with just over three million members in 2018 (HRSA, 2018). The field of nursing provides a diverse work environment, and nurses can be found in nearly every aspect of the U.S. healthcare system. For seventeen years in a row, nurses are considered the most "trusted" professionals in the U.S. In a 2018 Gallup poll, 84% of Americans responding rated the honesty and ethical standards of nurses as high or very high (AHA, 2019). It can easily be said that "nursing" has been around since the beginning of time, with family members or "healers" providing care to the sick. Florence Nightingale is attributed with the delivery of nursing service during the Crimea War in 1854 (see Chapter 1). Her principles of nursing education were considered groundbreaking. This led the U.S. to begin providing nursing education to women interested in caring for patients in the home. Later in 1873, professional nursing education began and by 1900, grew to over 400 programs across the U.S. (University of Pennsylvania School of Nursing, 2019). Today, nearly 1,000 programs offer baccalaureate nursing education in the U.S. (AACN, n.d.).

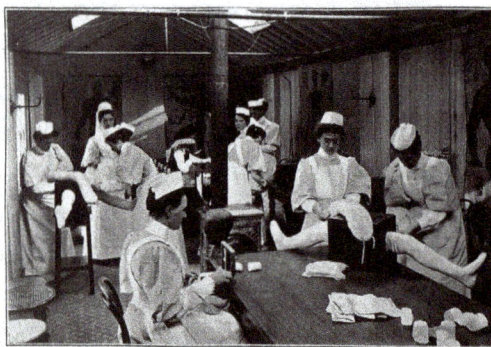

Figure 3.2: Nursing Training in the Late 19th Century

Source: Wikimedia Commons
Attribution: Science Museum Group
License: CC BY 4.0

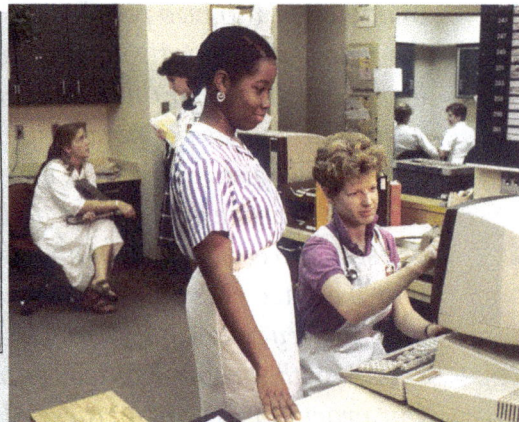

Figure 3.3: RNs in 1987, collaborating in teams

Source: Wikimedia Commons
Attribution: Bill Branson
License: Public Domain

3.6.1 Specialty

RNs work in a variety of clinical and non-clinical settings. While a majority of RNs work in hospital settings, there are many specialty areas within this environment, including medical-surgical, pediatrics, operating room, oncology, neurology, urology, quality assurance, nursing administration, and many more. Outside of the hospital, RNs work in community health, public health, schools, occupational health, and clinics. Nurses even provide consultation for insurance claims and court cases.

Following completion of entry-level nursing education, many nurses go on to seek certification in a specialty area. Specialty recognition is obtained by working in a specific area and passing a certification examination. The five most common nursing specialty certifications include the following: AIDS certified registered nurse (ACRN), certified pediatric nurse (CPN), oncology certified nurse (OCN), family nurse practitioner (FNP-BC), and certified registered nurse anesthetist (CRNA) (Nurse Journal, 2019). Table 3.2 shows the percentage of RNs per work environment (Bureau of Labor Statistics, 2020).

Table 3.2: Registered Nurse Work Environment, 2018	
Hospitals; state, local, and private	60%
Ambulatory healthcare services	18
Nursing and residential care facilities	7
Government	5
Educational services; state, local, and private	3

Source: US Bureau of Labor Statistics
Attribution: US Bureau of Labor Statistics
License: Public Domain

RNs typically work in a collaborative environment in most healthcare settings. Roles and responsibilities of RNs depend on the work setting and specialty. The four main categories of care for the RN include safe effective care, health promotion and maintenance, preventative healthcare, and psychosocial integrity (NCSBN, 2019). Below includes the responsibilities of the RN. Registered nurses who work in hospitals and nursing care facilities share the workload by working in shifts covering twenty-four hours a day, seven days a week. Shifts may be in eight or twelve-hour increments, depending on need.

- - - - - - - - - - - - - - - - - - -

General Responsibilities of the Registered Nurse

- Provide patient care (holistic approach)
- Assist physicians in providing treatment
- Monitor patients
- Record and report symptoms and changes in condition
- Maintain accurate patient reports and medical history
- Administer medications and treatments
- Perform diagnostic tests

- Prepare patients for examinations and treatments
- Supervise less skilled licensed nurses

3.6.2 Education

Nursing has multiple entries of education, all leading to a degree eligible for students to becoming registered nurses. Within the U.S., there are multiple entry points into nursing with diploma, associate degree, and baccalaureate degree nursing programs. Accelerated programs also are available for those with degrees in other fields or for those with healthcare experience, such as paramedics, licensed practical/vocational nurses, and surgical technicians. Graduates of any of the degree options from an accredited nursing program must take a national examination to earn the distinction of registered nurse. After successfully passing the National Council Licensure Examination for Registered Nurses (NCLEX-RN), the nurse must apply for licensure to practice in the desired state of employment. Each state has a board of nursing with rules for practice and continued licensure.

Generally, registered nurses will complete continuing education credits and seek continued licensure every two years. Nurses must seek a license in each state in which they wish to practice. However, they have the option to apply for a Nurse Licensure Compact (NLC) license, which ensures a uniform licensure requirement in all participating states. Nurses with the NLC license will not need to obtain an individual license from each of the thirty-four currently participating State Boards of Nursing.

Nursing schools have done a good job in creating several pathways to advanced education by offering bridge programs for an associate degree in nursing to a baccalaureate degree in nursing (RN-BSN); an associate degree in nursing to a master's degree in nursing (RN-MSN); and a baccalaureate degree in nursing to a doctorate in nursing practice degree (BSN-DNP). Also, master's degree programs offer advanced nursing education in areas of administration, informatics, and education. In addition, doctoral degree programs offer the Doctor of Philosophy (Ph.D.), Doctor of Nursing Science (D.N.S. or D.N.Sc), and Doctor of Nursing Practice (DNP) (Allnursingschools, 2020).

3.6.3 Projections for the Future

The Institute of Medicine (IOM) called for the nursing profession to increase the number of registered nurses with a bachelor's degree in nursing (BSN) to 80% by 2020 (IOM, 2010). This initiative is due to the increasing complexity of care and the need for more highly-educated nurses. As a result of the IOM report and studies showing that patient safety increases with level of education, many initiatives are underway. To increase the number of BSN graduates, hundreds of RN to BSN programs have been created, and "the percentage of RNs with a BSN or higher degree is now at an all-time high with the national average of approximately

56 percent" (AACN, n.d.). In 2017, the New York Governor signed into law a bill for "BSN in 10," requiring ASN graduate nurses who complete an ASN degree to earn a BSN degree within ten years after the initial license (Nurse.org, 2017). This initiative is gaining in popularity.

The RN profession is expected to grow 12% from 2018 to 2028 (BLS, 2020d). The demand continues for RNs because of the increased burden for healthcare services for seniors. However, the U.S. is expected to experience a continued shortage of RNs as the number of nurses entering retirement age grows (AACN, 2020).

3.7 LICENSED PRACTICAL/VOCATIONAL NURSES (LPN/LVN)

The first training programs for practical nurses date back to 1892 in New York City (The History of Practical Nursing, 2013). Licensed Practical Nurses (LPN) and Licensed Vocational Nurses (LVN) are a vital part of the healthcare team providing care to patients and working with the RN. LPN/LVNs have a variety of duties, and state regulations determine the extent to which they can practice. LPN/LVNs generally work under the supervision of an RN. In a 2018 HRSA survey, 852,420 LPN/LVNs worked in the U.S. Work environment primarily includes nursing and residential care facilities, but many LPN/LVNs work in hospitals, physician offices, home healthcare, and government settings.

3.7.1 Education

Educational requirements for the LPN/LVN include either a certificate or diploma and approximately one year of training from a technical school or community college. Some technical colleges have begun offering the LPN/LVN programs at an associate degree level. After completion of an accredited professional program, graduates must pass the NCLEX-PN examination and demonstrate competency in these four areas: safe effective care environment, health promotion and maintenance, psychosocial integrity, and physiological integrity (Practicalnursing.org, 2019). Following successful completion of the NCLEX-PN examination, an LPN/LVN will then be eligible to apply for licensure in the selected state for practice. Individual state boards of nursing will determine requirements for licensure. For LPN/LVN licensed nurses who want to advance their degree, many nursing programs are now offering a bridge to the professional nursing degree in an accelerated LPN/LVN to ASN-RN or the LPN/LVN to BSN-RN format (AACN, n.d.).

3.7.2 Projections for the Future

Licensed practical and licensed vocational nurses provide a majority of the needed nursing care of our elderly population. According to the Bureau of Labor

Statistics (2020d), LPN/LVNs can expect an 11% projected growth from 2018 to 2028. The added 78,100 jobs in this profession will help to ease the strain of caring for the aging population and ever-increasing chronic disease population.

3.8 OTHER ASSISTANT HEALTHCARE WORKERS

A large group of assistive personnel supports physicians and nurses in hospitals, home-settings, and long-term care facilities. However, they can also be seen in doctor's offices, surgical centers, and clinics which provide direct patient care. Nursing assistants, orderlies, home health aides, and personal care aides combined are numbered at 5,015,800 and offer basic care to patients through activities of daily living (BLS, 2020e). These support personnel may or may not be licensed, depending on the state in which they work. Average pay is upwards of $30,000 per year.

3.9 ALLIED HEALTH PROFESSIONALS

An entire book could be dedicated to describing the more than 80 allied health professional careers. Combined, allied health professionals make up 60% of the entire U.S. healthcare workforce (explorehealthcareers.org, 2019). According to the Association of Schools of Allied Health Professions (ASAHP) (2018), "allied health is defined as those health professions that are distinct from medicine and nursing" (p. 1). **Allied health professionals** work alongside other healthcare professionals to assess, diagnose, treat, and evaluate patients. The significance of these professionals in the overall healthcare system cannot be overstated. Table 3.3 lists other allied health professions not discussed in this chapter.

3.9.1 Physical Therapist (PT) and Physical Therapy Assistant (PTA)

Physical therapy assistants (PTAs) work in inpatient, outpatient, rehabilitation settings, home health, and nursing homes to assist patients recovering from injury, surgery, loss of mobility or functioning, and pain. The PTA works under the supervision of the licensed physical therapist (PT) with an earned doctoral degree (American Physical Therapy Association (APTA), 2019a). The physical therapist and physical therapy assistant work in collaboration with other health professionals within the hospital setting to help patients regain mobility, manage exercises to regain and maintain muscle strength, and receive instruction on the use of assistive devices, such as crutches, canes, and walkers. PTs and PTAs educate, monitor, and document the patient's progress, regardless of setting. PTs and PTAs also provide specialized wound care. Outpatient and rehabilitation settings will find the PT and PTA assisting patients with specific exercises, balance training, water therapy, and/or massage. The work of a PT and PTA is physically demanding.

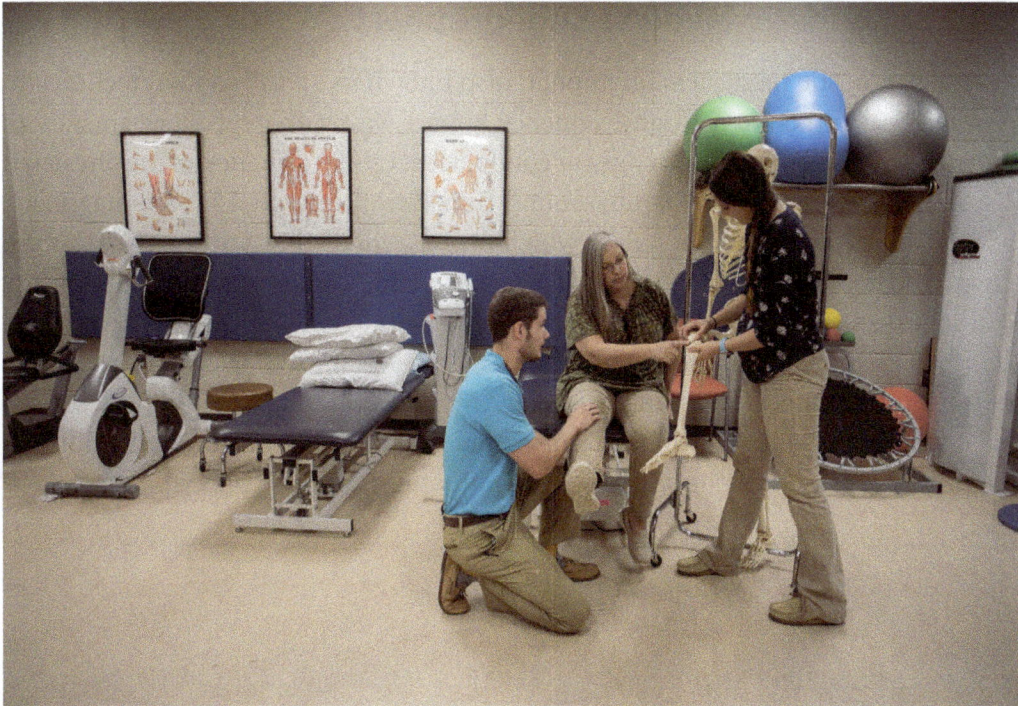

Figure 3.4: Physical Therapy

Source: University of North Georgia
Attribution: Peggy Cozart
License: Courtesy of the University of North Georgia

Education

Physical therapists receive a Doctor of Physical Therapy (DPT) degree from accredited educational programs and are required to successfully pass a national licensure examination to legally practice (American Physical Therapy Association [APTA], 2019b). PTA education includes successful graduation with an associate degree from an accredited physical therapy assistant program. Instruction for this degree includes education in anatomy, physiology, psychology, as well as program-specific training including hands-on clinical practicum training in a variety of hospital and outpatient settings. Graduates of PTA programs must pass the National Physical Therapy Exam for physical therapy assistants. A state application for licensure is required to practice. PTs and PTAs may also be required to complete continuing education credits for continued state licensure.

Projections for the Future

The employment for the physical therapy profession is healthy, with an expected growth of 18% for PT's and 29% for PTA's from 2018 to 2028 (BLS, 2020f). Work areas with the most expected jobs include nursing homes and home health. Elderly persons are at an increased risk for falls which can result in bone fractures. Rehabilitation services to promote optimal mobility and manage effects from injuries will be needed.

3.9.2 Diagnostic Medical Sonographer

The diagnostic medical sonographer, also known as an ultrasound technician, uses medical ultrasound (high-frequency sound waves that produce images of internal structures) to create images or conduct tests at the direction of the physician (CAAHEP, 2019, para 1). The ultrasound transducer, operated by the diagnostic medical sonographer, emits pulses which create echoes that are then sent to the ultrasound machine (BLS, 2020g). The ultrasound machine then processes the data and displays images for diagnosis. The several types of diagnostic medical sonographers include abdominal, breast, cardiac, musculoskeletal, pediatric, obstetric and gynecologic, and vascular. Similar to other health professions, diagnostic medical sonographers work predominantly in hospitals but also in doctor's offices, medical laboratories, and outpatient centers (BLS, 2020g).

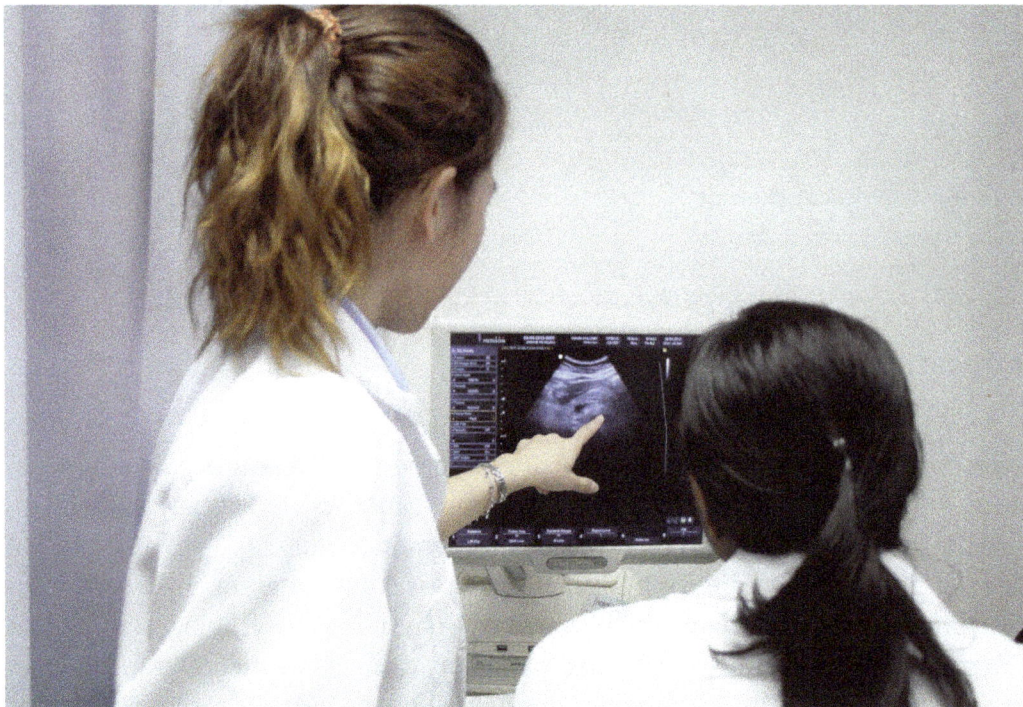

Figure 3.5: Sonographer

Source: Wikimedia Commons
Attribution: Vision College Siew Mun
License: CC BY-SA 4.0

Education

Accredited programs offer associate or bachelor degrees in Diagnostic Medical Sonography. Typical of most allied health professions, their education centers on anatomy and physiology, communication, psychology, and hands-on clinical experiences to develop skills needed for the career. Following successful completion of an accredited program, a certification examination in a generalized concentration is administered through the American Registry for Diagnostic

Medical Sonography (ARMDS, 2019). Many employers may expect certification, and many insurance providers only pay for procedures if certified sonographers have performed the diagnostic exam (BLS, 2020g). Annual renewal of certification is available through the ARMDS organization. Although few states require licensure to practice, individual state medical boards determine licensure requirements for Diagnostic Medical Sonographers. Certification is a major factor in earning the best positions and highest paid jobs.

Projections for the Future

The diverse field is important for early diagnostics and provides imaging without radiation. Elderly population growth will require an expanded use of services. Imaging professionals in the diagnostic medical sonographer, cardiovascular technologist and technician, and vascular fields is expected to grow 19% between 2018 and 2028 (BLS, 2020g).

3.9.3 Occupational Therapist (OA) and Occupational Therapy Assistant (OTA)

Occupational therapist (OT) and occupational therapist assistants (OTA) assist patients in maintaining or recovering those skills needed for activities of daily living, such as feeding oneself, bathing, and dressing. Patients may require help in relearning skills lost after suffering a stroke. These could include how to hold an eating utensil, how to button a shirt with one hand, or how to tie shoes. The OT and OTA may also assist children with autism to learn non-verbal skills to communicate with others. The OTA is supervised and directed by a state licensed occupational therapist (OT), with an earned master's or doctoral degree. Similar to physical therapy professionals, occupational therapy professionals work with patients in hospitals, therapy offices, and nursing homes.

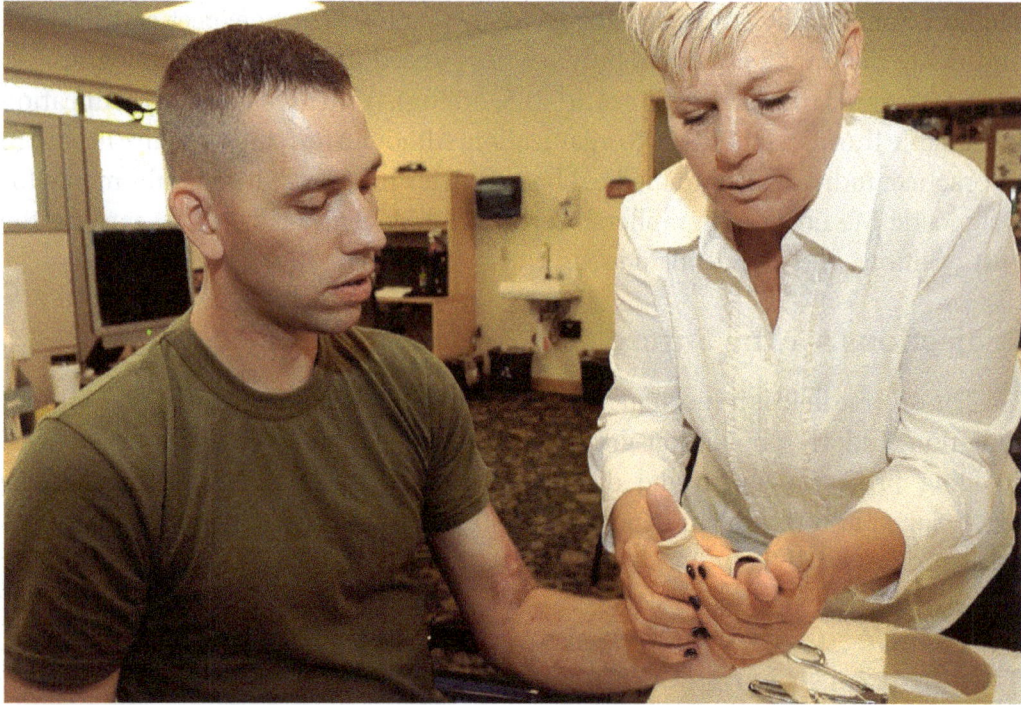

Figure 3.6: Occupational Therapy

Source: Wikimedia Commons
Attribution: User "Grazioso2"
License: CC BY-SA 4.0

Education

Education requirements for the occupational therapist include a master's degree or a doctoral degree in the discipline in order to be eligible to take the national certification examination (NCBOT). State licensure is required for practice (BLS, 2020h). The occupational therapy assistant must complete an associate degree from an accredited OTA program. The curriculum requirements depend on the program, but most include anatomy and physiology, psychology, and specific courses related to career focus. In addition, a clinical practicum must be completed. Following successful completion of the OTA program, candidates sit for an examination administered by the National Board of Certification in Occupational Therapy (AOTA, 2019). Successful passing of this exam results in certification as an occupational therapy assistant (COPA). State licensure must be made via application. Some states may require continuing education for licensure.

Projections for the Future

The need for occupational therapy services will grow as the aging population requires assistance related to Alzheimer's disease, arthritis, and other conditions that result from increased age. Occupational therapists will provide services that assist the elderly in maintaining independence and management of daily living tasks. According to the BLS (2020h), the job outlook for occupational therapy is projected to grow 31% from 2018 to 2028.

3.9.4 Respiratory Therapist (RT)

Respiratory therapists (RT) work with patients who have breathing difficulties. Certain chronic conditions, such as asthma or emphysema, require ongoing consultation and treatment for optimal respiratory functioning. Patients with cystic fibrosis will receive such treatments as chest physiotherapy that encourages coughing which thus removes mucus from the lungs. The RT performs diagnostic tests to evaluate patients and pulmonary treatments to increase lung functioning (BLS, 2020i). In addition, teaching and maintenance of ventilators may occur within many settings to include the hospital and home. Finally, RTs work in emergency settings to assist with maintenance of patient airway. Approximately 81% of the respiratory therapists work in a hospital setting (BLS, 2020i).

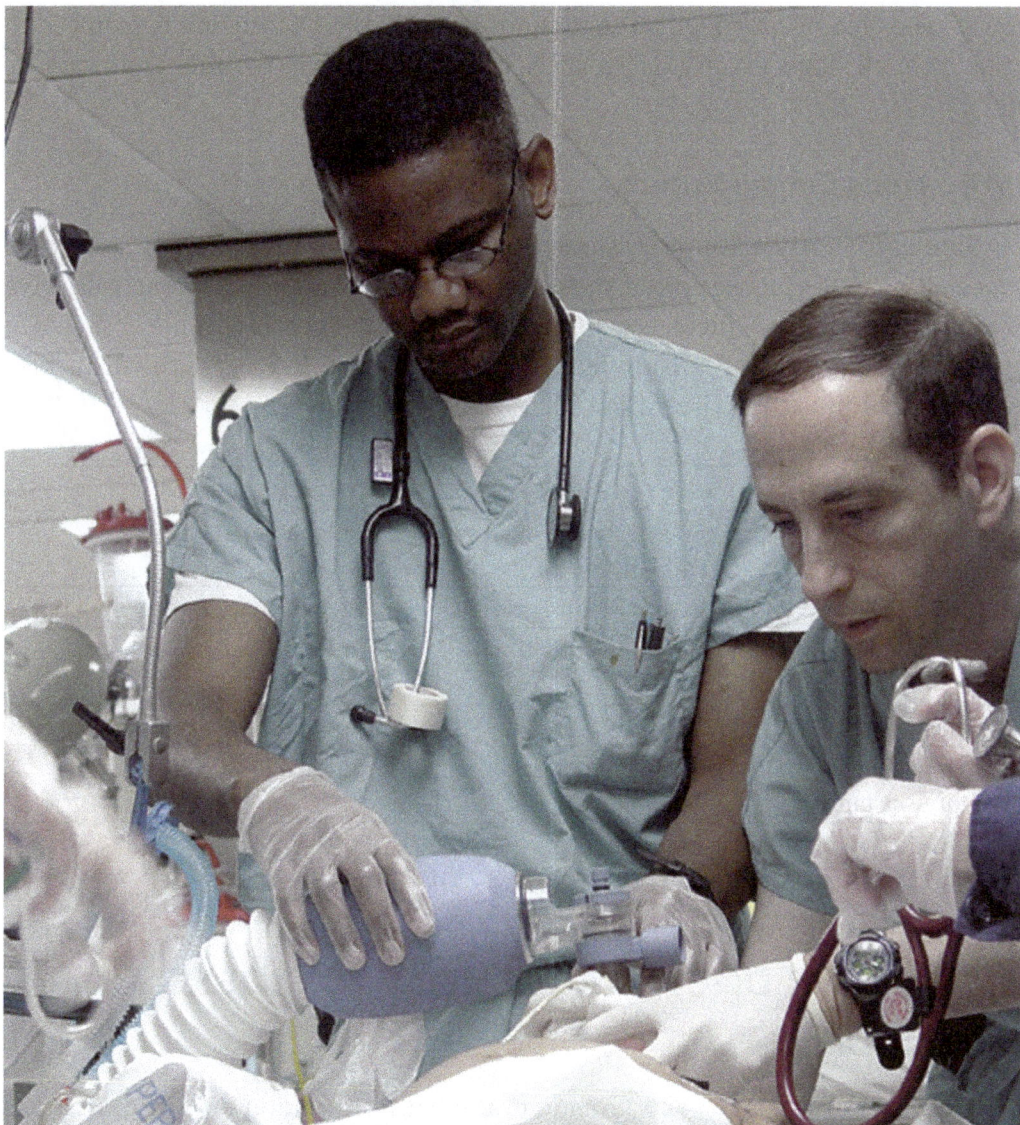

Figure 3.7: Respiratory Therapy

Source: Wikimedia Commons
Attribution: Journalist Seaman Erica Mater
License: Public Domain

Education

Respiratory therapy education requires a minimum of an associate degree from an accredited career program but may also be offered in an accredited bachelor degree program. Similar to most allied health programs, courses in basic anatomy and biology, algebra, psychology, and specific courses related to the career fulfill curriculum requirements. Additional training in clinics, hospitals, and home settings provide the hands-on training needed to develop necessary skills for the profession. Training may also include cardiopulmonary resuscitation (CPR), basic life support (BLS), advanced cardiac life support (ACLS), and pediatric advanced life support (PALS). Upon completion of educational program requirements, a national certification exam is administered by the National Board of Respiratory Care (NBRC). Other certification exams in specific specialties related to the career can also be obtained through an examination with NBRC. Licensure is required to practice in all states except Alaska (BLS, 2020i). Licensure requirements vary by state.

Projections for the Future

Similar to most health professions, demand for respiratory therapy services is expected to continue because of the aging population. Elderly persons will drive demand with increased incidence of chronic conditions such as chronic obstructive pulmonary diseases and pneumonia. There is an expected 19% growth in jobs between 2019 and 2028 (BLS, 2020i).

Table 3.3: Additional Professions in Health Sciences		
Athletic trainer	Emergency medical service and Paramedic	Phlebotomist
Audiology	Health administration	Radiation therapy technology
Cardiovascular perfusion technology	Health information management	Rehabilitation counselor
Cytotechnology	Medical technology	Speech-language pathology
Dental hygiene and Dental Assistant	Nuclear medicine technology	Surgical technology

Source: Original Work
Attribution: Deanna Howe
License: CC BY-SA 4.0

3.10 OTHER DOCTORAL LEVEL PROVIDERS

3.10.1 Dentist

Dentists are doctors who provide oral health promotion and care. Dentists typically remove decay from teeth, fill cavities, repair or remove damaged teeth, make models of teeth for dentures, and teach patients about good dental healthcare. Specialists in this field include dental anesthesiologists, public health specialists, endodontists, oral pathologists, orthodontists, pediatrics, and periodontists (American Dental Association [ADA], 2019). The typical work environment for the dentist is a dental office, private or multi-practice, which will include dental hygienists and dental assistants to aid in patient management. According to the Bureau of Labor Statistics (2020), there were about 155,000 dentists in 2018.

Education

According to the ADA (2019), most dentists have an earned bachelor's degree prior to entering dental school; many programs require a master's degree in public health, and many oral and maxillofacial surgeons earn a medical doctor (MD) degree in addition to the dental degree (para. 5). To become a dentist, one must complete course work for an earned Doctor of Dental Surgery (DDS) or Doctor of Medicine in Dentistry/Doctor of Dental Medicine (DMD). Any specialty practice will require additional postdoctoral preparation. Dental programs must be accredited by the Commission on Dental Accreditation (CODA). Dental programs typically last two-to-four years and mix classroom activities with hands-on training. Further, a written exam administered by the National Board of Dental Examinations as well as state clinical exams must be completed. Licensure to practice is approved with individual states, and requirements may include additional licensure for specialty dentistry (BLS, 2020j).

Projections for the Future

An incentive for ongoing dental care is the link between good oral health and overall health. As the aging population continues to grow, demand for dental services is expected to increase as well. According to BLS (2020j), overall employment is expected to grow 7% from 2018 to 2028. With more graduates entering the field, competition will increase. Those dentists willing to work in underserved areas will find jobs more readily (BLS, 2020j).

3.10.2 Optometrist

An **optometrist** specializes in care of the eyes and other parts of the visual system. Optometrists "examine, diagnose, treat, and manage diseases, injuries, and disorders of the visual system, the eye, and associated structures as well as identify related systemic conditions affecting the eye" (AOA, 2019, para 1). An optometrist is usually seen for a visual examination and testing for eyeglasses or contact lenses but may also provide treatment for certain eye conditions. However, a few states allow limited surgical procedures, such as removal of a foreign object from the eye and, in some cases, laser privileges (NCSL, 2019). Each state licensing board will dictate the practice, prescriptive, and surgical authority of the optometrist. An eye condition outside of the optometrist's scope of practice will be referred to an ophthalmologist. See Box 4 regarding differences in the careers of ophthalmologists, optometrists, and opticians.

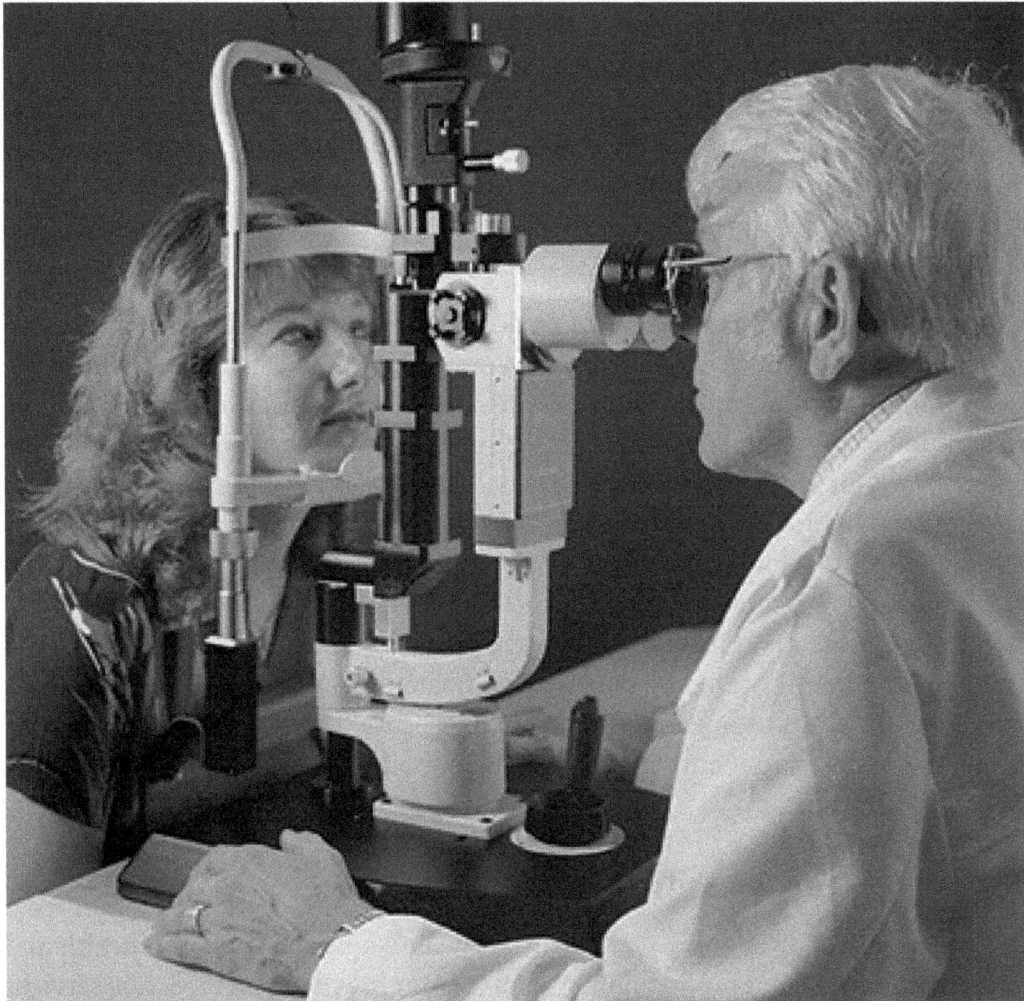

Figure 3.8: Optometry

Source: Wikimedia Commons
Attribution: US Government
License: Public Domain

Education

Educational requirements for the optometrist include completion of at least three years of postsecondary education and an earned doctoral degree as a Doctor of Optometry (OD). Programs generally take four years to complete, with education combining both classroom activities and supervised clinical experiences (BLS, 2020k). One-year residency programs are available for specialty focus areas. Licensure is required to practice in any state. To become state licensed to practice, the OD must obtain a degree from an accredited optometry program and successfully complete the National Board of Examiners in Optometry exam.

Projections for the Future

Vision problems can occur any time during life. However, a majority of people will have vision changes as they age. Difficulty reading close up can occur because of eye changes as we age and will require reading glasses to improve clarity. Other changes to the eyes may include cataract formation or macular degeneration. The aging population continues to increase the demand for optometry services. The projected growth of the optometrist profession is expected a 10% increase between 2018 and 2028 (BLS, 2020k).

- -

What is the difference?

An *ophthalmologist* is a physician with a medical degree (MD or DO), requiring eight years or more of education and training specializing in the eyes and visual structure. Ophthalmologists are also able to perform surgical procedures to the eyes and visual structures (AAPOS, 2019). Typical duties include conducting eye examinations, writing prescriptions, assessing eye conditions, and performing surgery.

An *optometrist* is a doctoral prepared (OD) professional with four years of formal education and training specializing in the eyes and visual structures. With few exceptions, optometrists do not have surgical privileges.

An *optician* is a professional who fits eyeglasses or contact lenses and fills prescriptions from either an ophthalmologist or optometrist. Education is typically an associate degree, technical school diploma, or on-the-job training.

- -

3.10.3 Pharmacist

A **pharmacist** specializes in filling prescriptions and educating customers on the safe use of prescription and over the counter medications. The primary responsibility for the pharmacist is determining if prescriptions will interact with other medicines a customer is prescribed. Other responsibilities may include conducting health screenings and providing immunizations, such as the flu vaccine. Pharmacists may also be trained to create personalized medicine through compounding. Compounding examples include adding special flavorings to medications, creating unique dosage forms, and customizing medicine strengths and dosage forms (Professional Compounding Centers of America [PCCA], 2019). According to the American Pharmacists Association (APhA) (2019), pharmacists can provide assistance with education on using medications safely, finding the correct over the counter medications, choosing supplements, providing smoking cessation resources, and monitoring blood pressure and blood glucose levels.

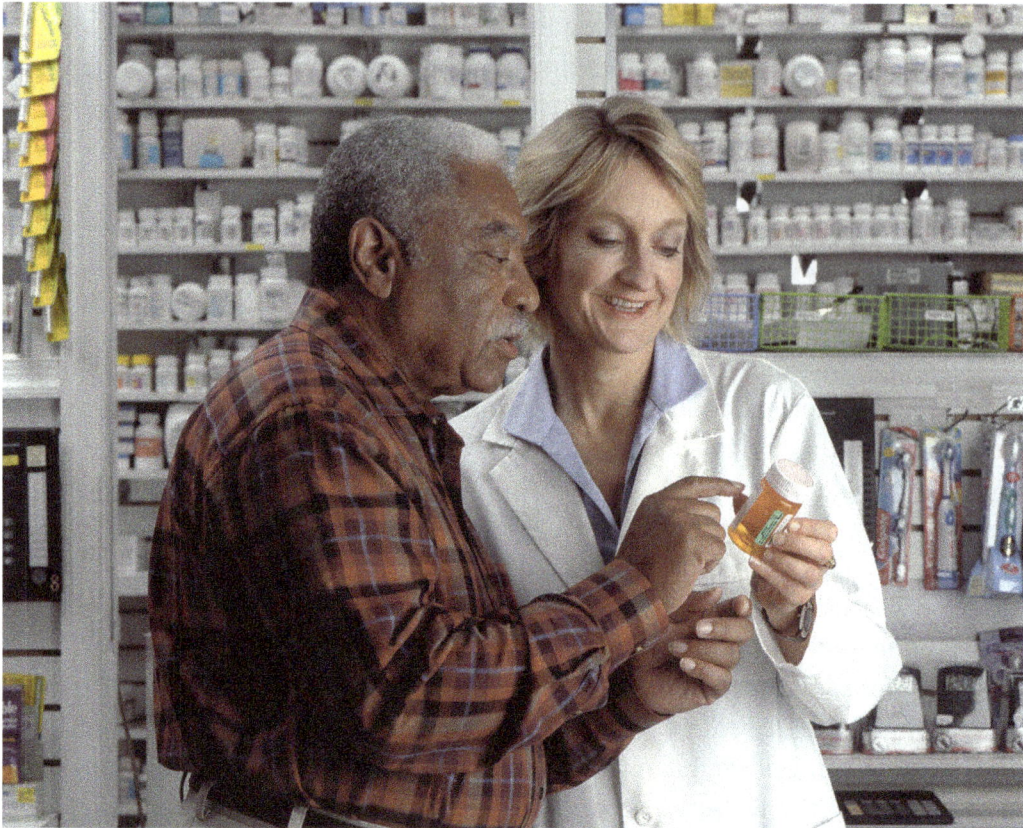

Figure 3.9: Pharmacist

Source: Wikimedia Commons/National Cancer Institute
Attribution: Rhoda Baer
License: Public Domain

Work Setting

There were 314,300 pharmacist jobs in 2018, with pharmacies and drug stores employing 43% of the workforce and hospitals employing another 26% of the workforce (BLS, 2020l). Pharmacists may also work in research and academics. Pharmacies can be located in major big box retailers, large grocery store chains, and neighborhood convenience stores.

Education

Educational requirements include two-to-four years of pre-pharmacy coursework completed at any accredited college or university. However, most pharmacy schools do not require a bachelor's degree as entry to a professional Doctor of Pharmacy (Pharm.D.) program (Pharmacyforme.org, 2020). Pharm.D. professional programs take approximately three or four years to complete. Career development can include an additional one-to-two years of postgraduate work in a specialty or fellowships. Upon graduation from an accredited professional pharmacy program, candidates must complete a licensure assessment examination (NAPLEX) administered by the National Association of Boards of Pharmacy

(NABP). A Multistate Pharmacy Jurisprudence Exam (MPJE) is also required. Licensure is required to practice pharmacy, and each state board of pharmacy may require additional assessment criteria. Continuing education courses are usually required for continued licensure. Additional education may be required for pharmacists who provide immunizations, vaccines, diabetes education, nutrition, and oncology (BLS, 2020l).

Projections for the Future

The jobs outlook for pharmacists is not expected to change in the next decade (2018–2028) (BLS, 2020l). While the growing aging population will help to keep pharmacists in need, specifically in hospitals, the burgeoning online purchase of medications may put many traditional brick-and-mortar pharmacies out of business. According to Farr (2019), Amazon recently purchased a company for $753 million which provides to consumers medications packaged in convenient white packets and delivered to their home. The convenience of quick delivery of prescriptions to homes may negatively impact this profession.

> **Pause and Reflect**
>
> Where do you get your information about medication? Have you ever talked to a pharmacist while picking up a prescription? What if pharmacies were put out of business because of big box stores? Will we miss a "live" professional with whom to talk to about medications?

3.10.4 Psychologist

A **psychologist** is a health professional who provides therapy and techniques to help people with a variety of health issues, such as depression, anger, stress, addiction, post-traumatic stress disorder (PTSD), marital problems, behavioral issues, attention deficit disorder (ADD), attention deficit hyperactivity disorder (ADHD), and many more. According to the American Psychological Association (APA) (2019), "common types of therapy are cognitive, behavioral, cognitive-behavioral, interpersonal, humanistic, psychodynamic, or a combination" (para. 6). Psychologists may also administer tests to assess intellectual skills, cognition, and personality traits. According to BLS (2020m), typical activities include observing, interviewing, and surveying individuals, diagnosing disorders, testing for patterns to predict behavior, discussing the treatment of problems with clients, and engaging in scholarly activity, such as writing articles and supervising other clinicians. Psychologists may work alone or collaborate with other health professionals as physicians and social workers. There were about 181,700 psychologist jobs in the U.S. in 2018. Psychologists work in a variety of settings, including schools, ambulatory settings, government, hospitals, industry, and private practice (BLS, 2020m).

Education

Educational requirements for becoming a psychologist include a completed bachelor's degree, preferably in psychology; an earned master's degree; and a doctoral degree (Doctor of Psychology (PsyD)) or a Ph.D. in psychology from accredited programs. A two-year internship in clinical and counseling psychology will prepare the psychologist and help meet some states' requirements for licensure (Allpsychologyschools.com, 2019). Clinical psychologists must complete supervised clinical experiences and pass the Examination for Professional Practice in Psychology administered by the Association of State and Provincial Psychology Boards (BLS, 2020m). Clinicians may seek specialty certifications through the American Board of Professional Psychology. All states require licensure to practice psychology independently.

Projections for the Future

Demand for psychologists is expected to grow as the awareness grows of the connection between mental health and overall well-being. Mental health services will be needed within school systems (cognitive and behavioral assessments), veteran populations (post-traumatic stress disorder and other war-time trauma), and aging populations (role changes and social isolation). Job growth is projected to increase 14% between 2018 and 2028 (BLS, 2020m).

3.10.5 Chiropractor

A **chiropractor** is a **complementary or alternative medicine (CAM) provider** who cares for patients with neuromusculoskeletal issues, such as back and neck pain. Box 3.5 describes the general duties of the chiropractor. According to the National Safety Council (NSC) (2019), "every 7 seconds a worker is injured on the job" (para. 1). Common types of work injuries include sprains, strains, tears, soreness or pain. Chiropractors perform hands-on treatments (or use a small instrument) called adjustments in which pressure is applied to a joint or spine to create proper alignment (National Institutes of Health [NIH], 2019). Chiropractors provide safe, drug-free, non-invasive therapy that complements other health professional treatments of musculoskeletal conditions.

General Duties of the Chiropractor

- Assess medical condition and history
- Analyze posture, spine, and reflexes
- Conduct tests and take x-rays
- Provide neuromusculoskeletal therapy
- Provide heat or cold therapy to injuries

- Encourage overall wellness
- Educate on exercise, nutrition, proper body mechanics

— — — — — — — — — — — — — — — — — — — —

Education

Educational requirements generally include a bachelor's degree in pre-medicine or related coursework for entry to an accredited chiropractic education program. Not all programs require a completed bachelor's degree for admission to Chiropractic programs. Chiropractor students complete four years of coursework and significant hands-on clinical training. The "curriculum includes a minimum of 4,200 hours of classroom, laboratory and clinical experience" (ACA, 2019). Following graduation, candidates must pass a national board exam managed by the National Board of Chiropractic Examiners (NBCE). Licensure is through application to an individual state which has varying requirements. Continuing education courses are usually required to maintain licensure.

Projections for the Future

The use of nonsurgical treatments for care of the body is appealing as complementary or alternative medicine becomes more accepted in the U.S. Similar to physical therapy and occupational therapy, chiropractic treatment enhances mobility and overall physical functionality as neuromusculoskeletal and joint problems occur as individuals age. Complementary care is increasing as Chiropractors and other health professionals collaborate in patient health plans. The chiropractic field is projected to grow 7% from 2018 to 2028 (BLS, 2020n).

3.11 OTHER HEALTHCARE OCCUPATIONS

In this chapter, we have only described a few of the professions in healthcare. Many more wonderful professionals need recognition; however, space does not allow for an in-depth review. Noted below are other recognizable professions you will see throughout the healthcare field (Table 3.4). The Bureau of Labor Statistics has an occupational outlook handbook which includes most healthcare occupations and can be located on their website.

Table 3.4: Other Notable Healthcare Occupations		
Athletic Trainers	Dental Assistants and Hygienists	Dietician and Nutritionists
Exercise Physiologists	Genetic Counselors	Massage Therapists
Medical Records and Health Information Technologists	Medical Transcriptionists	Orthotists and Prosthetists
Phlebotomists	Speech-Language Pathologists	Veterinary Technicians and Assistants
Source: Original Work Attribution: Deanna Howe License: CC BY-SA 4.0		

3.12 GENDER PAY GAP

A **gender pay gap** exists between men and women in the health profession careers. In a 2019 survey of 20,000 physicians, women reported a salary averaging 25% less than their male counterparts. This gender inequality of pay is slightly higher in specialty areas (Medscape Physician Compensation Report, 2019). Unfortunately, the pay difference between men and women physicians widens over time (Lagasse, 2020). In the nurse practitioner (NP) field, women hold a majority of positions (91.2%), yet pay differences by gender show males earned almost $13,000 per year more than females (AANP, 2018 National NP Sample Survey Results Released, 2019b). Similarly, a gender pay disparity for physician assistants (PA) is present in all specialties and for all levels of experience. The gender pay disparity continues in the registered nurse profession, with men earning on average $6,000 more annually than women (Nurse.com, 2018). According to Vujicic et al. (2017), women dentists make up nearly one-third of the profession yet are still earning 21-to-40% less than their male counterparts. Pay differences between men and women are seen throughout all healthcare professions.

> **Pause and Reflect**
>
> With all things being equal, should men and women earn the same rate of pay for the same work? What reasons can you think of that would justify the pay differences? Should the U.S. government initiate legislation to ensure equal pay for equal work among healthcare providers in regard to gender?

3.13 IMPACT OF COVID-19 ON THE HEALTHCARE WORKFORCE

The COVID-19 virus pandemic has created stress and mayhem within the healthcare sector. COVID-19 is a very contagious virus, spreading through droplets in the air, from sneezing and coughing (CDC, 2020). The very contagious nature of this virus requires the use of personal protective equipment (PPE) to protect healthcare workers. The healthcare industry was sent scrambling to protect themselves appropriately while caring for highly contagious patients. A lack of available personal protective equipment (PPE) for healthcare workers worldwide was broadcast on every television channel and a seeming panic began to be felt by those having to care for the sick without proper protection. PPE includes N95 respirators, gowns, gloves, and face masks. Initially PPE supplies were low. Many hospitals were not prepared and so were unable to provide adequate protection to their healthcare workers.

Physicians, nurses, and other frontline healthcare workers, like those discussed in this chapter, are put in danger of contracting the virus through patient care. For healthcare workers with underlying health conditions, such as diabetes and asthma, the exposure could be a death sentence. According to the CDC (2021), as of July 26, 2021, 513,130 healthcare providers have contracted COVID-19 virus with a reported 1,661 deaths.

In spite of great personal risk, healthcare workers continue to care for patients who are sick with COVID-19. Not readily highlighted is the emotional toll this pandemic is taking on healthcare staff. Healthcare workers have expressed feelings of betrayal, coercion, and moral injury as a result of an unprepared healthcare system (Gold, 2020). Many healthcare workers are socially isolating from their families to decrease the risk of exposure at home. The stress of long shifts and loss of patients will certainly have an effect for a long time to come. According to Rossi et al. (2020), healthcare workers during the pandemic "are exposed to high levels of stressful or traumatic events and express substantial negative mental health outcomes, including stress-related symptoms and symptoms of depression, anxiety, and insomnia" (para. 1).

For healthcare workers not willing to continue in the stressful environment under the current pandemic, quitting is seen as the only option. According to Masson (2020), in an NBC news report in which 1200 nurses from more than 400 hospitals were surveyed, 61% say they are planning to quit either their current job or the profession altogether. Consider the ramifications to the healthcare industry if this statistic were prevalent throughout healthcare professions.

Little discussed in the news has been the reduction in jobs within the healthcare sector. Large numbers of healthcare workers have been laid off or furloughed as operating rooms and doctor's offices delay seeing patients for non-emergent appointments or elective procedures. A case rarely ever before seen in healthcare is how many workers are now being forced to seek unemployment benefits as a result of changes due to the pandemic. According to the BLS (2020), during the time of COVID-19, employment in healthcare declined by 1.4 million jobs. Clearly, COVID-19 has affected professionals and other workers significantly through physical, emotional, and financial issues not often seen in the healthcare field.

3.14 SUMMARY

The strain of an ever-increasing aging population and baby boomers entering retirement age will have an impact on the growing need for new healthcare professionals in the U.S. workforce. This chapter highlighted the roles of physicians, advanced practice professionals, nurses, allied health professionals, and other doctoral level professionals. Individually, and often within teams, these professionals provide health expertise and care to the citizens of the nation. Work settings vary, including hospitals, clinics, private practice, prisons, government settings, private homes and elderly care homes. U.S. citizens rely on quick responses to health needs, requiring most health professionals to maintain flexible work schedules including nights, weekends and holidays. Individuals searching for complementary or alternative treatments to western medicine philosophy may seek out complementary and alternative medicine providers (CAM), such as chiropractors, acupuncturists, homeopaths and naturopaths to explore therapies for wellness, illness, or injury. All health professions presented in this chapter, with the exception of pharmacists, have a positive projected job growth and a need to fill positions to manage the health needs through the year 2028. This chapter noted differences in gender pay rates, with men earning more than women for the same education and work requirements. The COVID-19 pandemic and the impact on the healthcare professions is discussed.

3.15 REVIEW QUESTIONS

1. What is the current and expected role for nurse practitioners and physician assistants in the healthcare workforce? How are these two professions different?

2. What are the workforce projections for each healthcare professions through 2028?

3. How will the rising number of seniors impact the U.S. healthcare workforce?

4. What does gender pay inequality mean? How is it evident in the U.S. healthcare system?

5. What is the role of allied health professions within the healthcare workforce?

3.16 REFERENCES

Allnursingschools. (2020). Careers and degrees. Retrieved from https://www. allnursingschools.com/

All Psychology Schools.org. (2019). Learn how to become a psychologist. Retrieved from https://www.allpsychologyschools.com/clinical-psychology/how-to-become-a-psychologist/

American Academy of Physician Assistants (AAPA). (2019). History of the PA profession. Retrieved from https://www.aapa.org/about/history/

American Association of Colleges of Nursing (AACN). (n.d.). Baccalaureate education. Retrieved from https://www.aacnnursing.org/Nursing-Education-Programs/Baccalaureate-Education

American Association of Colleges of Nursing (AACN). (September 2020). Nursing shortage. Retrieved from https://www.aacnnursing.org/News-Information/Fact-Sheets/Nursing-Shortage

American Association of Nurse Practitioners (AANP). (2019a). NP Fact Sheet. Retrieved from https://www.aanp.org/about/all-about-nps/np-fact-sheet

American Association of Nurse Practitioners (AANP). (2019b, January 28). 2018 national NP sample survey results released. Retrieved from https://www.aanp.org/news-feed/nurse-practitioner-role-continues-to-grow-to-meet-primary-care-provider-shortages-and-patient-demands

American Association of Nurse Practitioners (AANP). (2018). State Practice Environment. Retrieved from https://www.aanp.org/advocacy/state/state-practice-environment

American Association for Pediatric Ophthalmology & Strabismus (AAPOS). (2019). Difference between an ophthalmologist, optometrist and optician. Retrieved from https://aapos.org/glossary/difference-between-an-ophthalmologist-optometrist-and-optician

Association of American Medical Colleges (AAMC). (2019, April 23). New findings confirm predictions on physician shortage. Retrieved from https://news.aamc.org/press-releases/article/2019-workforce-projections-update/

American Chiropractic Association (ACA). (2019). Chiropractic qualifications. Retrieved from https://www.acatoday.org/Patients/Why-Choose-Chiropractic/Chiropractic-Qualifications

American Dental Association (ADA). (2019). Dentists: Doctors of oral health. Retrieved from https://www.ada.org/en/about-the-ada/dentists-doctors-of-oral-health

American Hospital Association. (2019). For the 17th year in a row, nurses top Gallup's poll of most trusted profession. Retrieved from https://www.aha.org/news/insights-and-analysis/2019-01-09-17th-year-row-nurses-top-gallups-poll-most-trusted-profession

American Optometric Association (AOA). (2019). What is a doctor of optometry? Retrieved from https://www.aoa.org/about-the-aoa/what-is-a-doctor-of-optometry

American Physical Therapy Association (APTA). (2019a). Who are physical therapy assistants? Retrieved from http://www.apta.org/AboutPTAs/

American Physical Therapy Association (APTA). (2019b). Who are physical therapists? Retrieved from http://www.apta.org/AboutPTs/

American Psychological Association (APA). (2019). What do practicing psychologists do?

Retrieved fromhttps://www.apa.org/helpcenter/about-psychologists

Association of Schools of Allied Health Professions (ASAHP). (2018). What is allied health? Retrieved from http://www.asahp.org/what-is

Centers for Disease Control and Prevention (2021). COVID data tracker. Cases & deaths among healthcare personnel. https://covid.cdc.gov/covid-data-tracker/#health-care-personnel

Centers for Disease Control and Prevention (2020). What you should know about COVID-19 to protect yourself and others. Retrieved from https://www.cdc.gov/coronavirus/2019-ncov/index.html?CDC_AA_refVal=https%3A%2F%2Fwww.cdc.gov%2Fcoronavirus%2Findex.html

Commission on Accreditation of Allied Health Education Programs (CAAHEP). (2019). Diagnostic medical sonography. Retrieved from https://www.caahep.org/Students/Program-Info/Diagnostic-Medical-Sonography.aspx

Explorehealth careers.org. (2019). Allied health professions overview. Retrieved from https://explorehealth careers.org/field/allied-health-professions/

Farr, C. (2019, May 10). The inside story of why Amazon bought PillPack in its effort to crack the $500 billion prescription market. Retrieved from https://www.cnbc.com/2019/05/10/why-amazon-bought-pillpack-for-753-million-and-what-happens-next.html

Gold, J. (2020, April 3). The COVID-19 crisis too few are talking about: Health care workers' mental health. STAT. Retrieved from https://www.statnews.com/2020/04/03/the-covid-19-crisis-too-few-are-talking-about-health-care-workers-mental-health/

Health Resources and Services Administration (HRSA). (2018, September). The U.S. health workforce chartbook. Part 1: Clinicians. Retrieved from https://bhw.hrsa.gov/health-workforce-analysis/research

Henry, T. A. (2019). Employed physicians now exceed those who own their practices. American medical association. Retrieved from https://www.ama-assn.org/about/research/employed-physicians-now-exceed-those-who-own-their-practices

Institute of Medicine. (2010). The future of nursing, focus on education. Retrieved from http://www.nationalacademies.org/hmd/Reports/2010/The-Future-of-Nursing-Leading-Change-Advancing-Health/Report-Brief-Education.aspx

Kane, L. A. (2019, April 10). Medscape physician compensation report 2019. Retrieved from https://www.medscape.com/slideshow/2019-compensation-overview-6011286#2

Lagasse, J. (2020). Gender pay disparities in health care pronounced at the beginning of careers. Health care finance. Retrieved from https://www.health carefinancenews.com/news/gender-pay-disparities-health care-pronounced-beginning-careers

LPNtraining.org. (2013, Feb 6). The history of practical nursing. Retrieved from https://www.lpntraining.org/the-history-of-practical-nursing.html

Masson, G. (2020, May 12). Nurses say changing guidelines, unsafe conditions are pushing them to quit. Becker's Hospital Review. Retrieved from https://www.beckershospitalreview.com/nursing/nurses-say-changing-guidelines-unsafe-conditions-are-pushing-them-to-quit.html

Murphy, B. (2018, December 18). 3 misconceptions about what drives medicine's gender pay gap. Retrieved from https://www.ama-assn.org/practice-management/physician-diversity/3-misconceptions-about-what-drives-medicine-s-gender-pay

National Commission on Certification of Physician Assistants (NNCPA). (2019). 2018 Statistical profile of recently certified physician assistants. Annual report. Retrieved from https://www.nccpa.net/Research

National Conference of State Legislatures (NCSL). (2018). Optometrist scope of practice. http://www.ncsl.org/research/health/optometrist-scope-of-practice.aspx

National Institutes of Health (NIH). National center for complementary and integrative health. Spinal manipulation: What you need to know. Retrieved from https://nccih.nih.gov/health/pain/spinemanipulation.htm

Nurse.org. (2017). New York's "BSN in 10' law and the push for 80% of nurses to hold BSN by 2020. Retrieved from https://nurse.org/articles/BSN-initiative-80-2020/

Nurse Journal. (2019). 5 most common types of nursing certification you should have. Retrieved from https://nursejournal.org/articles/5-best-types-of-nursing-certifications-you-should-have/

Pharmacy is right for me (2020). Pharmacy FAQ. https://pharmacyforme.org/admissions-faqs/#1577989199316-03cb7e64-202f

PhysicianAssistantEDU.org. (2019). Everything you need to know about becoming a certified physician assistant. Retrieved from https://www.physicianassistantedu.org/certification/

Practical Nursing.org. (2019). NCLEX-PN Exam. Retrieved from https://www.practicalnursing.org/nclex-pn-exam

Professional Compounding Centers of America, Inc. (PCCA). (2019). What is compounding? Retrieved from https://www.pccarx.com/aboutus/whatiscompounding.aspx

Rossi, R., Socci, V., Pacitti, F., Di Lorenzo, G., Di Marco, A., Siracusano, A., & Rossi, A. (2020). Mental health outcomes among frontline and second-line health care workers during the Coronavirus disease 2019 (COVID-19) pandemic in Italy. JAMA Netw Open, 3(5). DOI: 10.1001/jamanetworkopen.2020.10185

The American Occupational Therapy Association, Inc. (2019). Occupational therapy assistants. Retrieved from https://www.aota.org/Practice/OT-Assistants.aspx

The National Organization of Nurse Practitioner Faculties. (2018, May). The doctor of nursing practice degree: Entry to nurse practitioner practice by 2025. v3_05.2018_NONPF_DNP_Stateme.pdf

Thompson, D. (2018, Jan 9). Health care just became the U.S.'s largest employer. In the American labor market, services are the new steel. The Atlantic. Retrieved from https://www.theatlantic.com/business/archive/2018/01/health-care-america-jobs/550079/

U.S. Bureau of Labor Statistics. (2020a). Occupational outlook handbook. Physicians and surgeons. Retrieved from https://www.bls.gov/ooh/health care/physicians-and-surgeons.htm

U.S. Bureau of Labor Statistics. (2020b). Occupational outlook handbook. Nurse anesthetists, nurse midwives, and nurse practitioners. Retrieved from https://www.bls.gov/ooh/health care/nurse-anesthetists-nurse-midwives-and-nurse-practitioners.htm#tab-1

U.S. Bureau of Labor Statistics. (2020c). Occupational outlook handbook. Physician assistants. Retrieved from https://www.bls.gov/ooh/health care/physician-assistants.htm#tab-6

U.S. Bureau of Labor Statistics. (2020d). Occupational outlook handbook. Registered nurses. Retrieved from https://www.bls.gov/ooh/health care/registered-nurses.htm

U.S. Bureau of Labor Statistics. (2020e). Occupational outlook handbook. Health care occupations. Retrieved from https://www.bls.gov/ooh/health care/home.htm

U.S. Bureau of Labor Statistics. (2020f). Occupational outlook handbook. Physical therapist assistants and aides. Retrieved from https://www.bls.gov/ooh/health care/physical-therapist-assistants-and-aides.htm#tab-4

U.S. Bureau of Labor Statistics. (2020g). Occupational outlook handbook. Health care occupations. Diagnostic medical sonographers. Retrieved from https://www.bls.gov/ooh/health care/diagnostic-medical-sonographers.htm#tab-2

U.S. Bureau of Labor Statistics. (2020h). Occupational outlook handbook. Occupational therapists. Retrieved from https://www.bls.gov/ooh/health care/occupational-therapists.htm

U.S. Bureau of Labor Statistics. (2020i). Occupational outlook handbook. Respiratory therapists. Retrieved from https://www.bls.gov/ooh/health care/respiratory-therapists.htm

U.S. Bureau of Labor Statistics. (2020j). Occupational outlook handbook. Health care occupations. Dentists. Retrieved from https://www.bls.gov/ooh/health care/dentists.htm#tab-4

U.S. Bureau of Labor Statistics. (2020k). Occupational outlook handbook. Health care occupations. Optometrists. Retrieved from https://www.bls.gov/ooh/health care/optometrists.htm#tab-4

U.S. Bureau of Labor Statistics. (2020l). Occupational outlook handbook. Pharmacist. Retrieved from https://www.bls.gov/ooh/health care/pharmacists.htm#tab-1

U.S. Bureau of Labor Statistics. (2020m). Occupational outlook handbook. Psychologists. Retrieved from https://www.bls.gov/ooh/life-physical-and-social-science/psychologists.htm#tab-2

U.S. Bureau of Labor Statistics. (2020n). Occupational outlook handbook. Health care occupations. Chiropractors. Retrieved from https://www.bls.gov/OOH/health care/chiropractors.htm#tab-1

U.S. Bureau of Labor Statistics. (2020o). Economic news release. Employment situation summary. Retrieved from https://www.bls.gov/news.release/empsit.nro.htm

U.S. News & World Report. (2019). U.S. news announces the 2019 best jobs. Retrieved from https://www.usnews.com/info/blogs/press-room/articles/2019-01-08/us-news-announces-the-2019-best-jobs

University of Pennsylvania School of Nursing. (2019). American nursing: An introduction to the past. Retrieved from https://www.nursing.upenn.edu/nhhc/american-nursing-an-introduction-to-the-past/

Vujicic, M., Yarbrough, C., & Munson, B. (2018). Time to talk about the gender gap in dentist earnings. Journal of American Dentist Association, 148(4), 204–206. http://dx.doi.org/10.1016/j.adaj.2017.02.004

WebMD. (2019). What are the different types of doctors? Retrieved from https://www.webmd.com/health-insurance/insurance-doctor-types#1

4 Healthcare Settings

4.1 LEARNING OBJECTIVES

By the end of this chapter, the student will be able to:
- Describe types of hospitals
- Discuss current statistics for hospital admissions, including number of admissions, length of stay, readmissions, payer sources, community income distribution, and geographical usage
- Differentiate types of long-term care facilities
- Explain the rise in outpatient healthcare resources
- Discuss how emergency departments are used
- Describe the role of public health and public health departments

4.2 KEY TERMS
- acute
- ambulatory care center
- assisted living
- home health
- hospice
- inpatient
- length of stay
- long-term care facility
- network
- outpatient
- skilled
- system

4.3 INTRODUCTION

This chapter will describe the different settings in which individuals receive healthcare services. An individual will need various healthcare services throughout their lifespan. This chapter discusses inpatient versus outpatient services, acute care settings, and long-term care settings. It describes statistics that impact hospitals' viability and how the healthcare system has evolved. And it discusses the role of public health in the care of the nation's population as a whole.

4.4 DEFINING HEALTHCARE SERVICES

Healthcare services may be provided to individuals in an inpatient or outpatient setting or at home. **Inpatient** services are provided in hospitals where patients are usually admitted for an **acute**, or unexpected, illness or a scheduled surgery and spend one or more nights there. **Outpatient** services are healthcare services provided where the patient enters a facility to receive healthcare and then returns to their home the same day. Examples of outpatient services where healthcare is provided and the patient returns home are free standing **ambulatory care centers**, where same-day surgical services or procedures are performed; clinics for non-urgent acute care (often called urgent care centers); specialty clinics for outpatient procedures such as wound care, diabetes education, or physical therapy; mental health clinics; adult day care centers; physician's offices; and health departments. Hospital emergency rooms are available for acute illnesses; the patient might return home or may be admitted as an inpatient. **Home health** services are services provided where the patient is considered homebound and services are provided within the patient's home. **Hospice care** is another service where the patient is seen in their home when death is expected within six months, although sometimes hospice services can now be provided in nursing homes and acute care settings.

Healthcare services are known as primary, secondary, or tertiary (see Figure 4.1). Usually, the first contact an ill person has with a healthcare provider is in a doctor's office. The healthcare provider is considered to provide primary, or basic, care (Johns Hopkins Medicine, n.d.). When additional healthcare services are needed, referrals are made to specialists, clinics, or to the local hospital for secondary healthcare. If more advanced specialization is needed, patients may be referred to large tertiary treatment centers, oftentimes a teaching hospital.

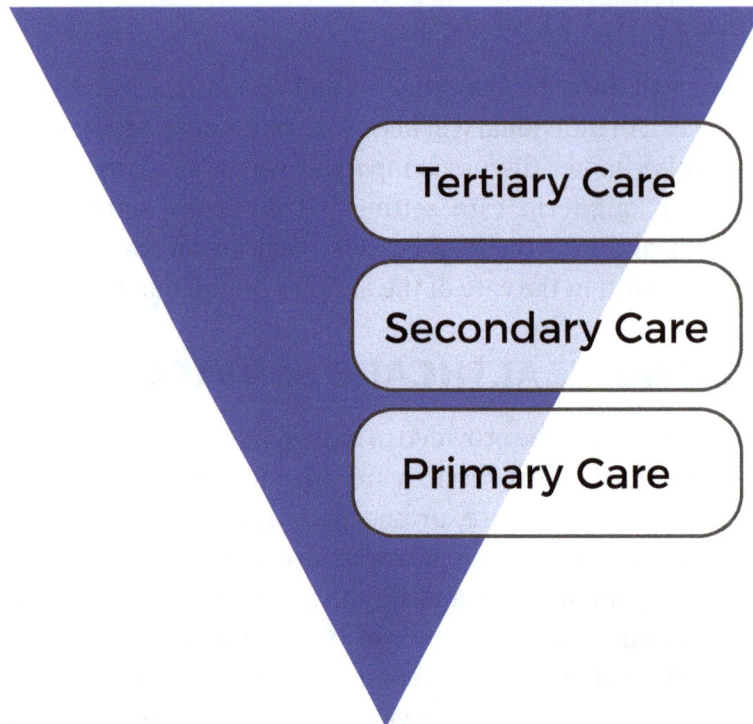

Figure 4.1: Healthcare Delivery Model

Source: Original Work
Attribution: Kristy Michelle Gamble
License: CC BY-SA 4.0

> **Pause and Reflect**
>
> If a person diagnosed with hypertension visits their physician for a blood pressure check, is the patient receiving primary, secondary, or tertiary care?

4.5 INPATIENT HEALTHCARE

4.5.1 Hospitals

Hospitals, sometimes called medical centers, are most known for admission to inpatient services for an acute illness or elective surgery. Other hospitals, such as rehabilitation hospitals and mental hospitals, are for protracted illnesses where the patient may stay for an extended period of time, or may not leave. There are 6,210 hospitals in the U.S. (American Hospital Association, [AHA], 2019). Most are community hospitals (5,262), nongovernmental, not-for-profit, and acute care facilities, providing secondary healthcare services. Community hospitals range from six to 500 beds (Liu & Kelz, 2018). Two hundred eight federal government hospitals treat those in the military and other military related department officials. Six hundred twenty nonfederal psychiatric hospitals admit patients for mental illnesses on a short-term or long-term basis. And there are 1,000 teaching hospitals. Teaching hospitals provide tertiary care for those needing advanced and specialized care, as well as training healthcare professionals and performing research (AHA, 2019). There remains a small number of both investor-owned (for-profit) and some state and local government community hospitals. There are 1,875 hospitals in rural communities and 3,387 in urban communities (AHA, 2019).

Community hospitals may have a range of services depending on the size, location, resources, and leadership. They may provide a variety of short-term inpatient and outpatient rehabilitation services and, possibly, urgent care clinics, depending on the size of the hospital. Some community hospitals provide long term acute care, and some partner with larger teaching hospitals to provide training for physician residents.

Hospitals used to be stand-alone organizations. Now, mainly due to reimbursement issues, many hospitals are in systems or networks. A multihospital arrangement is called a **system** (AHA, 2019). A single hospital system that also owns other services, such as a long-term care facility or an outpatient ambulatory surgical center or ambulatory healthcare clinic, is also called a system. A **network** includes hospitals, physicians, and possibly insurers and community agencies together to provide a broad range of services for the community (AHA, 2019). Approximately 68% of community hospitals are part of a system, whereas approximately a third of community hospitals are in a network (AHA, 2019).

Hospitals also provide acute care services with emergency rooms, around-the-clock nursing care, and physician or advanced healthcare provider care in most facilities. Other services provided include radiology, dietary, physical therapy, speech therapy, occupational therapy, social services, and other specialties to meet the needs of an acute care patient. Hospitals often coordinate the rehabilitation phase for a person who has suffered from an acute illness to either home with home health, a long-term care facility, or a rehab facility. Hospitals provide places of employment for healthcare workers, education for training healthcare workers, and facilities for research (WHO, n.d.).

Hospital inpatient healthcare is responsible for one-third of all U.S. healthcare expenditures, according to McDermott et al. (2017). Even with the growth of outpatient services, the number of inpatient hospital stays have remained relatively stable over the last twenty years (Agency for Healthcare Research and Quality, [AHRQ], 2021). Estimated data for inpatient hospital stays are retrieved from hospital discharges from participating states (forty-eight states and the District of Columbia). In 1998, there were 33,923,632 inpatient stays compared to 35,798,453 inpatient stays in 2017 (Figure 4.2).

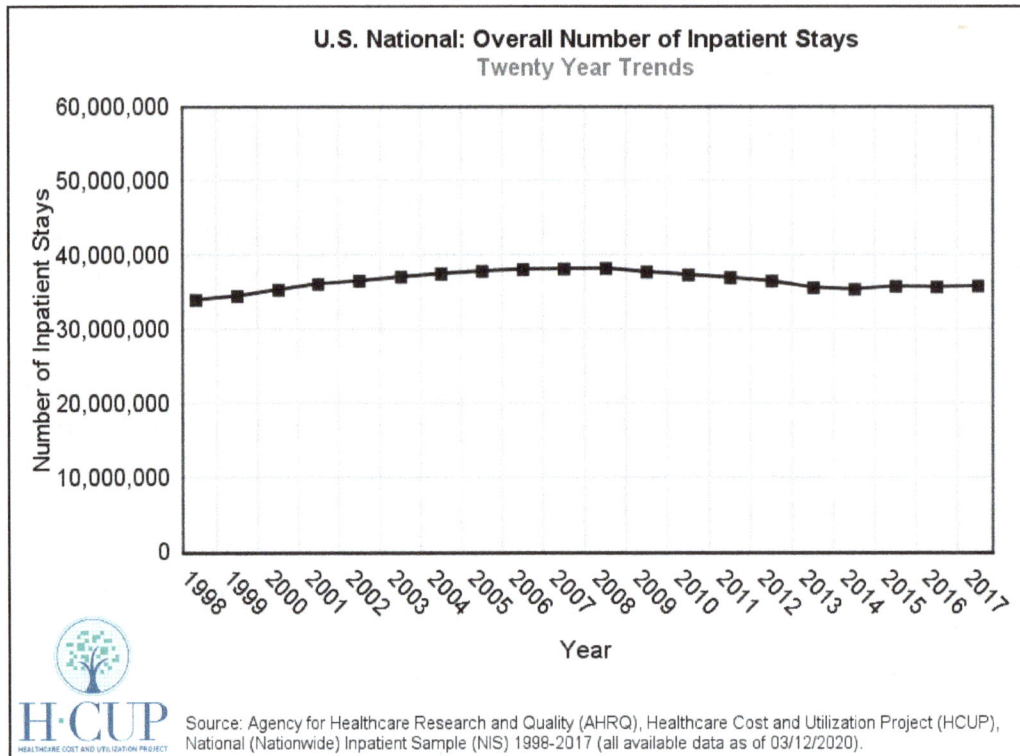

U.S. National: Overall Number of Inpatient Stays
Twenty Year Trends

Source: Agency for Healthcare Research and Quality (AHRQ), Healthcare Cost and Utilization Project (HCUP), National (Nationwide) Inpatient Sample (NIS) 1998-2017 (all available data as of 03/12/2020).

Figure 4.2: U.S. National: Overall Number of Inpatient Stays, 1998–2017

Source: Agency for Healthcare Research and Quality
Attribution: Agency for Healthcare Research and Quality
License: Public Domain

Comparing age groups of hospitalized patients, the twenty-year data reveals that the age group of 45–64 had the largest increase in hospital inpatient admissions, with slight increases in the older population groups of 65–74 and 75+, while the younger age groups of 0–17 and 18–44 had slight decreases (AHRQ, 2021). The overall U.S. population is aging, and patients with chronic diseases are living longer. Sun et al. (2018) report that market forces and changes in population attributes may affect inpatient admission rates. Moreover, projections indicate that by the year 2030, approximately 20% of the population, 71 million people, will be 65 years or older (CDC & Merck Co. Foundation, 2007). See Figure 4.3 for age distribution inpatient admissions.

Pause and Reflect

The 45 to 64 age group had the largest increase in admissions in the twenty-year data presented. What accounts for this specific group having more hospitalizations? What specific health factors affects this age group?

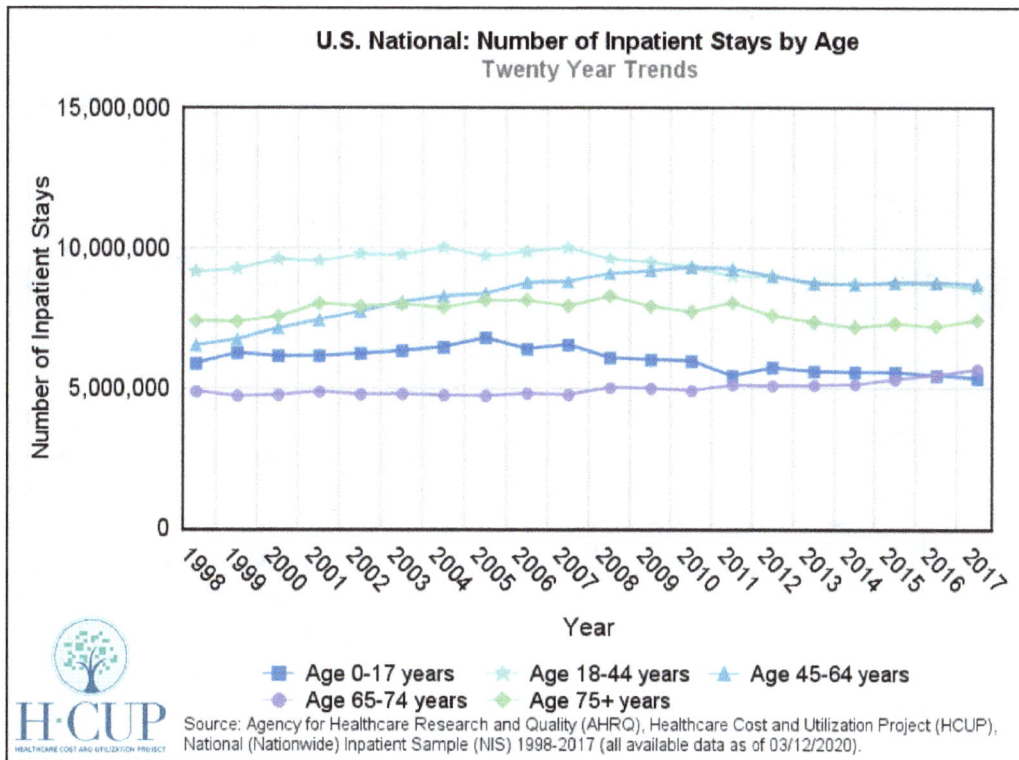

Figure 4.3: U.S. National: Number of Inpatient Stays by Age, 1998–2017

Source: Agency for Healthcare Research and Quality

Attribution: Agency for Healthcare Research and Quality

License: Public Domain

Evaluating data concerning the causes of inpatient hospitalizations from 1997 to 2016 reveals no meaningful changes. For both years, 1998 and 2017, the most common cause of admission is from a medical condition, followed by surgical problems, maternal issues, neonatal issues, mental health or substance abuse, and injury (AHRQ, 2021) (Figure 4.4).

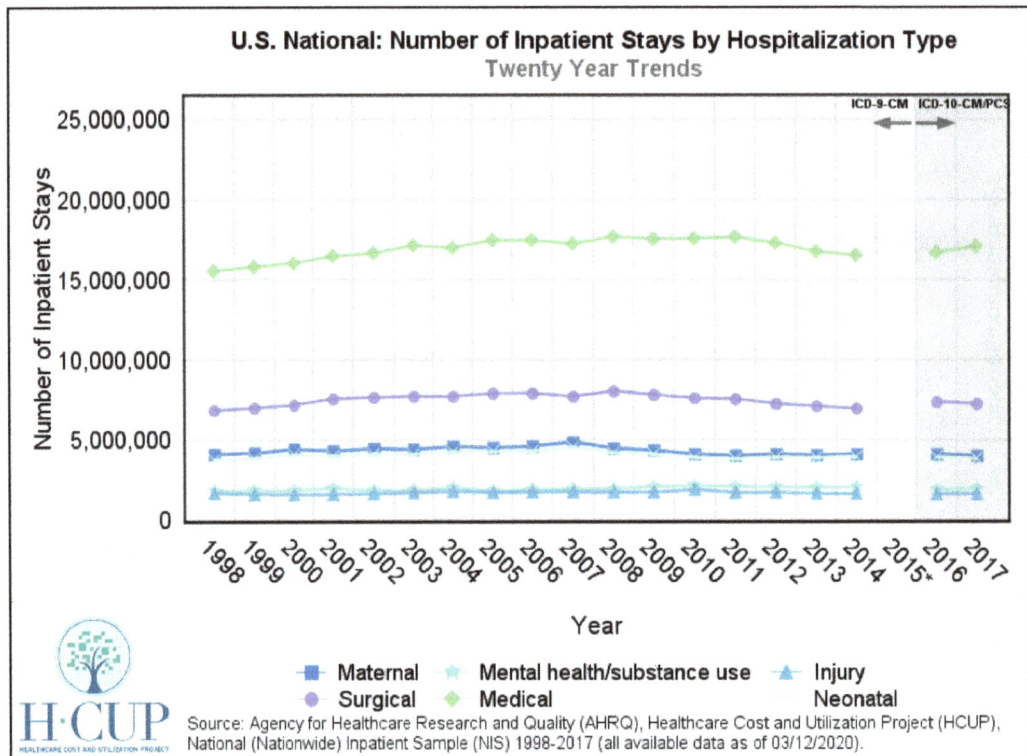

Figure 4.4: U.S. National: Number of Inpatient Stays by Hospitalization Type, 1998–2017

Source: Agency for Healthcare Research and Quality
Attribution: Agency for Healthcare Research and Quality
License: Public Domain

McDermott et al.'s (2017) report, completed in 2014, found that the top two most common diagnoses for inpatient hospital stays were pregnancy with childbirth and newborns/neonates in 2005 and 2014. The rest of the top ten common diagnoses causing inpatient hospital admissions were ranked slightly differently in occurrence in 2005 compared to 2014. In 2005, the most common diagnoses causing hospital admissions after the maternal/newborn admissions, in order, were pneumonia, coronary atherosclerosis, congestive heart failure, nonspecific chest pain, osteoarthritis, mood disorders, cardiac dysrhythmias, and acute myocardial infarction. In 2014, beginning with the third most common diagnosis for causing inpatient hospital admission, in order, were septicemia, osteoarthritis, congestive heart failure, pneumonia, mood disorders, cardiac dysrhythmias, and complication of a device/implant/graft. Again, this data reveals that, besides maternal care, diagnoses of conditions common in the elderly population are most often seen with inpatient hospitalizations.

Payer sources is a variable that affects the viability of hospitals and services the hospital provides to the community. Private insurance generally pays more for services, while Medicare payments from the federal government have changed over the years but continue to pay less than private insurance. In the literature review by Lopez et al. (2020), evaluating Medicare payments compared to private insurance payments since 2010, private insurance companies on average paid hospitals almost twice the rate of Medicare. Medicaid, from federal and state monies, also pays less than private insurance companies (Cunningham et al., 2016). Comparing payer sources for inpatient admissions from 1998 to 2017-6 (AHRQ, 2021), data reveals an increase in patients who are insured by Medicare and Medicaid, while admissions of patients with private health insurance and those with no insurance decreased. Of note, hospitals with greater numbers of admissions of patients with private pay insurance are on stronger financial footing. Also noteworthy is the fact that the **Affordable Care Act** of 2010 provided additional coverage from Medicaid to those of low income, and Medicare also expanded as the population has aged (Figure 4.5).

Pause and Reflect

From 1997 to 2016, there was a decrease in reimbursement to hospitals from private insurance and the uninsured but an increase in Medicare and Medicaid payments to hospitals. Why do you think this changed?

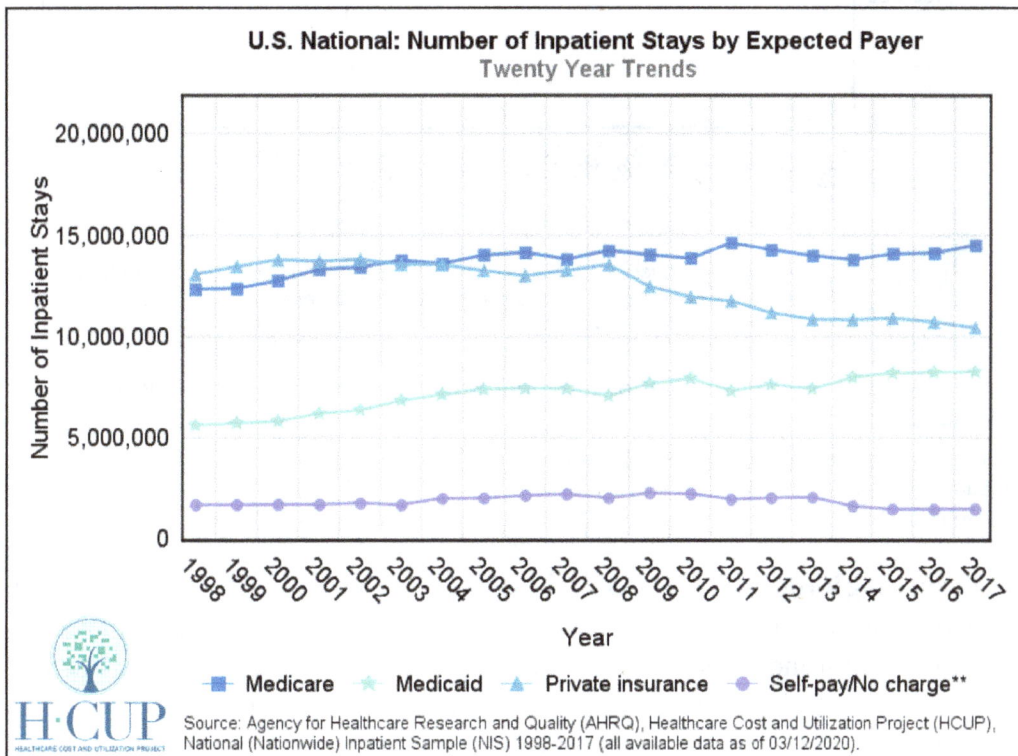

U.S. National: Number of Inpatient Stays by Expected Payer
Twenty Year Trends

Source: Agency for Healthcare Research and Quality (AHRQ), Healthcare Cost and Utilization Project (HCUP), National (Nationwide) Inpatient Sample (NIS) 1998-2017 (all available data as of 03/12/2020).

Figure 4.5: U.S. National: Number of Inpatient Stays by Expected Payer, 1998—2017
Source: Agency for Healthcare Research and Quality
Attribution: Agency for Healthcare Research and Quality
License: Public Domain

Community-level income of inpatient hospital admissions, obtained from the median household income using the zip codes of patient data, was also evaluated from 2002 to 2016 (AHRQ, 2021). Data evaluating community-level income by quartiles indicate that persons living in lower income areas have increased hospital admission rates compared to persons in the higher income quartile (10,297,216 admissions to 7,344,105, respectively, in 2002, and 10,680,030 to 6,946,894, respectively, in 2017). Factors associated with lower income and healthcare outcomes are being evaluated with the 2020 Healthy People initiative. (See Figure 4.6.).

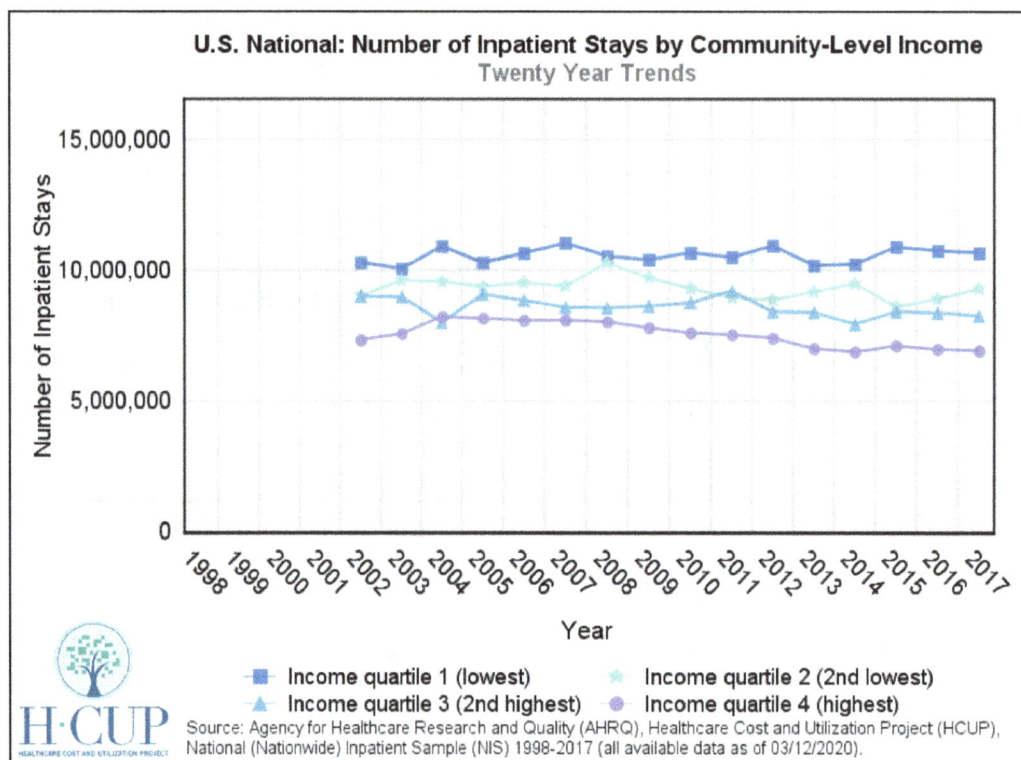

Figure 4.6: U.S. National: Number of Inpatient Stays by Community-Level Income, 1998–2017

Source: Agency for Healthcare Research and Quality
Attribution: Agency for Healthcare Research and Quality
License: Public Domain

Evaluating **length of stays** in the hospital, Freeman et al. (2018) found that in 2016, there were 104.2 hospitalizations per 1,000 persons with a mean, or average, length of stay for individuals at 4.6 days. The mean cost was $11,700 per hospital stay. Freeman et al. compared different groups related to age, income, housing location (rural vs suburban), and types of insurance groups. Freeman et al. found that the groups with the greatest number of hospital stays were females in the 65–84 age group, were of the lower income quartiles, lived in rural areas, and had Medicare coverage. Generally, longer lengths of stays are more costly for hospitals.

Looking at the U.S. geographically (see Figure 4.7), the South Atlantic area had one-fifth of all hospital stays in 2016. The proportion of hospital stays compared to the percentage of the U.S. population was greatest in the East, South-Central area (6.8% of all hospital stays compared to 5.9% of the U.S. population) and least in the Mountain division (6.2% of all hospital stays compared to 7.4% of the population). The most expensive cost for a hospital stay was greatest in the Pacific areas at $15,600 per stay, and the least expensive cost of stay was $9,900 in the East, South-Central area.

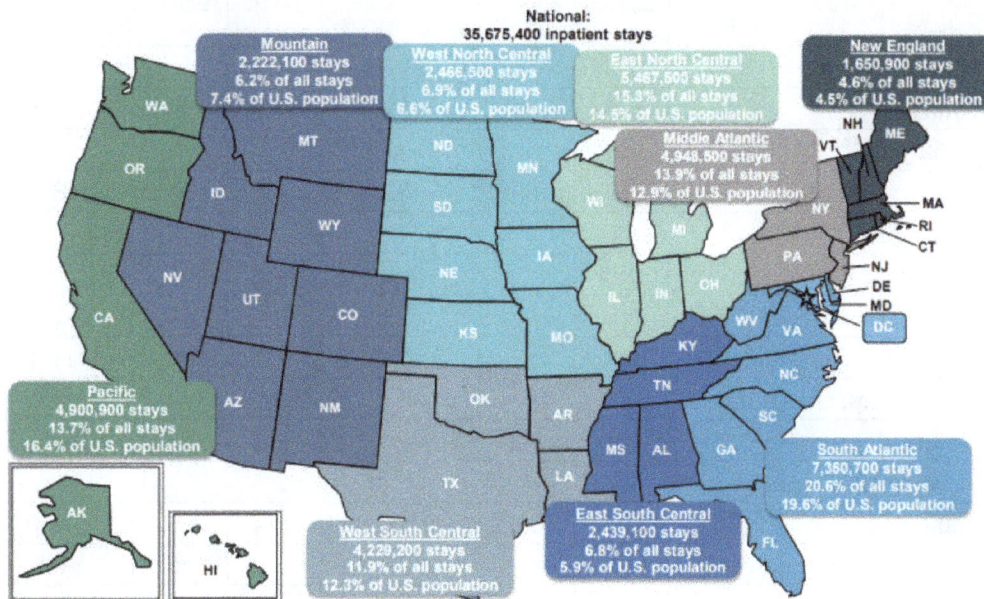

Source: Agency for Healthcare Research and Quality (AHRQ), Center for Delivery, Organization, and Markets, Healthcare Cost and Utilization Project (HCUP), National Inpatient Sample (NIS), 2016

Figure 4.7: Number and Percentage of Inpatient Stays by U.S. Census Division (Geographic Distribution), 2016

Source: Agency for Healthcare Research and Quality
Attribution: Agency for Healthcare Research and Quality
License: Public Domain

Readmissions are also a concern for patients, healthcare administrations, and payers. Hospital reimbursement may be denied if a patient is readmitted within a short period of time after hospital discharge. Due to the costliness of readmissions, hospitals are incentivized to prevent readmissions (Bailey et al., 2019). According to Bailey et al., a 6.7% decline in readmissions of total Medicare recipients occurred from 2010 to 2016. Comparing all payers (Medicare, Medicaid, private insurance, and the uninsured) and age groups reveals the greatest percentage increase of readmissions in these six years (28.7%) was the 1–20 years of age, non-maternal, uninsured population (Table 4.1).

Table 4.1: Rate and Number of 30-day All-cause Readmissions by Expected Payer and Age Group, 2010 and 2016

Expected payer and age group	Readmission rate			Number of Readmissions[b] (thousands)		
	2010	2016	% change 2010-2016	2010	2016	% change 2010-2016
Medicare						
Total	18.3	17.1	-6.7	2,615	2,447	-6.4
21-64 years	21.8	21.2	-2.7	627	626	-0.2
65 years and above	17.4	16.0	-8.1	1,985	1,818	-8.4
Medicaid						
Total	13.7	13.7	0.1	804	862	7.2
1-20 years, non-maternal	11.4	12.3	7.8	111	105	-4.9
21-44 years, non-maternal	19.0	17.8	-6.6	241	276	14.5
45-64 years, non-maternal	21.9	20.4	-6.9	347	395	14.0
Maternal	5.1	4.4	-14.1	104	84	-18.9
Private insurance						
Total	8.8	8.6	-1.3	735	641	-12.8
1-20 years, non-maternal	9.4	10.8	15.7	62	58	-6.6
21-44, non-maternal	9.6	10.2	6.2	173	153	-11.9
45-64 years, non-maternal	11.0	11.0	0.2	434	378	-13.0
Maternal	3.4	2.8	-17.7	67	54	-18.3
Uninsured						
Total	10.4	11.8	13.7	169	137	-18.7
1-20 years, non-maternal	6.1	7.9	28.7	5	4	-30.8
21-44 years, non-maternal	9.9	11.8	18.7	75	64	-14.3
45-64 years, non-maternal	11.9	13.0	9.4	85	67	-21.2
Maternal	4.8	3.8	-20.5	3	2	-35.2

The top five principal diagnoses with the highest readmissions and rate of readmission over the six years, in order, were blood diseases (25.3 %), neoplasms (17.9%), infectious/parasitic diseases (17.7%), endocrine/metabolic diseases (17.5%), and respiratory system diseases (16.9%) (Bailey et al., 2019). Again, innovations in new treatments and medications have increased the length of survival of patients who would previously have succumbed to complications of illnesses in past years.

4.5.2 Long-Term Care Facility

A **long-term care facility (LTCF)** may also be known as a skilled nursing home, a nursing home, or an assisted living facility. A long-term care facility is a non-acute facility that provides around-the-clock nursing services to patients, usually for rehab or recuperation after a hospitalization or as a permanent residence when loved ones can no longer care for the aged or disabled person. A nursing home may only provide basic custodial care, such as meals and activities of daily living, whereas the term **"skilled"** nursing home indicates a higher level of care that professionals provide, like sterile dressings by registered nurses or speech, physical, and occupational therapy services (U.S. Centers for Medicare and Medicaid Services, n.d.). Medicare will only pay for a skilled nursing facility, whereas Medicaid will pay based on the patient's income. Advanced healthcare providers usually evaluate each nursing home resident monthly. According to the CDC (2019), the annual census of nursing and skilled nursing facilities is four million people, while assisted living homes have approximately one million residents.

Assisted living facilities are often associated with nursing homes. Assisted living facilities provide housing. They usually also provide meals, while medications may or may not be provided. The resident, however, is lucid and able to provide their own activities of daily living and, in some places, may come and go as they please. Often, insurance will not cover assisted living costs.

4.6 OUTPATIENT HEALTHCARE

Today, many healthcare services that once were provided to a hospitalized (inpatient) individual are now provided on an outpatient basis. Hospital costs account for the majority of healthcare spending (Torio & Moore, 2016), and with the emphasis on decreasing costs and increasing satisfaction, outpatient procedures are increasing. Outpatient surgeries and procedures can now be done in an ambulatory setting, thus decreasing healthcare costs and increasing the chance of a quick recovery with less complications as well as positive experiences by the patient (Steiner et al., 2018).

4.6.1 Physician's Offices

The healthcare or primary care provider may be a general or family physician, internist, pediatrician or physician caring for geriatric patients. Physician assistants and nurse practitioners (registered nurses with advanced degrees and extensive training) are also included as office-based primary care providers (Hing & Hsiao, 2014). A primary care provider is responsible for health promotion and preventive care, as well as identifying and treating disease. When a patient experiences complex issues or multiple conditions or disease processes, a referral to a specialist is often made.

The number of primary care physicians (PCP) in 2012 was 46.1 per 100,000 persons, while there were 65.5 specialists for the same population. Northeastern states had a larger supply of primary care physicians than had southern states. In 2012, over half of the PCPs partnered with physician assistants (PA) or nurse practitioners (NP) (Hing & Hsiao, 2014).

4.6.2 Urgent Care Centers

Urgent care centers are clinics or centers that provide treatment for non-life-threatening conditions (Mount Sinai, 2020). They are staffed with physicians, nurse practitioners, or physician's assistants and provide ambulatory services, but not for emergencies. Urgent care centers are convenient because they are easily accessible, and most remain open later than do the offices of regular doctors on weeknights and weekends.

4.6.3 Ambulatory Surgery

Ambulatory surgery centers may be associated with a hospital or medical center, owned by physicians, or independent centers where same day surgery or procedures are performed. Patients usually are admitted in the morning and discharged the same day. Many invasive surgeries performed for therapeutic reasons and noninvasive surgeries usually performed for diagnostic or exploratory reasons are now mostly performed in ambulatory settings rather than requiring inpatient admission (Steiner et al., 2018). Steiner et al.'s report on surgical procedure statistics from the 2016 American Hospital Association for participating community hospitals indicate an increase in the number of invasive surgeries completed in ambulatory locations from 57% in 1994 to 66% in 2014. In 2014, the top five invasive, therapeutic surgeries performed in an ambulatory setting were lens and cataract procedures; procedures on muscles, tendons, or soft tissue; joint lesion destruction or incision or fusion of joint; cholecystectomy and common duct exploration; and excision of semilunar cartilage of the knee (Steiner et al., 2018).

4.6.4 Home Health

Home healthcare can be provided at home and paid for by Medicare and, usually, private insurance—if skilled services are required and ordered by healthcare providers. Skilled services include skills performed by registered nurses and rehab specialists, such as occupational therapists, physical therapists, and speech therapists. Services can include physical therapy after a joint replacement or sterile dressing changes after an abdominal surgery. Additional services from nursing assistants, such as assisting with bathing and position changes, also are often covered when skilled nursing services are provided. Medicaid covers some services as well. According to the National Center for Health Statistics (2019), 3.7 million persons utilized home health services between 2015 and 2016. Moreover, adults 65 years of age and older utilized home health services more than any other long-term care service during that time period.

4.6.5 Hospice

Hospice services are available for patients with terminal conditions that are expected to survive less than six months. Hospice services can be provided at home, in the nursing home, and even in the hospital. A physician must order hospice services. Medicare usually pays for hospice services, while Medicaid may or may not pay for the services, depending on the state. In 2015–2016, hospice was the second most-used long-term care service, caring for 1.3 million patients, and nursing home services was the third most-used long-term care service, with 1.2 million residents (Figure 4.9).

4.6.6 Adult Day Care

Adult day care services are utilized to provide respite for caregivers or supervised care for senior adults while the family or caregivers maintain employment (National Adult Day Services Association [NADSA], n.d.) Most adult day care centers are available during regular working hours, Monday through Friday; some may provide evening and weekend services. Most adult day care centers provide social activities, custodial care, meals, and medications, if needed. According to the NADSA, there are three different types of adult day care centers. Each center's primary focus is social interaction, medical/health, or specialized for persons with dementia or disabilities.

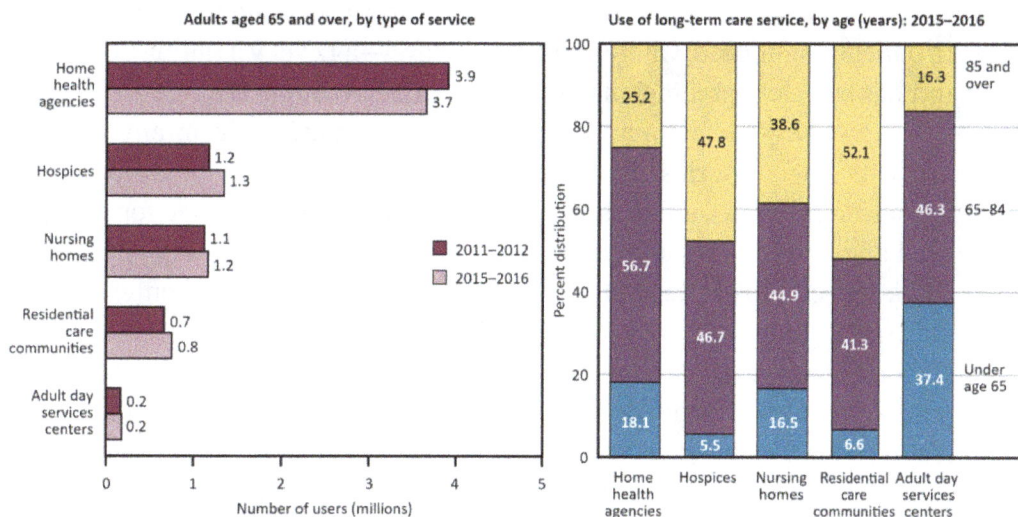

Figure 4.9: Use of Long-term Care Services, By Type of Service and Age: United States, 2011–2012 and 2015–2016

Source: Centers for Disease Control and Prevention
Attribution: National Center for Health Statistics
License: Public Domain
NOTE: Number of users were rounded to the nearest 100. Percentages were based on the unrounded numbers and may not sum to 100 because of rounding. People may use more than one service per year and were counted in each service used.

4.6.7 Emergency Services

The emergency department (ED) is a part of a hospital established for patients experiencing emergencies that could result in life alterations, such as an injury, an acute illness, or an exacerbation of a chronic disease process. Often, EDs are crowded with patients who are not experiencing true emergencies. Because of this, many EDs have added "fast tracks" for the patient to be seen by healthcare providers other than ED physicians. It is common for persons without health insurance to seek care in the ED rather than have a primary healthcare provider. Because of the Emergency Medical Treatment and Labor Act established by Congress in 1986, it is unlawful for hospitals to turn anyone away, regardless of insurance or any means of payment (CMS, 2012). As a result, emergency departments can become crowded, creating long wait times for those with emergencies, especially if the ED does not have a "fast track" program which sorts out emergent from non-emergent conditions.

Pause and Reflect

How would you devise an education plan to encourage individuals with non-emergent health conditions or injuries to seek care with a primary healthcare provider instead of the emergency department?

Levels of Care Provided in Emergency Rooms

Emergency departments may also be designated as Trauma Centers. A Level I Trauma Center is considered a tertiary center—the top level—and provides any type of care a patient might need, whereas the lowest level—a Level V Trauma Center—is basic and has transfer agreements with other Trauma Centers (American Trauma Society, n.d.). A Level I Trauma Center may receive patients from anywhere in the state with such injuries as extensive burns or extensive neurological or musculoskeletal injuries from massive automobile injuries. Coverage for all types of medical and surgical specialty is available twenty-four hours every day. Often, Level I Trauma enters are teaching hospitals. A Level V Trauma Center is what most local hospitals are with basic emergency room coverage.

Many emergency rooms, regardless of their status as a Trauma Center, use a guide similar to the one below (Figure 4.10), to assess the acuity level of a patient and resources needed to provide care to the patient. This guide has levels one-through-five, where levels one-through-three are considered minor problems requiring brief periods of time and minimal resources. Levels four and five require intravenous fluids, extensive testing, more nursing care, and other healthcare professionals assisting.

Level 1	Minor medical issue. Rare.
Level 2	The base charge when patients visit the ER.
Level 3	More complex problems that involves limited testing. Common.
Level 4	More serious issue that may involve medication, IVs, testing, etc.
Level 5	Critical care. Life-threatening illness or injury. Usually arrives by ambulance.

Figure 4.10: Assigning Acuity Level to Patients Seen in the Emergency Room

Source: Mercy, ProMedica, UTMC, and The Blade
Attribution: Corey Parson, Adapted from Mercy, ProMedica, UTMC, and The Blade
License: Fair Use

Sun et al. (2018) provided the 2013 CDC information that ED usage is increasing. In the report, 20% of the total population had visited the ED in the previous year examined. Most of the ED patients during that time had Medicaid coverage compared to those with private insurance or those uninsured.

ED visits increased for all age groups between the years 2006–2015, with 2015 reaching a ten-year high for all (Sun et al., 2018). The age group with the highest increase in ED visits is between 45 and 64 years of age. However, those 65 years and older had the highest number of visits for any age group each of these years (Figure 4.11).

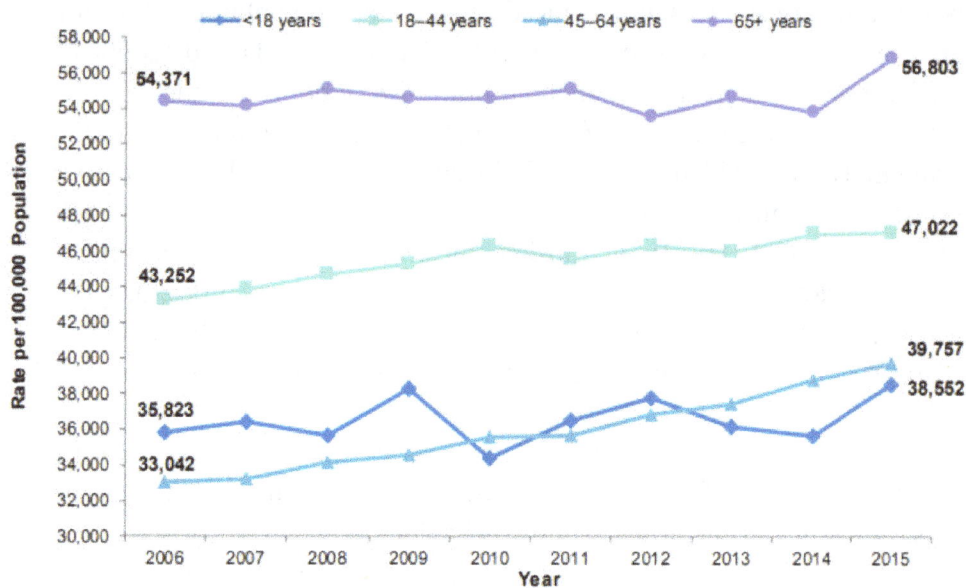

Figure 4.11: Rate of ED Visits, Per 100,000 Population by Age Group, 2006–2015

Source: Agency for Healthcare Research and Quality
Attribution: Agency for Healthcare Research and Quality
License: Public Domain

Page | 95

Moore et al. (2017) evaluated the causes of ED visits in the years 2006 and 2014. The top diagnoses for an ED visit fell into four categories: injury, medical condition, mental health/substance abuse, and maternal/neonatal condition. Medical conditions, specifically abdominal pain, was the leader in diagnoses, followed by injuries (specifically, sprains and strains), mental health or abuse problems (specifically, mood disorder in 2006, but alcohol-related disorders in 2014), and maternal/neonatal issues (specifically, hemorrhage during pregnancy, abruptio placentae, and placenta previa). Of note, mental health issues had increased by 44.1% in 2014; significantly, suicidal ideation increased 414.6% (Moore et al., 2017).

Emergency department visits often result in hospitalization. However, Sun et al. (2018b) reported that hospital admissions from 2006 to 2015 decreased in every age group. For this nine-year period, the greatest decrease was a 27% decrease in the under 18 years of age population; followed by those over 65 years of age, with a 20% decrease; 45–64 years of age, with a 17% decrease; and 18–44 years of age, with a 12% decrease.

4.6.8 Public Health, Health Departments

Public health, as an entity, is population rather than individual focused. Usually, when thinking of public health, what comes to mind are environmental prevention services (such as sanitation), safe water assessment, evaluation of restaurant safe food handling, and lead poisoning identification. Emergency preparedness, as in disaster relief with 9/11 or during hurricanes, and prevention or eradication of diseases in large populations (through immunizations or vaccinations) are other services that are readily acknowledged as public health services. Individual-focused healthcare services at a reduced rate can also be obtained at local health departments. Some of the services provided for individuals and families at the local health department usually include immunizations; tuberculosis skin tests; clinics such as Women, Infant, and Children (WIC), where mothers and infants are evaluated and provided milk; well-baby clinics; women's clinics, where female exams are performed and tests given, such as those for sexually transmitted infections, including HIV; tuberculosis clinics, where individuals are monitored and a medication regimen is created; high blood pressure clinics; and diabetes clinics. Home visits for premature or high-risk infants and some high-risk patients are also provided. Birth records and immunization records are housed at local health departments, also.

According to the CDC (2014), the purpose of public health is to "prevent epidemics and spread of disease, protect against environmental hazards, prevent injuries, promote and encourage healthy behaviors, respond to disasters and assist communities in recovery, and assure the quality and accessibility of services" (slide 3). The CDC (2020a) states that "we work 24/7 to protect the safety, health and security of America from threats here and around the world" (para. 1). The CDC assures the public that they are equipped with up-to-date lab capabilities and the highest caliber of public health officials and workers and can provide quick response to outbreaks in the U.S. and other nations (CDC, 2020a).

Public health is not only one agency's responsibility, however. As a community, every member is responsible for the health of the community, thus creating a public health community composed of public, private, and voluntary organizations. See the CDC's image of how public health is intertwined with every aspect of the community (Figure 4.12).

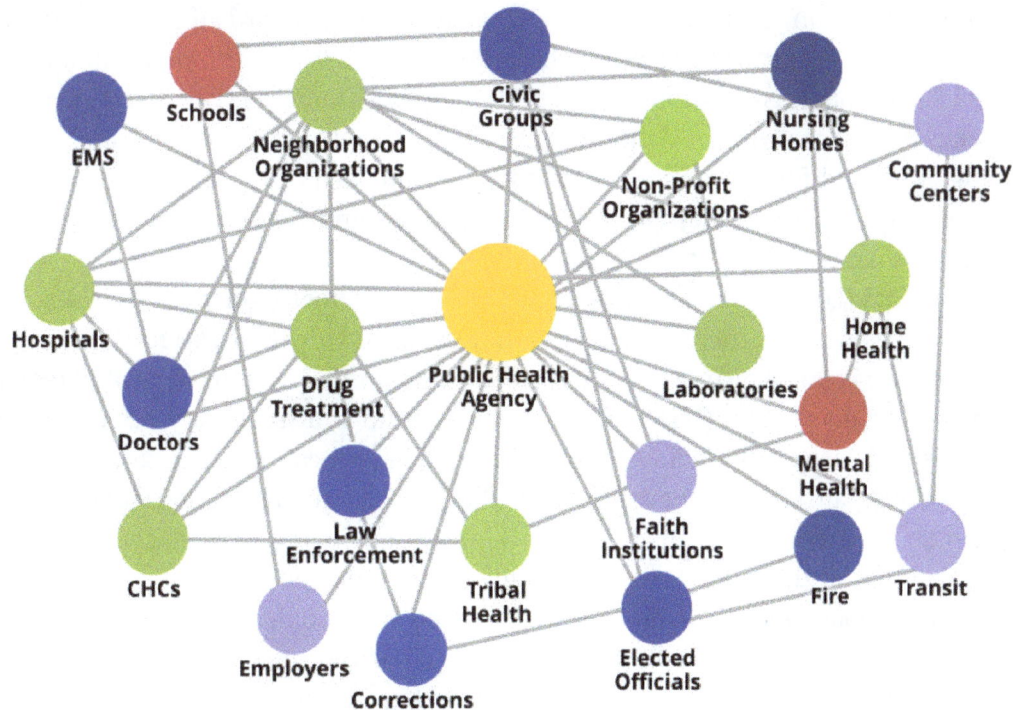

Figure 4.12: The Public Health System

Source: Centers for Disease Control and Prevention
Attribution: Public Health Professionals Gateway
License: Public Domain

Working together, the ten essential public health services should be accomplished. The CDC's (2018) ten essential public health services are as follows:

1. Monitor health status to identify and solve community health problems.
2. Diagnose and investigate health problems and health hazards in the community.
3. Inform, educate, and empower people about health issues.
4. Mobilize community partnerships and action to identify and solve health problems.
5. Develop policies and plans that support individual and community health efforts.
6. Enforce laws and regulations that protect health and ensure safety.

7. Link people to needed personal health services and assure the provision of healthcare when otherwise unavailable.

8. Assure competent public and personal healthcare workforce.

9. Evaluate effectiveness, accessibility, and quality of personal and population-based health services.

10. Research for new insights and innovative solutions to health problems.

Each state—and even each county within the state—is given latitude to organize, function, and regulate according to the local board of health (Public Health Law Center, 2015). In 2019, there were 2,459 local health departments in the U.S. (National Association of County & City Health Officials [NACCHO], 2019). Resources for local health departments also vary and include federal and state funds; Medicaid funds; county appropriations; and such others as environmental fees, grants, fees or partial fees for some services, and possibly some Medicare reimbursements (Moore et al., 2012).

The COVID-19 pandemic has brought renewed focus on public health. A pandemic is an occurrence of a disease or illness worldwide (CDC, 2020b), whereas an epidemic is an occurrence of a disease or illness in a large number of persons in a specific population (NIHa, 2020). An endemic is a frequently occurring or sustained disease or illness in a specific population or location (NIH, 2020b). The CDC is the organization responsible for leading the charge in any type of pandemic, epidemic, or endemic. During the COVID-19 pandemic, the CDC is working with the president of the U.S.; a task force; governors; and the directors of the FDA, HHS, and department of defense concerning recommendations for citizens. Each person is responsible for staying up to date with current information and abiding by recommendations made by the White House task force and the CDC.

- -

First Person Perspective

Nurse B., R.N., is a registered nurse with a Georgia county Public Health Department.

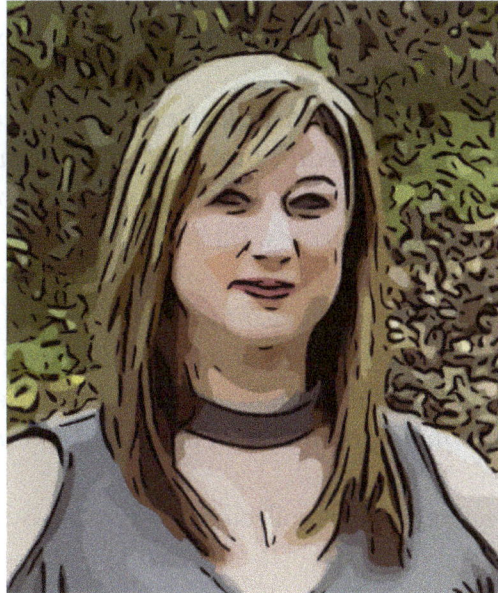

Figure 4.8: First Person Perspective

Source: Original Work
Attribution: Deanna Howe
License: CC BY-SA 4.0

I have had the pleasure of working in various fields in nursing, ranging from the emergency room to wound care, but none have afforded me the autonomy that Public Health provides. Public Health in my state allows registered nurses to work within an expanded role. We perform health physicals, hearing and vision exams, women's preventative health examinations, screenings for certain cancers, and prescribe medications following state guidelines. In addition to offering all of these services, the health department offers diagnostic and laboratory tests, vaccinations, and health education services at a discounted rate. This is especially important in creating equal access for clients who may not otherwise be able to obtain these services in other medical facilities.

The health department offers many programs such as Family Planning and Women's Health program, which is an essential community operation; the Child Health program, which has more extensive developmental screening than provided at a pediatrician's office; and the Blood Pressure/ Diabetes Program, which provides critical screening, education, and medications based on a safe program protocol. Other services people are most familiar with include our shot clinic, which provides vaccinations to children and adults; sexually transmitted infections (STI) clinic, which provides screening and medications; and the Women, Infants, and Children (WIC) program, which provides special supplemental nutrition. We also treat clients from multiple social-economic backgrounds with a broad range of services. We are able to file insurance claims for services with patients who have health insurance but also are able to provide no fee service through grant funding to aid our patients who do not have insurance.

Prior to working at the health department, I was unaware of the depth of services Public Health provided in the community. As a health department, we try to provide outreach into our local community and educate clients on our programs. During the last few challenging months, we have been actively involved in providing COVID-19 testing to various community areas that may have difficulty reaching a physician's office for testing. This is a true testament of how Public Health evolves and excels within the community during difficult times. Public health will continue to strive to provide quality care to our clients and communities.

First person perspective vignette collected and created by Deanna Howe, 2020

For your consideration: Nurse B. notes several programs her local health department offers. There is often a perception that the health department is just for underprivileged clients. What was your knowledge about health department services prior to this perspective? After reading about Nurse B.'s work at the health department, are you surprised at the extensive number of services provided? How does Public Health contribute to the health of the community population they serve? How might a health department campaign best highlight the important services they provide? Is there a need to destigmatize seeking healthcare at a health department?

4.7 SUMMARY

This chapter has provided information concerning where healthcare services are available. It discussed inpatient and outpatient services and provided statistics that affect the functioning of hospitals, including admissions, payers, length of stays, readmission rates, and causes of admissions. It discussed public health services and the importance of working together as a community for our overall public health.

4.8 REVIEW QUESTIONS

1. Explain the different types of hospitals.

2. Compare and contrast trends of hospital admissions related to patient age, hospitalization type, payer source, community level income, and length of stays; and readmissions related to payer source and patient age, payer sources, and principal diagnosis.

3. What differentiates a skilled nursing facility from a non-skilled nursing facility?

4. What are types of outpatient services available in the U.S., and why has the number and availability of outpatient services increased?

5. What is the purpose of public health, according to the CDC?

4.9 REFERENCES

Agency for Health care Research and Quality. (2019a). HCUP fast stats: Trends in inpatient stays. Retrieved February 22, 2021 from https://www.hcup-us.ahrq.gov/faststats/NationalTrendsServlet

American Hospital Association. (2019, November 2). Fast facts on U.S. hospitals, 2019. Retrieved from https://www.aha.org/statistics/fast-facts-us-hospitals

American Trauma Society. (n.d.). Trauma center levels explained. Retrieved from https://www.amtrauma.org/page/traumalevels

Bailey, M. K., Weiss, A. J., Barrett, M. L., & Jiang, H. J. (2019). Statistical brief #248/ Characteristics of 30-day all-cause hospital readmissions, 2010–2016. Retrieved October 31, 2019, from Agency for Health care Research and Quality.

Center for Disease Control and Prevention. (2020a, May 19). A bold promise to the nation. Retrieved from https://www.cdc.gov/about/24-7/index.html

Center for Disease Control and Prevention. (2020b, May 19). Pandemic influenza. Retrieved from https://www.cdc.gov/flu/pandemic-resources/

Center for Disease Control and Prevention. (2019, November 1). Nursing homes and assisted living (Long term care facilities [LTCFs]). Retrieved from https://www.cdc.gov/longtermcare/index.html

Center for Disease Control and Prevention. (2018). The 10 essential public health services. Retrieved from https://www.cdc.gov/publichealthgateway/publichealthservices/essentialhealthservices.html

Center for Disease Control and Prevention. (2014). The 10 essential public health services: An overview PowerPoint. Retrieved from https://www.cdc.gov/publichealthgateway/publichealthservices/pdf/essential-phs.pdf

Center for Disease Control and Prevention and The Merck Company Foundation. (2007). The state of aging and health in America 2007. Whitehouse Station, NJ: The Merck Company Foundation; 2007. Retrieved November 2, 2019, from https://www.cdc.

gov/aging/pdf/saha_2007.pdf

Centers for Medicare and Medicaid Services. (2012). Emergency medical treatment and labor act (EMTALA). Retrieved from https://www.cms.gov/Regulations-and-Guidance/Legislation/EMTALA

Cunningham, P., Rudowitz, R., Young, K., Garfield, R., & Foutz, J. (2016, June 09). Understanding Medicaid hospital payments and the impact of recent policy changes. Kaiser family foundation. Retrieved from https://www.kff.org/medicaid/issue-brief/understanding-medicaid-hospital-payments-and-the-impact-of-recent-policy-changes/view/footnotes/#footnote-190356-1

Freeman, W. J., Weiss, A. J, & Heslin, K. C. (2018). Overview of U.S. hospital stays in 2016: Variation by geographic region Agency for Healthcare Research and Quality. Retrieved October 31, 2019, from https://www.hcup-us.ahrq.gov/reports/statbriefs/sb246-Geographic-Variation-Hospital-Stays.pdf

Hing, E. & Hsiao, C. (2014). State variability in supply of office-based primary care providers: United States, 2012. NCHS data brief, no. 15. Retrieved November 2, 2019, from https://www.cdc.gov/nchs/data/databriefs/db151.pdf

Johns Hopkins Medicine. (n.d.) Patient care. Retrieved February 1, 2020, from https://www.hopkinsmedicine.org/patient_care/billing-insurance/insurance_footnotes.html

Liu, J. B. and Kelz, R. R. (2018). Types of hospitals in the United States. Journal of American Medical Association, 320(10), 1074. DOI:10.1001/jama.2018.9471

Lopez, E., Neuman, T., Jacobson, G., & Levitt, L. (April 15, 2020). How much more than Medicare do private insurers pay? A review of the literature. Kaiser Family Foundation Retrieved from https://www.kff.org/medicare/issue-brief/how-much-more-than-medicare-do-private-insurers-pay-a-review-of-the-literature/

McDermott, E., & Sun, R. (2017). Trends in hospital inpatient stays in the United States, 2005–2014. Agency for Health care Research and Quality. Retrieved November 1, 2019, from https://www.hcup-us.ahrq.gov/reports/statbriefs/sb225-Inpatient-US-Stays-Trends.pdf

Moore, B. J., Stocks, C., & Owens, P. L. (2017). Trends in emergency department visits, 2006–2014. Agency for Health care Research and Quality. Retrieved October 31, 2019, from https://www.hcup-us.ahrq.gov/reports/statbriefs/sb227-Emergency-Department-Visit-Trends.pdf

Moore, J. D., Berner, M. M., & Wall, A. N. (2012). How are local public health services financed? The University of North Carolina at Chapel Hill. Retrieved from https://www.sog.unc.edu/resources/faqs/how-are-local-public-health-services-financed

Mount Sinai. (2020, September 30). What is urgent care and when should you use it? Retrieved from https://www.mountsinai.org/locations/urgent-care/what-is-urgent-care

National Adult Day Services Association. (2020, June 11). About adult day services.

Retrieved from https://www.nadsa.org/learn-more/about-adult-day-services

National Association of County & City Health Officials. (2019). 2019 National profile of local health departments. Retrieved from https://www.naccho.org/resources/lhd-research/national-profile-of-local-health-departments

National Center for Health Statistics. (2019, November 2). Health, United States, 2018. Hyattsville, MD. Retrieved from https://www.cdc.gov/nchs/data/hus/hus18.pdf

National Institutes of Health. (2020a, May 19). Epidemic. Retrieved from https://search.nih.gov/search?utf8=%E2%9C%93&affiliate=nih&query=epidemic

National Institutes of Health. (2020b, May 19). Endemic. Retrieved from https://search.nih.gov/search?utf8=%E2%9C%93&affiliate=nih&query=endemic

Public Health Law Center. (2015). State and local public health: An overview of regulatory authority. Retrieved from https://www.publichealthlawcenter.org/sites/default/files/resources/phlc-fs-state-local-reg-authority-publichealth-2015_0.pdf

Steiner, C. A., Karaca, Z., Moore, B. J., Imshaug, M. C., & Pickens, G. (2018). Surgeries in hospital-based ambulatory surgery and hospital inpatient settings. Agency for Health care Research and Quality. Retrieved November 1, 2019, from https://www.hcup-us.ahrq.gov/reports/statbriefs/sb223-Ambulatory-Inpatient-Surgeries-2014.pdf

Sun, R., Karaca, Z, & Wong, H.S. (2018a). Trends in hospital inpatient stays by age and payer, 200-2015. Agency for Health care Research and Quality. Retrieved October 31, 2019, from https://www.hcup-us.ahrq.gov/reports/statbriefs/sb235-Inpatient-Stays-Age-Payer-Trends.pdf

Sun, R., Karaca, Z, & Wong, H. S. (2018b). Trends in hospital emergency department visits by age and payer, 2006-2015. Retrieved October 31, 2019, from https://www.hcup-us.ahrq.gov/reports/statbriefs/sb238-Emergency-Department-Age-Payer-2006-2015.pdf

Torio, C. M., & Moore, B. J. (2016). National inpatient hospital costs: The most expensive conditions by payer, 2013. (Statistical Brief #204). In healthcare cost and utilization project statistical briefs, Rockville, MD: Agency for Health care Research and Quality; 2006 Feb

U.S. Centers for Medicare and Medicaid Services. (n.d.) Nursing home care. Retrieved November 1, 2019, from https://www.medicare.gov/coverage/nursing-home-care

World Health Organization. (n.d.) Hospital role in health system. Retrieved November 1, 2019, from https://www.who.int/hospitals/hospitals-in-the-health-system/en/

5

Federal and State Funded Healthcare

5.1 LEARNING OBJECTIVES

By the end of this chapter, the student will be able to:
- Compare Original Medicare and the different parts (Part A and Part B) and Medicare Part D with Medicare Advantage, also known as Part C
- Describe the two trust funds that pay for or support Medicare
- Discuss Medicaid and the Children's Health Insurance Program (CHIP)
- List two objectives of the Patient Protection and Affordable Care Act
- Discuss four healthcare delivery reforms of the Affordable Care Act (ACA)
- Describe the breakdown of costs for federally-funded healthcare services proposed for federal year (FY) 2020

5.2 KEY TERMS

- Basic Health Program
- Centers for Medicare and Medicaid Services
- Children's Health Insurance Program (CHIP)
- Medicaid
- Medicare
- Medicare Part A
- Medicare Part B
- Medicare Advantage (Part C)
- Medicare Part D
- Medigap

- Original Medicare
- Patient Protection and Affordable Care Act (Affordable Care Act, ACA, Obamacare)

5.3 INTRODUCTION

Healthcare is paid for by federal or state funds, private insurance, or private pay. Health insurance is important to assist with the costs of healthcare but, arguably, most important to provide individuals easier access to healthcare. Most persons aged 65 and older are covered by **Medicare**, having paid into the Social Security system during employment for at least ten years or forty quarters (U.S. Department of Health and Human Services [HHS], n.d.). For individuals under 65 years of age and noninstitutionalized, the Congressional Budget Office (CBO, 2018) projected that the majority of individuals (89%) would also have health insurance. Most health insurance for individuals under 65 years of age is from employment-based plans (two thirds). Government and state-subsidized **Medicaid** or **Children's Health Insurance Program (CHIP)** accounts for about one fourth of those with insurance. Others are insured with Medicare, nongroup policies, or other forms (about 4%), leaving 29 million people (11%) uninsured (CBO, 2018). The total cost for government-subsidized healthcare insurance—Medicare, Medicaid, and CHIP—was $1.3 trillion in 2016, comprising 38% of all healthcare expenses (Klees et al., 2018). In this chapter, we will explore federal and state-funded health insurance in greater detail. We also look at the U.S. Department of Health and Human Services (HHS) and identify services provided by the federal government for the health of all citizens.

5.4 FEDERALLY-FUNDED HEALTHCARE

The **Centers for Medicare & Medicaid Services (CMS)** is a federal agency within the U.S. government's Health and Human Services department (HHS). CMS administers and operates the Medicare program. Medicaid, although administered by individual states, also receives oversight by CMS (CMS, n.d.a).

5.4.1 Medicare

Medicare is subsidized health insurance for persons aged 65 or older who are eligible for Social Security, for some individuals who are disabled, and for all patients diagnosed with end-stage renal disease (Congressional Budget Office [CBO], 2018; Klees et al., 2018). Medicare insurance is not automatic for those aged 65 and older; certain actions must be taken and criteria met. For individuals receiving social security benefits, an information packet is sent three months prior to the individual's 65th birthday, and specific actions must be taken by certain deadlines to obtain Medicare insurance (CMS, n.d.b).

The federal government offers Medicare insurance coverage in two main ways. The choice for the qualified recipient is Original Medicare or Medicare Advantage. Original Medicare is provided directly through Medicare, whereas Medicare Advantage is provided by private insurance companies (CMS, n.d.b).

Original Medicare includes Part A and Part B. **Medicare Part A** covers hospitalizations, skilled nursing homes, some skilled nursing home health services after hospitalization, and hospice. **Medicare Part B** covers physician's office visits, outpatient care, home health visits without prior hospitalization, medical supplies, and preventive services. Individuals with original Medicare, Part A and Part B, can choose any doctor or healthcare provider and any hospital who accepts Medicare in the U.S., without limitations. Original Medicare pays approximately 80% of costs incurred, and recipients aren't required to pay a premium for Part A. Premiums aren't required for Part A because eligible recipients or their spouses paid payroll taxes for Medicare during their working years. A monthly premium is required for part B Medicare, however (CMS, n.d.c).

Medicare Part D, effective as of 2006, provides coverage for prescription drugs (Kirchhoff, 2018). This is a separate plan, and beneficiaries pay a monthly premium. Low-income individuals are eligible for additional assistance (Kirchhoff, 2018). The prescription drug plans have a formulary, and the Medicare Part D beneficiary may have to pay full price if the medication prescribed is not on the formulary or has not received a qualifying formulary exception. Prices have been negotiated to obtain the best prices. Importantly, individuals applying for Medicare Part A and Part B should also apply for Medicare Part D concurrently to avoid a late penalty charge.

Medigap supplemental insurance is an optional insurance bought from private companies for persons with Original Medicare Part A and Part B. Medigap supplemental insurance may pay for some of the costs not covered by Original Medicare—such as copayments, coinsurance, and deductibles—after Original Medicare has paid its part (CMS, n.d.d). Each person with Original Medicare A and B must have their own policy and pay individual monthly premiums for Medigap insurance. Of note, several important healthcare services are not covered by Medigap, such as prescription drug costs (provided under Part D Medicare), purchases of eyeglasses or hearing aids, dental or vision care, private-duty nursing, or long-term care.

Medicare Advantage (also known as Part C or MA Plans) is the second main option for receiving Medicare. With Medicare Advantage, Part A, Part B, and usually Part D are bundled (CMS, n.d.b). Additional benefits, such as dental, hearing, and vision, are also usually offered. Individuals with Medicare Advantage must choose healthcare providers and hospitals within a specific network; using outside providers will result in additional costs. There are monthly premiums. There are several plans to choose from, including the following: Health Maintenance Organization (HMO) plan, Preferred Provider Organization (PPO) plan, Private Fee-for-Service (PFFS) plan, and a Special Needs plan (SNP).

Medicare Advantage Health Maintenance Organization (HMO) plan

With this plan, a primary care provider is chosen within a given network and all services are provided within the network. The exception is emergency care and two out of area services: urgent care and dialysis treatment. A referral is required for any type of specialist. Usually, out of network care may be allowed but may cost more or the beneficiary may be required to pay all the costs. Prescription drugs are usually covered. Prior approval for tests and some services are required and rules must be followed (CMS, n.d.b). There are also HMO Point of Service (HMOPOS) plans within this plan. These HMOPOS plans allow out of network services with the beneficiary paying higher copayments or having coinsurance (CMS, 2020).

Medicare Advantage Preferred Provider Organization (PPO) plan

This plan is very similar to an HMO but may have a little more flexibility with choosing healthcare providers and agencies within the network, including specialists; a primary care physician is not required. Using providers outside of the network is possible but usually it will cost more. Extra benefits are usually provided, but there are extra costs associated with the benefits (CMS, n.d.b).

Medicare Advantage Private Fee-for-Service (PFFS) plans

With the PFFS plans, the plan dictates the fees for the healthcare providers at the time of service. Choosing a primary care provider is not required and referrals for specialists are not required. Drug costs may or may not be covered. Prior to each healthcare provider visit, the beneficiary must check with the provider to ensure acceptance of the insurance, and copayment is due when the service is provided (CMS, n.d.b).

Special Needs plan

With this plan, persons who have specific healthcare needs, disabilities or diseases with limited income have benefits customized to meet their needs (CMS, 2020). Examples of persons eligible for this type of Medicare plan are persons in nursing homes or other types of institutions, persons eligible for both Medicare and Medicaid, and persons with debilitating conditions, such as chronic heart failure, diabetes, dementia, end-stage renal disease, and HIV/AIDs. A primary care doctor is usually required, and referrals to specialists are also usually required. The plan may or may not cover out-of-network services. Prescription drugs are covered with this plan.

Cost of Medicare

The U.S. Treasury holds two trust funds solely for paying for Medicare; these are a Hospital Insurance (HI) trust fund and a Supplementary Medical Insurance

(SMI) trust fund (CMS, n.d.e). The HI trust fund receives money in several ways. Monies are received for the fund through payroll taxes of working individuals, income taxes of those receiving Social Security benefits, interest earned through trust fund investments, and Medicare Part A premiums from those who have purchased Medicare Part A but did not meet the eligibility requirements (paying into the system while working) for premium-free Medicare Part A. The SMI trust fund receives the premium payments from recipients of Part B and Part D and funds allocated from Congress and other sources, such as trust fund investment interest (CMS, n.d.e).

According to the Congressional Budget Office (CBO, 2018, April), Medicare costs in 2017 were $702 billion and accounted for 3.7% of the gross domestic product (GDP); in comparison, defense spending was $590 billion, accounting for 3.1% of the GDP. In 2017, there were over 58 million enrollees in Part A; over 53 million enrollees in Part B; and over 44 million in Part D with the following beneficiary payments in billions: $293.3, $308.6, and $100.1, respectively (Klees et al., 2018).

Costs to the Medicare Part A recipient in 2020 for a hospitalization of one-to-60 days is a $1408 deductible (CMS, 2020). Medicare Part A also pays for a skilled nursing facility after hospitalization, if needed. If care in a skilled nursing facility is required following hospitalization after 20 days and up to 100 days, Part A pays, but the beneficiary must pay a coinsurance of $176 daily (CMS, 2020). After 100 days, the beneficiary is responsible for all costs (CMS, 2020).

Costs for most of the Medicare Part B recipients in 2020 is $144.60 monthly with an additional monthly cost if the beneficiary's modified adjusted gross income tax is greater than $87,000 (individual) or $174,000 (joint), for the year 2018 (CMS, 2020). The 2020 annual deductible is $198 for all Part B recipients. There is a statutory provision for Social Security recipients called "hold harmless." This provision prevents the government from charging higher Part B premiums than the Social Security cost of living increase received in that same year. Medicare Part B is paid for by beneficiary premiums (25%) and U.S. Treasury (75%). Calendar year (CY) 2020 spending is expected to total $220 billion (HHS, n.d.).

There are monthly premiums for Medicare Part D, with additional monthly fees based on the same income tax numbers as with Part B. Part D yearly deductibles are no more than $435 in 2020 (CMS, n.d.f). There may be a copayment or coinsurance payment for medications after the deductible is met. There is also a coverage gap—"donut-hole"—a temporary limit after $4020 of covered drugs have been spent in 2020. However, after reaching the limits, a large percentage of generic drug prices will be covered by Medicare (in 2020, 75%). As stated previously, individuals who do not sign up for Part D when first eligible are charged. As explained, the costs for Original Medicare have several different parts and programs for seniors to extrapolate, whereas Medicare Advantage has most of these services bundled so may possibly be less confusing.

According to the HHS 2020 budget, Medicare Advantage enrollment is increasing and is expected to total 24 million beneficiaries in calendar year (CY) 2020 (HHS, n.d.a.). This estimated enrollment number will be around 42% of the amount of Medicare beneficiaries enrolled in Original Medicare, Part A and Part B. HHS reports that access to Medicare Advantage is available to almost all individuals nation-wide and the premiums have remained steady while benefits have increased. Total budget costs for Medicare Advantage are expected to be around $286.5 billion in federal year (FY) 2020.

5.5 JOINT FEDERAL/STATE FUNDED HEALTHCARE

Medicaid, also known as Title XIX of the Social Security Act, was signed into law in 1965 (Klees et al., 2018). Medicaid is funded by the state and federal government jointly with each state administering the program and with the federal government, through the Center for Medicare and Medicaid Services, providing oversight. Medicaid is health insurance for the poor, some elderly, and some disabled persons (CBO, 2018). With Medicaid being administered by states, each state's eligibility and services covered are different (CMS, n.d.a). Certain benefits are mandatory for each state, however, while others are optional and may vary from state to state. Basic costs such as inpatient or outpatient hospitalization, home health services, and family planning services are some of the mandatory benefits covered. Optional benefits include various occupational, physical, or speech therapies, preventive screenings and rehabilitation services, and hospice. For a full list of mandatory and optional benefits, see Medicaid.gov. For FY 2018, 36,287,063 children were covered by Medicaid (CMS, n.d.e).

Children's Health Insurance Program (CHIP), also known as Title XXI of the Social Security Act, was signed into law in 1997. CHIP is another jointly-funded program that provides health insurance to those who are poor but whose income is not low enough to meet the Medicaid threshold (CBO, 2018, April). The CHIP and Medicaid programs have been successful in enrolling over 87% of children who are eligible (HHS, 2015). Various acts and laws have been passed by Congress to provide federal allocation of funds through FY 2027 (Klees et al., 2018). For FY 2018, 9,632,367 children were enrolled in CHIP (CMS, n.d.g).

5.5.1 Enrollment in Medicaid and CHIP

As of August 2019, 71,969,720 individuals were enrolled in Medicaid and CHIP nationally, with children representing 50.5% of the total enrollment for both programs. Medicaid enrollment (adults and children) was 65,331,188 individuals. 6,638,532 individuals were enrolled in CHIP. 35,317,330 individuals were enrolled in CHIP or were children in the Medicaid program (CMS, n.d.a).

In federal fiscal year (FFY) 2017, there were 46,405,189 children receiving Medicaid and CHIP funds (unduplicated enrollment numbers) compared to 45,919,430 in FFY 2018, reflecting a 1% decline from 2017 to 2018 (CMS, n.d.e).

5.5.2 Patient Protection and Affordable Care Act

The **Affordable Care Act (ACA)**, signed into legislation in 2010 under President Obama (and therefore often called **Obamacare**), primarily provided monies (tax credits) to subsidize health insurance coverage for individuals through federal or state government marketplaces as well as expanded Medicaid coverage for individuals with low-income (CBO, May 2018). The ACA also created the **Basic Health Program**, also known as Medicaid expansion, a program granting states an option to expand Medicaid coverage to individuals in the 138th to 200th percent of the federal poverty guidelines. Through the ACA, states received federal funding "equal to 95% of the subsidies for which those people would otherwise have been eligible through a marketplace" (CBO, 2018, May). Thirty-nine states have chosen to accept this option and are considered Healthcare.gov states (HHS, 2018). The states of Missouri and Oklahoma have adopted the plan but have not yet implemented it; the federal district of Washington, D.C., has implemented the plan (KFF, 2020) (Figure 5.1).

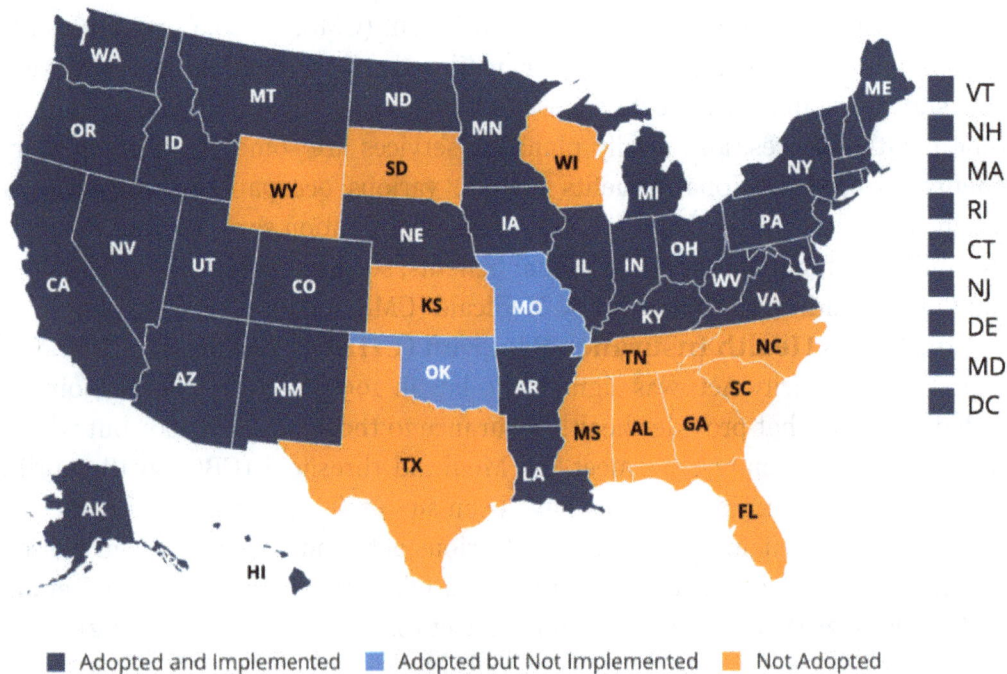

Figure 5.1: Status of State Action on Medicaid Expansion, November 2020

Source: Kaiser Family Foundation
Attribution: Kaiser Family Foundation
License: © Kaiser Family Foundation. Used with permission.

Within the Healthcare.gov states, state level issuers for health plans, essentially insurance companies, received subsidies from the ACA to provide care for the people in the state. In the plan year 2014, there were 187 insurance carriers for the entire conglomerate of Healthcare.gov states; in plan year 2015 and plan year 2016, there were 217 insurance carriers. However, in plan year 2017, there were only 152 carriers; 121 in plan year 2018; and 144 in plan year 2019, thus decreasing. The number of issuers of health plans for each state ranged from one to six, thereby limiting choice of insurance carriers for states with only one insurance carrier. There are also a wide range of costs.

The HHS Assistant Secretary for Planning and Evaluation (ASPE) (2018) provided the following information: premiums will increase up to 85% higher in 2019 ($405) compared to 2014 ($218) monthly for the silver plan. The silver plan is the second lowest cost plan and is considered the benchmark plan. Nebraska, the state that has adopted but not implemented the plan, had only one insurance carrier and would have the highest percentage increase ($686 in 2019 compared to $205 in 2014), whereas Indiana, a state with more than one insurance carrier, was slated to have the lowest percentage increase ($280 in 2019 compared to $270 in 2014) (HHS, 2018). Levitt (2020) reports that the ACA is structured so that the highest premium cannot increase above 9.5% of a person's income, with federal subsidies paying any costs over that amount.

Perception of the enactment of the ACA was and remains controversial. The Kaiser Family Foundation (KFF) tracking poll conducted in October 2020 investigated the favorability view of ACA (Hamel et al., 2020). Participants (1106 voters) show a larger favorable view than unfavorable view (Figure 5.2).

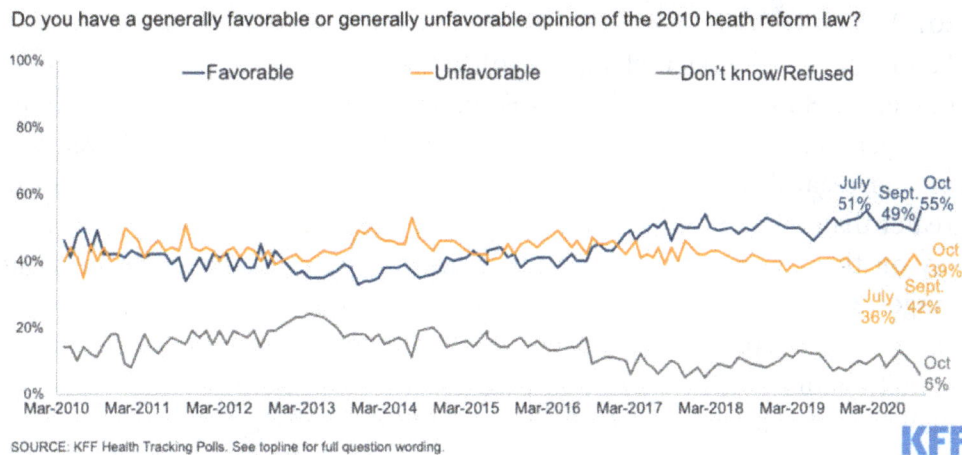

Do you have a generally favorable or generally unfavorable opinion of the 2010 heath reform law?

SOURCE: KFF Health Tracking Polls. See topline for full question wording.

Figure 5.2: Clear Majority of Public View the ACA Favorably

Source: Kaiser Family Foundation
Attribution: Kaiser Family Foundation
License: © Kaiser Family Foundation. Used with permission.

According to Blumenthal et al. (2015), benefits of the ACA include allowing young adults to be added to their parent's health insurance policies until the age of 26 years old; providing availability of insurance to young adults, minorities, and the poor; providing quicker access to healthcare providers; and having less complaints about access to care and medical expenses. In addition to expanding health insurance, healthcare delivery reforms were another major component of the ACA (Blumenthal et al., 2015). The reforms include value-based healthcare rather than volume-based healthcare, promotion of healthcare services integration, efforts to boost numbers of and payment to primary care providers, and a responsiveness to the constantly-evolving healthcare environment.

Value-based incentives include decreasing hospital reimbursement for thirty-day readmission rates or occurrence of hospital-acquired infections, with increased funds if certain cost and quality measures were obtained for hospitals as well as physician practices. For promotion of healthcare services integration, organizational arrangements with all parties involved in the care of a patient's inpatient or outpatient experience are combined, and the organization receives bundled payments for the care episode. By organizing the providers in this manner, the burden of keeping costs low and the quality high is on the healthcare providers within the organization. For those caring for patients with Medicare, savings can be accomplished and then passed on to the providers within the organization. To boost numbers and payment for primary care providers, states were mandated to pay primary care providers Medicare rates when seeing Medicaid patients. Also, funds were provided for scholarships and forgiveness of loans for primary care providers willing to work in underserved areas. In response to the continually-evolving healthcare milieu, the Center for Medicare and Medicaid Innovation (CMMI) was created to devise and investigate various measures and plans to improve the quality of healthcare and reduce the associated costs (Blumenthal et al., 2015).

According to Kirzinger et al. (2019), a health tracking poll conducted in November 2018 by the Kaiser Family Foundation (KFF) indicated that although the ACA plan remains controversial, many of the ACA provisions are desired by all Americans, regardless of their political persuasion. Those ACA provisions desired by greater than 60% of those surveyed included the following: allow young adults to stay on their parents' insurance plans until age 26; create health insurance exchanges where small business and people can shop for insurance and compare prices and benefits; provide financial help to low- and moderate-income Americans who don't obtain insurance through their jobs to help them purchase coverage; gradually close the Medicare prescription drug "donut hole" so people on Medicare will no longer be required to pay the full cost of their medications when they reach the gap; and eliminate out-of-pocket costs for many preventive services (Kirzinger et al., 2019).

Interestingly, overall physician visits have not increased since enactment of the ACA, although there have been more Medicaid patient visits (Gaffney et al., 2019; Johansen & Richardson, 2019). Klein et al. (2017) found similar results with emergency department visits in Maryland. Although the Medicaid population increased by 20% after the implementation of the ACA, there was no significant change in emergency department visits. Expectations were that patients would utilize the new coverage to seek primary healthcare providers.

Kobayashi et al. (2019), assessed patients' feeling of well-being after receiving greater access to affordable healthcare and found that feelings of well-being did not improve. However, Blumenthal et al. (2015) reported those recently insured were happy with their new coverage. Moreover, 75% of those surveyed had promptly obtained appointments with appropriate healthcare providers and received those appointments in a timely manner within a four-week time period. The costs of healthcare were also reported as a problem less frequently.

Pause and Reflect

Do you know anyone who has received health care through the ACA? Consider that the Supreme Court heard arguments regarding the constitutionality of ACA, in November 2020. The decision was 7-2 opinion that the challenge to the individual mandate had no standing. Thus, ending the case. Consider how a different opinion could have affected the outcome. Or if, in the future, the ACA is repealed. How should the U.S. government protect those who are uninsured or who lose health insurance? How can the ACA better protect people with pre-existing conditions? Name two advantages and two disadvantages of the Affordable Care Act.

First Person Perspective

Ms. W., M.S.W., has a Concentration in Administration and Public Policy and is a Healthcare Advocate in her community.

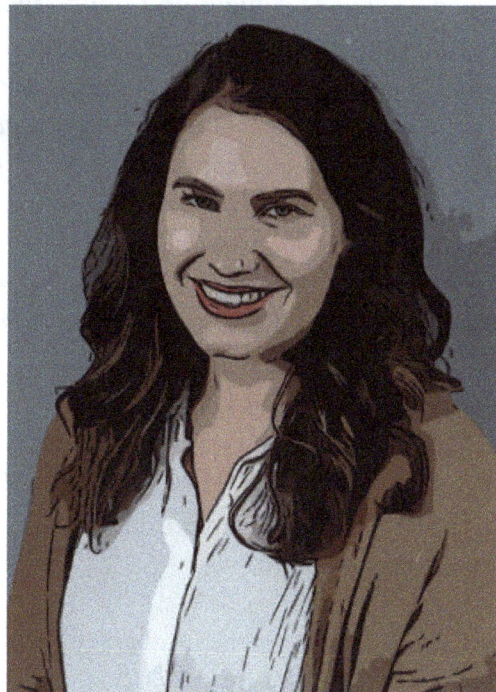

Figure 5.3: First Person Perspective

Growing up in America, my insurance status was always tied to my father's employment. He was the one to hold the steady job with all the benefits. My mother cycled through employment after having my younger brother and then spent a few years as a caregiver for my ailing grandmother. In my senior year of high school, everything changed. At fifty years old, my father was diagnosed with terminal cancer. It was an immense shock to my family; my parents had one child about to head to college and the other was just twelve years old. They did all they could to continue working and providing for our family, but a year later, my father needed to step away from working to commit himself to the costly and demanding experimental treatment he was undergoing. My father opted into the COBRA program, a costly alternative to ultimate loss of coverage, but my father had a whole treatment team in place within his current network and feared losing his place in the experimental trial he was in. My parents were forced to have a difficult conversation with me about how my mother, brother, and I were all about to lose our health coverage.

At nineteen, I was terrified trying to navigate healthcare on my own, but thankfully my state had just expanded care under the Affordable Care Act. I was one of the many first-time enrollees in the state's Apple Health through their Health Benefit Exchange. By this time, I was a full-time college student, working part time, and trying to afford a place on my own. Being able to qualify for state Medicaid gave me peace of mind that access to medical care wasn't something I had to worry about. The same month my insurance coverage began, I came down with the norovirus. I fell ill very quickly while receiving treatment, and I was transported from the urgent care facility to a nearby hospital via ambulance where I was admitted for overnight observation. When I left the hospital, I was terrified of the medical bill I would receive in the mail. I knew I could never afford it, but thankfully that bill never came. To this day, I am grateful for the access to needed services that the expansion of the Affordable Care Act has afforded me. I was able to access coverage through a job for a few years, but when I decided to go back to school for my master's degree, I had comfort knowing that I would once again be able to access care. No one should have to choose between getting the medical care they need and being able to provide a clear path for their future. Thanks to Washington state's commitment to expand Medicaid under the ACA ten years ago, I am able to share this with you today.

First person perspective vignette collected and created by Deanna Howe, 2020

For your consideration: Ms. W. describes the fear of having to navigate the unfamiliar territory of finding health insurance. Her state is one of many which provide access to expanded Medicaid health services.

If you were a voter, would you vote in favor or against ACA Medicaid expansion? Why or why not? For college students who are unable to remain covered under a parent's plan, should the government offer an insurance protection benefit under the ACA? Consider what would have happened to Ms. W. had ACA insurance coverage not been available to her during the illness she described. What financial implications might Ms. W. face?

5.6 FEDERALLY FUNDED ORGANIZATIONS FOR THE PROMOTION OF HEALTH

5.6.1 The U.S. Department of Health and Human Services (HHS)

The mission of Health and Human Services (HHS) is "to enhance and protect the health and well-being of all Americans by providing for effective health and human services and by fostering sound, sustained advances in the sciences underlying medicine, public health, and social services" (HHS, n.d., p. 2). There are nine divisions and more than 100 programs provided by HHS. The nine divisions are as follows: the Administration for Children and Families, the Administration for Community Living (ACL), the Centers for Disease Control and Prevention (CDC) (which has subsumed the previous stand-alone Agency for Toxic Substances and Disease Registry), the Centers for Medicare and Medicaid Services (CMS), the Food and Drug Administration (FDA), the Health Resources and Services Administration (HRSA), the Indian Health Service, the National Institutes of Health (NIH) (which has subsumed the previous stand-alone Agency for Healthcare Research and Quality [AHRQ]), and the Substance Abuse and Mental Health Services Administration (SAMHSA).

The FY 2020 Budget allocates $1,286 billion for all of HHS programs and services. The $1,286 billion is divided as follows: 53% for Medicare; 32% for Medicaid; 8% for discretionary programs; 3% for children's entitlement programs; 3% for other mandatory programs; and 1% for temporary assistance for needy families (TANF) (HHS, n.d., p. 2) (Figure 5.4).

$1,286 Billion in Outlays

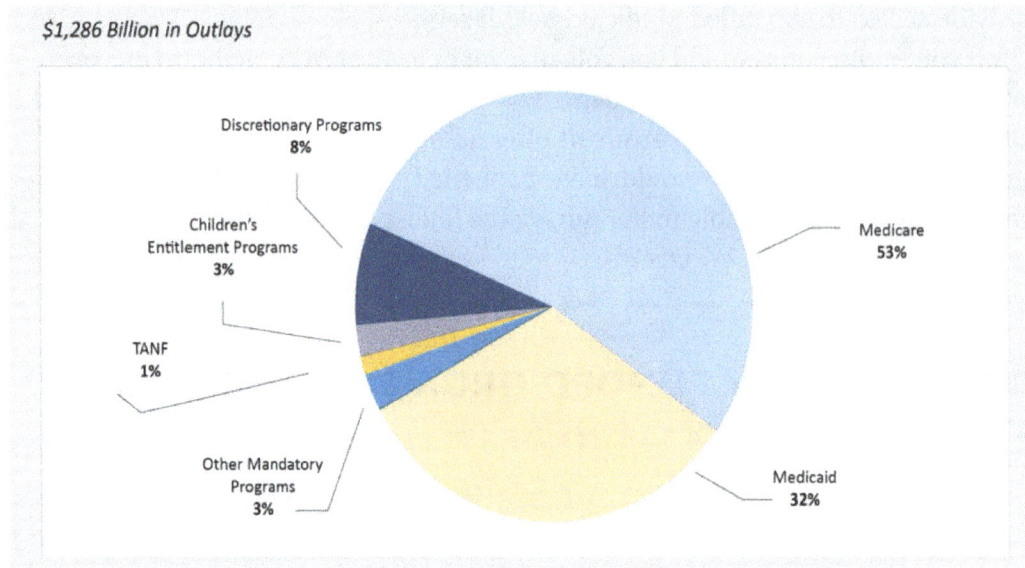

Figure 5.4: Composition of the FY 2020 Budget

Source: US Department of Health and Human Services
Attribution: US Department of Health and Human Services
License: Public Domain

5.6.2 Centers for Medicare and Medicaid Services (CMS)

The mission of the CMS is as follows: "The Centers for Medicare and Medicaid Services supports innovative approaches to improve quality, accessibility, and affordability" (HHS, n.d., p. 49). As stated previously, the CMS funds, administers, and operates the Medicare program and the Center for Medicare and Medicaid Innovation agency. Medicaid and CHIP, although administered by individual states, also receives funds and is overseen by CMS (HHS, n.d.). The FY 2020 budget proposal requests $60.5 billion over the 2019 budget and is expecting a savings of $954.1 billion due to changes made and being made. The priorities for the CMS as outlined in the 2020 budget (HHS, n.d.) are reducing prescription drug costs, transforming the healthcare system to one that pays for quality and outcomes (value-based care), combating the opioid crisis, and reforming America's health insurance system (pp. 65–67). To decrease drug costs, reforms are focused on improving competition, negotiating for better prices, providing incentives for lower list prices, and lowering out-of-pocket costs for patients (HHS, n.d.).

To transform the healthcare-system to one that pays for quality and outcomes, some of the reforms include allowing accrediting bodies of hospitals and other healthcare facilities to release accrediting surveys. Also, several hospital-required quality programs will be consolidated to one program, thus decreasing regulatory burden. There is an effort throughout the plan to provide equitable payments to all parties involved in healthcare who provide the same type of services. To reform America's health insurance system, several proposals make Medicare payments more equivalent to the private pay market, provide greater choices for beneficiaries, and encourage innovation at the consumer and state level. Consolidation of medical school payments for physicians and reforms for medical liability are also planned.

5.6.3 The Food and Drug Administration

The Food and Drug Administration's (n.d.) mission statement is as follows:

> *The Food and Drug Administrations' (FDA) is responsible for protecting the public health by assuring the safety, efficacy, and security of human and veterinary drugs, biological products, medical devices, the nation's food supply, cosmetics, and products that emit radiation. FDA also advances the public health by helping to speed innovations that make medicines more effective, safer, and affordable; and by helping the public get the accurate, science-based information they need to use medicines and foods to maintain and improve their health. Furthermore, FDA has responsibility for regulating the manufacturing, marketing, and distribution of tobacco products to protect the public health and to reduce tobacco use by minors. Finally, FDA plays a significant role in the nation's counterterrorism capability by ensuring the security of the food supply and fostering development of medical products to respond to deliberate and naturally emerging public health threats.* (Para. 1)

Advancing innovations for effective, safe, and affordable medications and medical devices; foods safety; management of tobacco products; and counterterrorism are priorities for the FDA. A highlight for FY 2018 was setting a record for approving the most generic medications in a single year (971), compared to a five-year average of 771 generics approved per year. In addition, the FDA provided for the emergency approval and authorization for COVID-19 vaccines in 2020. This action paved the way for an early campaign to provide protection to millions of U.S. citizens as well as persons throughout the world.

5.6.4 The Health Resources and Services Administration

The mission of the Health Resources and Services Administration (HRSA) is the following:

> *The Health Resources and Services Administration (HRSA) is the primary federal agency for improving healthcare to people who are geographically isolated, economically or medically vulnerable. HRSA works to improve health through access to quality services, a skilled health workforce and innovative programs.* (HHS, n.d., p. 16)

Funds are provided for primary health centers, increasing the healthcare workforce in areas of shortage, funds for reducing maternal mortality and child health, and HIV/AIDs programs. Healthcare systems, such as Poison Control and Organ Transplant, and healthcare systems in rural areas are also provided funds.

5.6.5 The Indian Health Service

"The mission of the Indian Health Service is to raise the physical, mental, social, and spiritual health of American Indians and Alaska Natives to the highest level" (HHS, n.d., p. 22). Funds are provided to expand healthcare and provide facilities for the American Indian population. Preventive health services and special programs, such as for diabetes education, are examples of other areas receiving funds. Indian Health Services is expanded upon in Chapter 7.

5.6.7 The Centers for Disease Control and Prevention

The mission statement for the Centers for Disease Control and Prevention is multifaceted. The mission statement is as follows:

> *The Centers for Disease Control and Prevention (CDC) works 24/7 to protect America from health, safety, and security threats, both foreign and in the United States. Whether diseases start at home or abroad, are chronic or acute, curable or preventable, human error or deliberate attack, CDC fights disease and supports communities and citizens to do the same. CDC increase(s) the health security of our nation. As the nation's health protection agency, CDC saves lives and protects people from health threats. To accomplish its mission, CDC conducts critical science and provides health information that protects our nation against expensive and dangerous health threats, and responds when these arise.* (HHS, n.d., p. 27)

Some of the funds provided are for such preventative strategies as immunizations; prevention of such diseases as HIV/AIDS, viral hepatitis, and sexually transmitted diseases and tuberculosis; and health promotion. Some funds are for management of chronic diseases, such as high blood pressure and diabetes. Recently, because of the rise in opioid addictions and overdoses in the U.S., the opioid epidemic has been a focus of the CDC. More recently and presently, viruses such as the coronavirus have taken center stage. Occupational safety and health, environmental health, overall public health preparedness, and global health are also critical areas of emphasis.

5.6.8 The National Institutes of Health

According to HHS, *"The National Institutes of Health's (NIH) mission is to seek fundamental knowledge about the nature and behavior of living systems and the application of that knowledge to enhance health, lengthen life, and reduce illness and disability"* (HHS, n.d., p. 37). Some of the research priorities for 2020 include the opioid crisis, neonatal abstinence syndrome, chronic pain, and childhood cancer. The quality and safety of healthcare, precision medicine, and health services research are other priorities.

5.6.9 The Substance Abuse and Mental Health Services Administration

The mission statement of the Substance Abuse and Mental Health Services Administration is the following: *"The Substance Abuse and Mental Health Services Administration (SAMHSA) reduces the impact of substance abuse and mental illness in America's communities"* (HHS, n.d., p. 45). Funds for this department support community mental health services, children's mental health services, and behavioral health clinics. The mental health needs of students, substance abuse prevention and treatment, and suicide prevention programs are also priorities.

5.6.10 The Administration for Children and Families

According to HHS, *"The mission of the Administration for Children and Families promotes the economic and social well-being of children, youth, families, and communities, focusing particular attention on populations such as children in low-income families, refugees, and Native Americans"* (HHS, n.d., p. 100). The Administration for Children and Families' proposed 2020 budget provides funds for the following in descending order: temporary assistance for needy families; Head Start; Child Care and Development Fund; foster care and permanency; child support enforcement; and refugee and entrant assistance. These departments provide monies for vulnerable populations, such as those needing temporary financial assistance, child abuse victims, human trafficking victims, runaways and homeless individuals, and for foster care. Funds are provided with goals to improve the lives of low-income families, especially through early childhood programs and childcare.

5.6.11 The Administration for Community Living (ACL)

The mission of the Administration for Community Living is: *"The Administration for Community Living maximizes the independence, well-being, and health of older adults, people with disabilities across the lifespan, and their families and caregivers"* (HHS, n.d., p. 116). The ACL provides monies for nutritious meals to senior centers and homebound individuals. Monies are also provided to fight elder abuse and neglect, Alzheimer's disease, and disability programs.

5.6.12 The Office of the Secretary

The Office of the Secretary, though not a division, is responsible for oversight of all HHS programs. These several staff divisions, agencies, and programs report directly to the Secretary for HHS:

1. Office of the Secretary, General Departmental Management. *"The General Departmental Management budget line supports the Secretary's role as chief policy officer and general manager of the department"* (HHS, n.d., p. 120).

2. Office of the Secretary, Opioids and Serious Mental Illness. This is a new office and was developed as a result of 64,000 deaths to drug overdoses in 2016 (HHS, n.d.).

3. Office of the Secretary, Office of Medicare Hearings and Appeals. The Office of Medicare Hearings and Appeals provides a forum for the adjudication of Medicare appeals for beneficiaries and other parties. *"This mission is carried out by a cadre of Administrative Law Judges exercising decisional independence under the Administrative Procedures Act with the support of a professional, legal, and administrative staff"* (HHS, n.d., p. 124).

4. Office of the Secretary, Office of the National Coordinator for Health Information Technology (ONC). The mission of this office is *"To help lower healthcare costs, empower consumer choice, and improve provider satisfaction, ONC will work to make health information more accessible, decrease the documentation burden, and support electronic health records' usability"* (HHS, n.d., p. 126).

5. Office of the Secretary, Office for Civil Rights (OCR). The mission of this office is as follows: *"The Office for Civil Rights is the Department's chief law enforcer and regulator of civil rights, conscience and religious freedom, and health information privacy and security"* (HHS, n.d., p. 128).

6. Office of Inspector General. *"The mission of the Office of Inspector General is to protect the integrity of Department of Health and Human Services programs as well as the health and welfare of the people they serve"* (HHS, n.d., p. 130).

7. Public Health and Social Services Emergency Fund (PHSSEF). The mission of this office is as follows: *"The Public Health and Social Services Emergency Fund directly supports the nation's ability to prepare for, respond to, and recover from the health consequences of naturally occurring and man-made threats"* (HHS, n.d., p. 133).

5.7 SUMMARY

This chapter has explored federally funded healthcare (Medicare) and jointly federal/state funded healthcare (Medicaid and CHIP). It looked at the costs of the programs. It described the Affordable Care Act and it has discussed other federally funded programs provided through the HHS.

5.8 REVIEW QUESTIONS

1. How would you explain the difference between the Medicare choices to someone close to retirement age?

2. How is Medicare funded?

3. During what circumstances can Medicaid and the Children's Health Insurance Program be utilized?

4. What are two objectives of the Patient Protection and Affordable Care Act?

5. What are four healthcare delivery reforms of the Affordable Care Act?

6. How are the FY 2020 HHS budget funds allocated?

5.9 REFERENCES

Blumenthal, D., Abrams, M., & Nuzum, R. (2015). The affordable care act at 5 years. New England Journal of Medicine, 372, 2451-2458. DOI: 10.1056/NEJMhpr1503614

Center for Medicare and Medicaid Services (CMS). (2020, January). 2020 Medicare costs. CMS product No. 11579. Retrieved from https://www.medicare.gov/Pubs/pdf/11579-Medicare-Costs.pdf

Center for Medicare and Medicaid Services (CMS). (2019). The official U.S. government Medicare handbook: Medicare & you 2020. CMS product no. 10050. Retrieved from https://www.medicare.gov/Pubs/pdf/10050-Medicare-and-You.pdf

Center for Medicare and Medicaid Services. (n.d.a). Medicaid and you: Frequently asked questions. Medicaid.gov., Centers for Medicare and Medicaid services, An official site of the U.S. government. Retrieved November 21, 2019, from https://www.medicaid.gov/medicaid-and-you/index.html

Center for Medicare & Medicaid Services. (n.d.b). Get started with Medicare, Medicare.gov., The official U.S. government site for Medicare. Retrieved November 21, 2019, from https://www.medicare.gov/sign-up-change-plans/get-started-with-medicare

Center for Medicare & Medicaid Services. (n.d.c). How is Medicare funded? Medicare.gov, The official U.S. government site for Medicare. Retrieved November 21, 2019, from https://www.medicare.gov/about-us/how-is-medicare-funded

Center for Medicare & Medicaid Services. (n.d.d). What's Medicare supplemental insurance (Medigap)? Medicare.gov, The official U.S. government site for Medicare. Retrieved November 22, 2019, from https://www.medicare.gov/supplements-other-insurance/whats-medicare-supplement-insurance-medigap

Center for Medicare and Medicaid Services. (n.d.e). Federal fiscal year (FFY) 2018 statistical enrollment data system (SEDS) reporting. Medicaid.gov., Centers for Medicare and Medicaid services. Retrieved November 23, 2019, from https://www.medicaid.gov/chip/downloads/fy-2018-childrens-enrollment-report.pdf

Center for Medicare and Medicaid Services. (n.d.f). Costs for Medicare drug coverage. Medicare.gov, Centers for Medicare and Medicaid services. Retrieved November 23, 2019, from https://www.medicare.gov/drug-coverage-part-d/costs-for-medicare-drug-coverage

Center for Medicare and Medicaid Services. (n.d.g). August 2019 Medicaid & CHIP enrollment data highlights. Medicaid.gov, Centers for Medicare and Medicaid services. Retrieved November 23, 2019, from https://www.medicaid.gov/medicaid/program-information/medicaid-and-chip-enrollment-data/report-highlights/index.html

Congress of the United States Congressional Budget Office. (2018, May). Federal subsidies for health insurance coverage for people under age 65: 2018 to 2028. Retrieved November 20, 2019, from https://www.cbo.gov/system/files?file=2018-06/53826-healthinsurancecoverage.pdf

Congress of the United States Congressional Budget Office. (2018, April). The budget and economic outlook: 2018 to 2028. Retrieved November 20, 2019, from https://www.cbo.gov/system/files/2019-04/53651-outlook-2.pdf

Gaffney, A., McCormick, D., Bor, D., Woolhandler, S., & Himmelstein, D. (2019). Coverage expansions and utilization of physician care: Evidence from the 2014 Affordable Care Act and 1966 Medicare/Medicaid expansion. American Journal of Public Health, 109(12), 1694–1701.

Hamel, L., Kirzinger, A. Muñana, C., Lopes, L., Kearney, A., & Brodie, M. (2020, October 16). 5 Charts About Public Opinion on the Affordable Care Act and the Supreme Court. Kaiser Family Foundation. Retrieved from https://www.kff.org/health-reform/poll-finding/5-charts-about-public-opinion-on-the-affordable-care-act-and-the-supreme-court/

Johansen, M. E. & Richardson, C. R. (2019). Annals of family medicine, 17(6), 526–537. https://doi.org/10.1370/afm.2462

Kaiser Family Foundation (KFF). (2020, November 2). Status of state Medicaid expansion decisions: Interactive map. Retrieved from https://www.kff.org/medicaid/issue-brief/status-of-state-medicaid-expansion-decisions-interactive-map/

Kirchhoff, S. M. (2018). Medicare part D prescription drug benefit. Congressional research service. 7-5700 R40611. Retrieved from https://fas.org/sgp/crs/misc/R40611.pdf

Kirzinger, A., Muñana, C., & Brodie, M. (2019, October 4). Six charts about public opinion on the Affordable Care Act. Retrieved November 27, YEAR, from https://www.kff.org/health-reform/poll-finding/6-charts-about-public-opinion-on-the-affordable-care-act/#

Klees, B. S., Eckstein, E. T., and Curtis, C. A. (2018). Brief summaries of Medicare and Medicaid: Title XVIII and Title XIX of the Social Security act. Centers for Medicare and Medicaid services, Department of health and human services. Retrieved from https://www.cms.gov/Research-Statistics-Data-and-Systems/Statistics-Trends-and-Reports/MedicareProgramRatesStats/Downloads/MedicareMedicaidSummaries2018.pdf

Klein, E., Levin, S., Toerper, M. F., Makowsky, M. D., Xu, T., Cole, G., & Kelen, G. D. (2017). The effect of Medicaid expansion on utilization in Maryland emergency departments. Annals of emergency medicine, 70(5), 607–614. DOI: 10.1016/j. annemergmed.2017.06.021

Kobayashi, L. C., Altindag, O., Truskinovsky, Y. & Berkman, L. F. (2019). Effects of Affordable Care act Medicaid expansion on subjective well-being in the US adult population, 2010–2016. American Journal of Public Health, 109(9), 1236-1242.

Levitt, L. (2020). The Affordable Care Act's enduring resilience. Journal of Health Politics, Policy and Law, 45(4), 609–616. DOI 10.1215/03616878-8255529.

U.S. Department of Health and Human Services (HHS). (2018). 2019 Health plan choice and premiums in Health care.gov states. Assistant secretary for planning and evaluation (ASPE) research brief. Retrieved November 25, 2019, from https://aspe. hhs.gov/system/files/pdf/260041/2019LandscapeBrief.pdf

U.S. Department of Health and Human Services (HHS). (2015). Certification of comparability of pediatric coverage offered by qualified health plans. Center for Medicare & Medicaid services. Retrieved from https://www.medicaid.gov/sites/ default/files/2019-12/certification-of-comparability-of-pediatric-coverage-offered-by-qualified-health-plans.pdf

U.S. Department of Health and Human Services (HHS). (n.d.). Putting America's health first: FY 2020 President's budget for HHS. Retrieved November 23, 2019, and February 2, 2020, from https://www.hhs.gov/sites/default/files/fy-2020-budget-in-brief.pdf

6

Private Insurance

6.1 LEARNING OBJECTIVES

By the end of this chapter, the student will be able to:
- Define managed care
- List the pros and cons of managed care
- Distinguish the primary types of health maintenance organizations
- Discuss how managed care impacts healthcare
- Explain private insurance
- Explain problems associated with Fee-for-Service healthcare plans
- State questions to consider before deciding on a healthcare plan
- Discuss the benefits of worker's compensation insurance for employees

6.2 KEY TERMS

- Health Maintenance Organization (HMO)
- Exclusive Provider Organization (EPO)
- managed care
- medical underwriting
- Point of Service plan (POS)
- Preferred Provider Organization (PPO)
- provider networks
- worker's compensation insurance

6.3 INTRODUCTION

Healthcare coverage for average Americans has been much discussed over the years. Private insurance and **managed care** organizations are often confusing to consumers. This chapter will provide a brief summation of private insurance and four major types of managed care organizations. These four major types of managed care organizations are as follows: Preferred Provider Organizations (PPOs), Point of Service plans (POS), Health Maintenance Organizations (HMOs), and Exclusive Provider Organizations. The chapter will include discussion on the advantages and disadvantages of managed care options. Finally, there is discussion of worker's compensation insurance.

6.4 FEE-FOR-SERVICE

Fee-for-Services plans were the staple of healthcare service plans in the U.S. before the advent of private insurance and managed care organizations. Fee-for-service is a method for which healthcare providers are paid for each individual service rendered. Payment can be from an individual or through a health insurance plan. Treatments or procedures that were deemed necessary by the healthcare provider were often conducted without approval from insurance agencies (U.S. Legal, 2019). This caused discord between healthcare providers and insurance companies who frequently disagreed on prescribed healthcare treatments. This conflict often resulted in delayed consumer medical care. Private healthcare insurance and managed care organizations would eventually change the way healthcare services were offered and payments for services were received.

6.5 PRIVATE INSURANCE

Healthcare coverage not sponsored by the government is known as **private insurance**. Many individuals have private insurance through their employers. In fact, approximately 60% of non-elderly Americans do so (Anderson, 2018). An employer sponsored private insurance policy charges employees a fee for their insurance coverage. However, many companies cost share and pay a significant amount of employee premiums. This fee is usually deducted from the employee's paycheck. There is often an open enrollment time frame whereby employees can choose the desired health insurance coverage options. New employees are offered the opportunity to gain healthcare coverage upon their hiring date as well. The option of private insurance is very important to a lot of employees and their families, so many people investigate private insurance benefits when job seeking.

While the employer-sponsored private health insurance is quite popular, some individuals can purchase private insurance without an employer. For instance, self-employed individuals may purchase private healthcare plans from insurance companies. Before the **Affordable Care Act (ACA)**, the acquisition of individual private insurance was a bit more complicated. For one thing, individual market insurance companies could decide the costs of premiums and whether to accept or deny individual healthcare coverage based on pre-existing conditions. This process is known as **medical underwriting** and is no longer used because of the Affordable Care Act (Healthinsurance.org, 2020). The ACA now prohibits discrimination against an individual based on pre-existing conditions, and the cost of the coverage is no longer a factor in determining the premium (Norris, 2019).

The cost of healthcare coverage depends on several factors. For example, the cost of private insurance may be influenced by the number of individuals the plan covers. The price may differ between the employee only having coverage for themselves versus the employee having healthcare coverage for their immediate family members. Additionally, components of private insurance healthcare plans may include options for medical, vision, dental, and short-term, long-term, and disability care coverage. Further, an overwhelming majority of U.S. residents have health insurance plans that are a part of a managed care program (Speights, 2018).

6.6 MANAGED CARE BACKGROUND

According to the U.S. National Library of Medicine (2019), managed care insurance plans consist of contractual agreements between medical facilities and healthcare providers to render healthcare at lower consumer costs. The providers are known as the managed care network. Managed care systems help provide organization, quality, and cost containment to healthcare services for clients.

Managed care has historical beginnings from the late 1920s (National Council on Disability, n.d.). Dr. Michael Shadid launched a small Oklahoma hospital to provide needed medical care for farmers who had limited access to such care. An annual fee schedule covered the care this hospital provided. This type of medical service with yearly fees or prepaid contracts by physicians began to expand both in Oklahoma and such other places as California. Through the years, the term *managed care* became associated with this type of contractual healthcare coverage. Managed-care plans helped curtail increasing healthcare costs by discouraging participating physicians from needless patient hospitalizations. Physicians were also required to provide healthcare at lower costs.

With managed care, healthcare providers receive predetermined fee-for-service rendered to clients. Unnecessary medical treatments are often avoided because of the insurance company's refusal to pay without preauthorization. This helps decrease consumer healthcare costs.

6.7 MANAGED CARE ORGANIZATIONS

Given that employers pay a considerable portion of U.S. healthcare insurance costs, the introduction of **managed care organizations** provides a more systematic guideline for healthcare providers to follow, which helps cut those costs (U.S. Legal, 2019). Physicians and statisticians usually work together to devise generalized guidelines for clients based on their symptoms or conditions. When this is done, the managed care organizations can prescribe what treatments and procedures are most beneficial to applicable clients based on client diagnoses and symptoms. Managed care organizations also predetermine the cost of these treatments and procedures, including hospital stays (if needed).

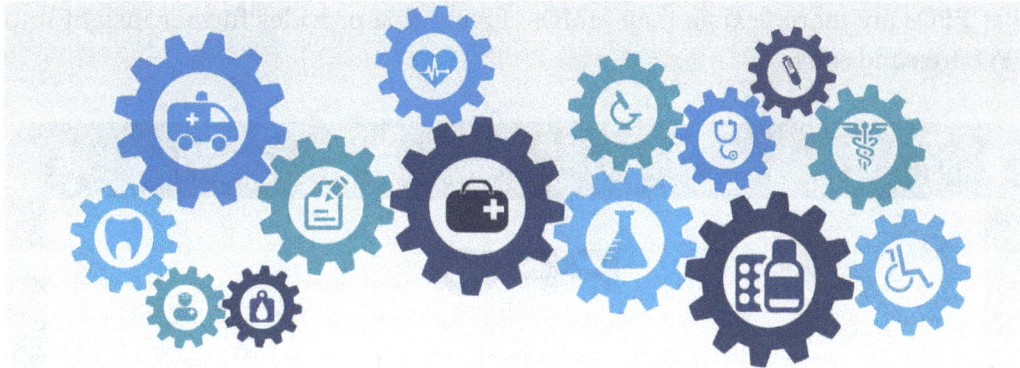

Figure 6.1: Healthcare

Source: Pixabay.com
Attribution: User "ar130405"
License: Pixabay License

Provider networks are a pivotal component of managed care systems. Members of provider networks may include hospitals, advanced healthcare practitioners, and doctors who work together to provide the most efficient, cost-effective care for consumers. There are two types of provider networks: in-network providers and out-of-network providers. As the names indicate, in-network providers work with insurance plans to provide services, while out-of-network providers opt not to participate in contractual agreements. Providers choosing to become part of a managed care system agree to work with networks in attempts to contain costs of healthcare services. Additionally, providers that opt to become part of a managed care system are expected to comply with specified quality standards and predetermined healthcare costs to decrease the amount clients are expected to pay (U.S. National Library of Medicine, 2018).

6.8 TYPES OF MANAGED CARE ORGANIZATIONS

6.8.1 Preferred Provider Organizations (PPO)

Preferred provider organizations (PPOs) are a prevalent type of managed care organization. PPOs have a **Preferred Provider Arrangement**, which serves as a contractual agreement with a group of large healthcare providers to keep the cost down for clients. Costs associated with client care are predetermined, which prohibits physicians from charging higher client fees (Medical Mutual, 2020). Enrollees within PPOs have a choice to use providers and hospitals within the network or not. Incentives, such as decreased deductibles and lower copayments, are used to encourage consumers to use in-network doctors. If the enrollee chooses to use a provider that is not part of the network, the cost of the rendered healthcare service is higher. In other words, enrollees can opt to save their cost by choosing a provider within the network. Nevertheless, no referral is needed if the client selects a provider outside of the network. The premium of a PPO is often higher than an HMO, which means the costs to the client is higher. However, it should be noted that PPOs are more flexible than HMOs. Figure 6. 2 provides further insight into PPO pros and cons.

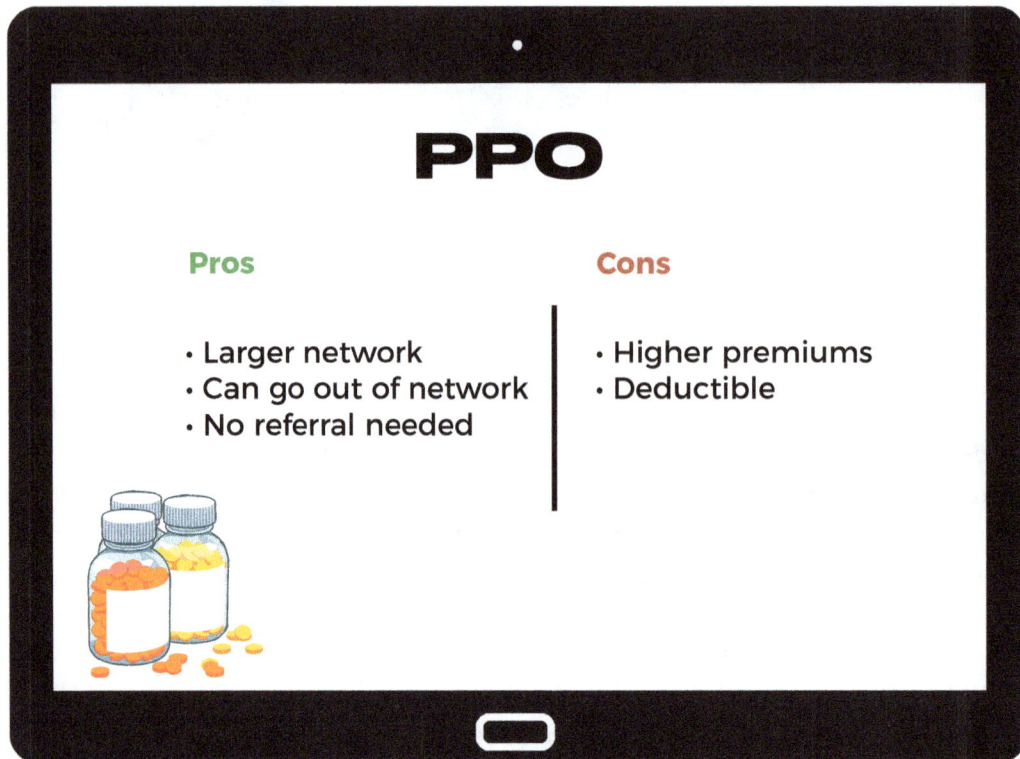

Figure 6.2: Pros and Cons of Preferred Provider Arrangements

Source: Original Work
Attribution: Kristy Michelle Gamble
License: CC BY-SA 4.0

6.8.2 Point of Service Plan (POS)

Point of Service (POS) plans are like PPOs except when the client chooses a provider outside of the network and has a referral from their primary healthcare provider, the cost of services is covered by the medical insurance (Small Business Majority, 2019). However, if the client chooses to see an out-of-network provider without a physician referral, the client is responsible for a portion of the bill. The client will also have to meet their deductible and copayment. A **deductible** is a cost the consumer is required to prepay to receive the benefits indicated in the health insurance policy (WiseGeek, 2020). Consumers may have high or low deductible plans depending on their preferences. A high deductible requires the consumer to pay more out of pocket expenses, while a low deductible requires consumers to pay less. Once the deductible is met, the insurance company will cover the cost of the services. The healthcare premium cost is often influenced by the type of deductible an individual selects. Figure 6.3 shows the pros and cons of the POS plan.

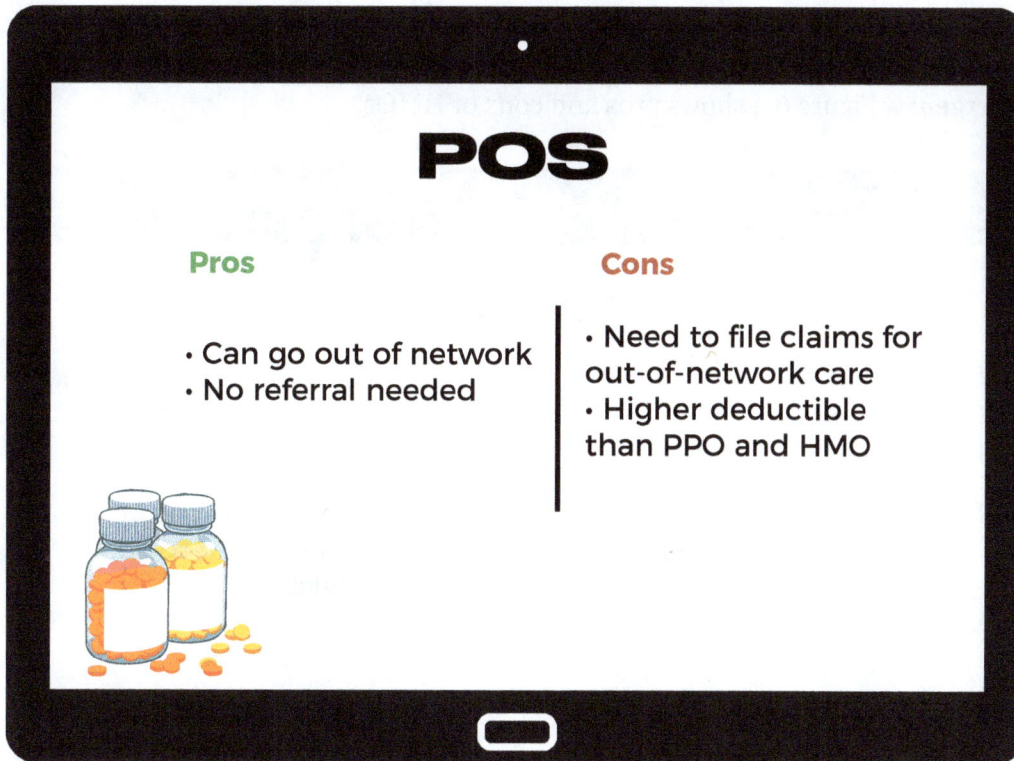

Figure 6.3: Pros and Cons of Point of Service

Source: Original Work
Attribution: Kristy Michelle Gamble
License: CC BY-SA 4.0

6.8.3 Health Maintenance Organizations (HMO)

In contrast to PPOs, HMO enrollees do not have the same level of flexibility when choosing a provider. Yet, HMOs are associated with lower premiums. Additionally, while a primary care physician is not required in a PPO, a primary care provider must be selected in an HMO. Named by Dr. Paul Elwood, the purpose of HMOs was to offer prepaid group practices, which meant lower cost and improved utilization of healthcare services for consumers (Yesalis et al., 2013). Not surprisingly, the advent of HMOs was met with resistance from physicians who preferred more flexibility when providing care under the fee-for-service plan.

HMOs generally cover treatment costs if care is rendered within the network. However, it should be noted that treatments for emergency care, out-of-area urgent care, or out-of-area dialysis care services are excluded from provider networks, which means patients can receive these services from providers outside of the network without penalty (U.S. Centers for Medicare & Medicaid Services, n.d.). With this type of plan, it is recommended that approval for services is obtained before services are rendered to decrease the client's cost (U.S. Centers for Medicare & Medicaid Services, n.d.). Except for yearly screening, referrals are needed for specialist visits. HMOs usually do not provide coverage for services rendered outside of the network unless it is a service that the listed providers are not conducting. Individuals receiving care from providers outside of the network may ultimately be responsible for the cost of care received unless in the case of an emergency. Figure 6.4 shows pros and cons of HMOs.

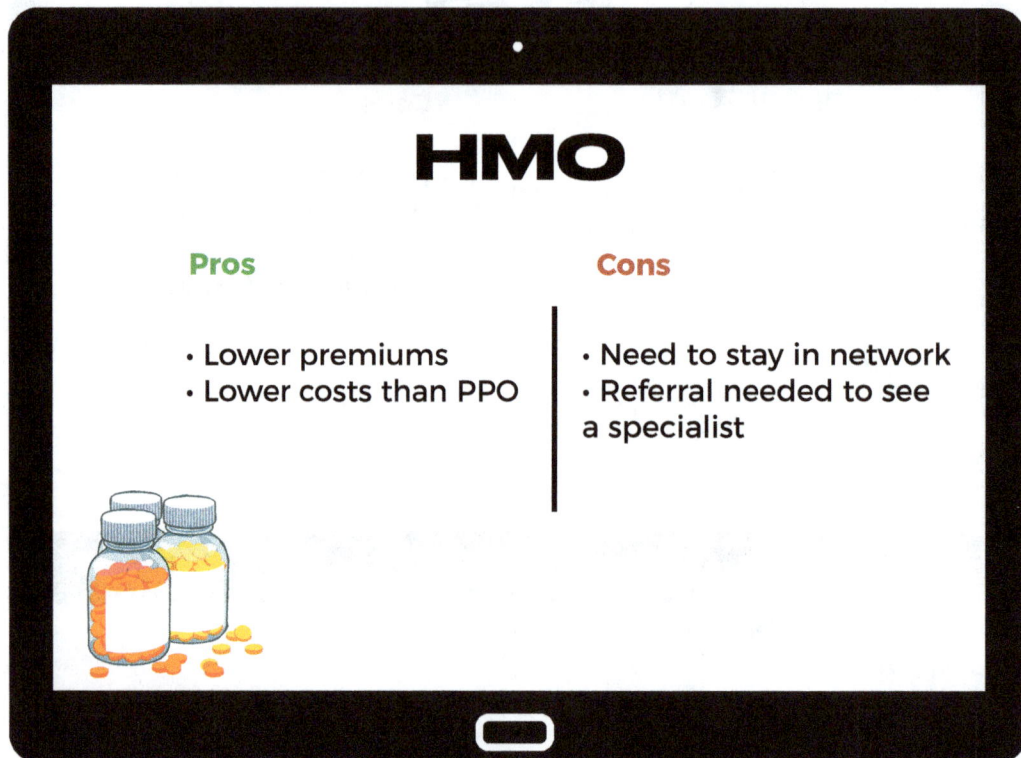

Figure 6.4: Pros and Cons of Health Maintenance Organizations

Source: Original Work
Attribution: Kristy Michelle Gamble
License: CC BY-SA 4.0

6.8.4 Exclusive Provider Organizations (EPO)

Consumers opting for an **exclusive provider organization (EPO)** managed care plan receive insurance coverage when they receive care from in-network providers (Silva, 2019). However, if an out-of-network provider is chosen, the services are not covered by the health insurance plan, unless in an emergency. Consumers with the EPO plan have a primary care physician who provides comprehensive care. It should be noted that unlike other types of insurance plans, EPO clients have a limited network from which to choose. An advantage of EPOs is that referrals are not needed for a specialist visit. Figure 6.5 shows the pros and cons of EPO.

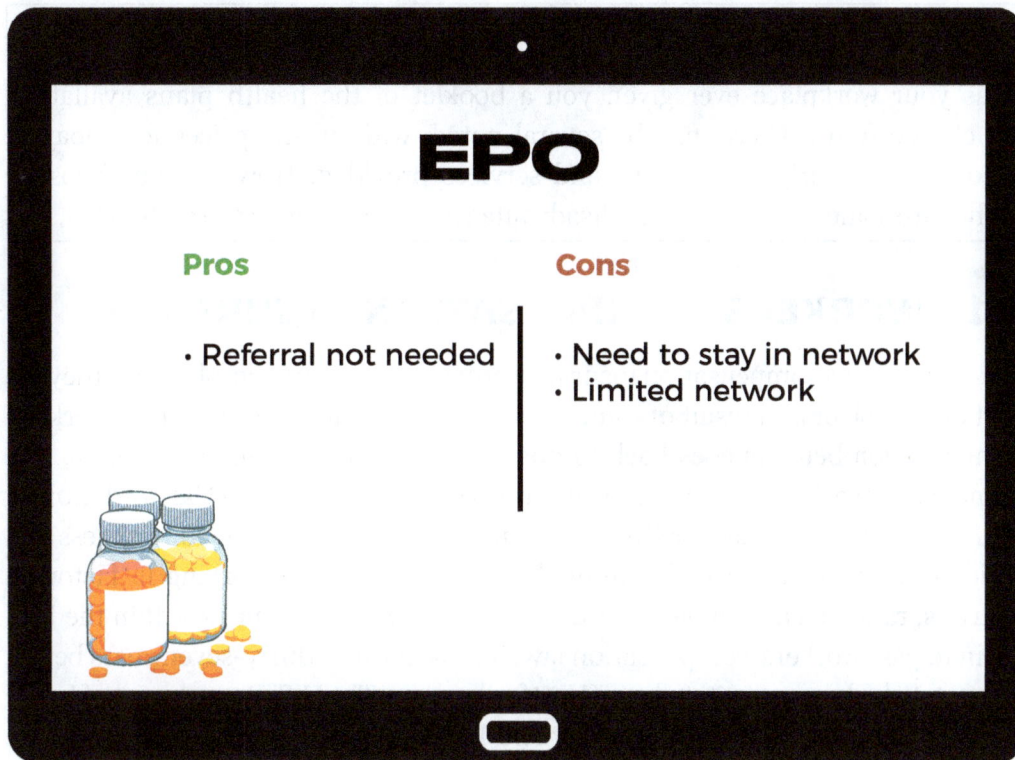

Figure 6.5: Pros and Cons of Exclusive Provider Organizations

Source: Original Work
Attribution: Kristy Michelle Gamble
License: CC BY-SA 4.0

6.9 WHICH TYPE OF HEALTHCARE PLAN IS RIGHT FOR YOU?

Many managed care plans are available and which plan fits you and your family's needs is a personal choice. Individuals should be knowledgeable about the options of each plan based on several factors. Some general questions to think about when deciding include the following:

- Do you have a preferred primary care provider? If so, are they participating in a managed care organization?

- How much are you willing to contribute to healthcare premiums monthly?

- How much flexibility do you desire regarding healthcare provider choices?

- Do you often visit a specialist? If so, are they members of a managed care group?

- Are you willing to pay a copayment or coinsurance if required?

> **Pause and Reflect**
>
> Has your workplace ever given you a booklet of the health plans available to choose from? There may be several noted, with all the prices for copays, deductibles, yearly maximums, and services provided. How do you choose? What are some advantages and disadvantages of a managed care system?

6.10 WORKERS' COMPENSATION INSURANCE

Workers' compensation insurance provides benefits to employees if they are hurt on the job or as a result of some work-related activity. The genesis of workers' compensation benefits goes back to 2050 B.C. in Ancient Sumeria, Greece, and China when workers were paid for injuries suffered on the job (Hartford, 2020). In 1887, Prussian Chancellor Otto von Bismarck, created laws called "sickness and accident laws" which provided limited protection to those working in factories, quarries, railroads and mines. Not until 1911 did individual states within the U.S. begin to pass workers' compensation law; it took another thirty-seven years before every state had compensation laws (Hartford, 2020). The U.S. Department of Labor (n.d.) created the Occupational Safety and Health Act (OSHA) of 1970 "to ensure safe and healthful working conditions for working men and women by setting and enforcing standards and by providing training, outreach, education and assistance" (para. 1). OSHA mostly covers private sector employers and workers. The U.S. Department of Labor, Office of Workers' Compensation Programs oversees federal workers and claims for work related injuries.

Some work settings and occupations are more dangerous than others. In the U.S., logging workers, fishers, aircraft pilots, and roofers have the highest rates of fatal injuries (Kiersz & Hoff, 2020). However, non-fatal injuries account for a majority of cases. In 2019, there were 888,220 injuries or illness resulting in days off of work (Bureau of Labor Statistics (BLS), 2020). In 2019, ten occupations accounted for 33.2% of days away from work as a result of injury or exposure (BLS, 2020) (Figure 6.6). Examples of injury or exposure are employees working in manufacturing harmed as a result of machinery, toxins, or cramped settings; employees working in mining harmed from breathing in dirty air or a sudden collapse of a mine; and healthcare workers in the hospital setting being hurt physically by moving patients or by contracting diseases, such as hepatitis, HIV, or COVID-19. Injuries do not have to be permanent or life-threatening. For example, the most common causes of non-fatal workplace injuries in 2019 were overexertion, falls, slips, trips, contact with objects of equipment, violence or injuries caused by people or animals, and transportation accidents (BLS, 2020). Compensation insurance ensures funds are available to pay for medical care; rehabilitation services; lost wages; and, potentially, funeral expenses.

■ 2018 ■ 2019

Incidence rates per 10,000 FTE workers

Nursing assistants

Heavy and tractor-trailer truck drivers

Laborers and freight, stock and material movers, hand

Light truck drivers

Construction laborers

Maintenance and repair workers, general

Stockers and order fillers

Janitors and cleaners, except maids and housekeeping cleaners

Registered nurses

Retail salespersons

0   50   100   150   200   250   300

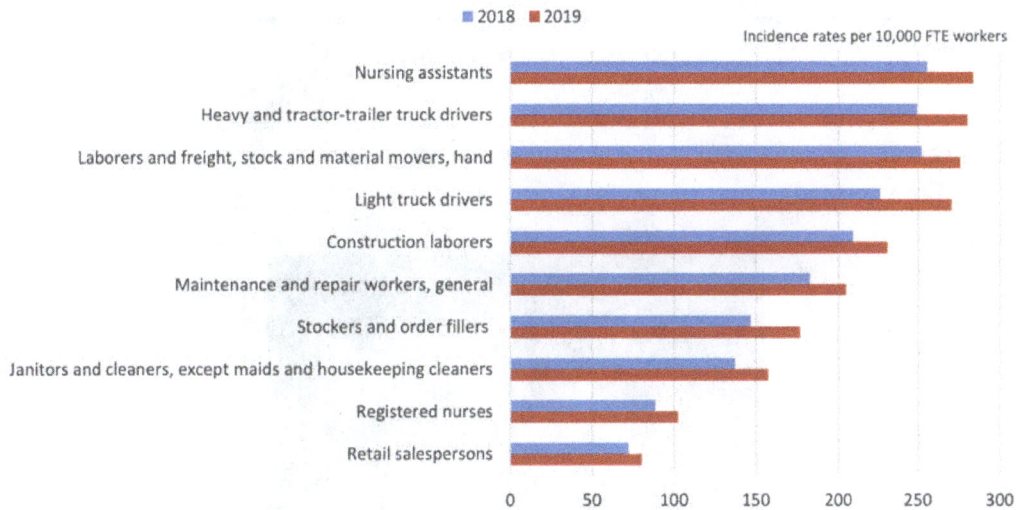

Figure 6.6: Incidence Rates Of Cases Involving Days Away From Work Selected Occupations

Source: US Bureau of Labor Statistics
Attribution: US Bureau of Labor Statistics
License: Public Domain

In addition to state laws, many large companies whose employees are at a higher chance of injury have implemented health and safety teams who are able to respond at the time of injury. These teams also study and create policies and work procedures which protect employees on the job. These same organizations may provide employee health clinics and first responders in the case of injury. The ultimate goals are to have healthy, injury free employees and maintain productivity.

- -

First Person Perspective

Nurse M, RN-eNLC, CCM, has thirteen years of experience as a nurse, seven years certified in case management, and works as a Workers Compensation Nurse Case Manager for her company.

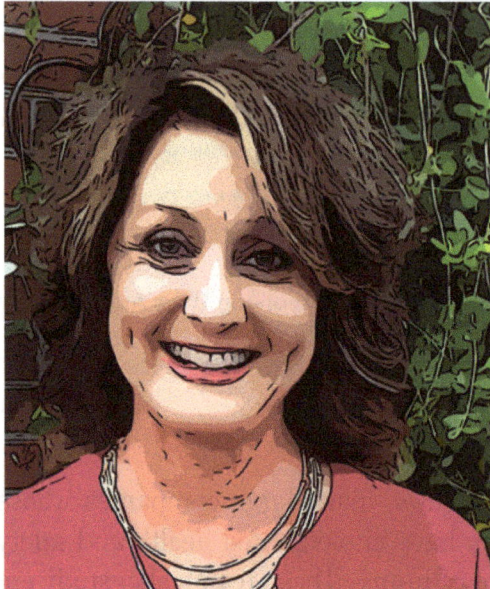

Figure 6.7: First Person Perspective

Source: Original Work
Attribution: Deanna Howe
License: CC BY-SA 4.0

As a worker's compensation Nurse Case Manager, I act as a liaison between the employee, their medical team, employers, insurance carriers, and other stakeholders involved in the management of a worker's comp claim. Work injuries can range from minor to catastrophic and often are very stressful events for the injured worker and their families. Nurse Case Managers educate and advocate for the injured worker and guide them through the entire process so they know what to expect. My involvement in a worker's compensation claim tends to benefit injured workers by streamlining the process for faster, more complete access to care, improved care quality, and better recovery outcomes. Employers, insurance carriers, and other stakeholders benefit from improved communication flow, faster returns to work, quicker claims closure, and lower overall workers' compensation costs.

Providing worker's comp case management during the worldwide COVID-19 pandemic has brought new challenges as many physicians have moved to telemedicine formats. Case managers are now coordinating and educating injured workers on how to connect with their physicians virtually rather than in person. I am also beginning to receive cases involving injured workers who most likely contracted COVID-19 while at work, including those involved in healthcare and factory workers. While many who contract COVID-19 have mild cases with no known lasting effects following their recovery, others are not so lucky.

Although I no longer provide bedside nursing, it is my nursing foundation learned during nursing school that instilled in me that it is the nurse who upholds patient's rights and serves as liaison with their physicians, families, and other involved parties—because we are advocates. Worker's comp case management can be very challenging and not all nurses can be successful case managers. Collaboration, well-supported clinical judgement, and negotiation are key skills for a case manager to possess. I do not see myself leaving the field of worker's comp case management; I enjoy the challenges. Knowing my presence on the case was instrumental in the injured worker having a favorable outcome and returning to his pre-injury condition is very rewarding.

First person perspective vignette collected and created by D. Howe, 2020.

For your consideration: Nurse M. describes her role as a nurse advocating for the worker. Have you ever known someone who was injured on the job? Did they have worker's compensation insurance available? If not, how does worker's compensation insurance protect the worker? How does this insurance protect the employer? If you were injured on the job, how could a nurse case manager help you through the process of seeking treatment and recovery? What laws should be in place to protect workers who do not have access to worker's compensation insurance?

6.11 SUMMARY

Private insurance and managed care organizations provide consumers the opportunity to receive healthcare services at a reduced cost. Many individuals have healthcare insurance from their employers. Self-employed individuals can obtain healthcare coverage from the individual's health insurance marketplace without discrimination against preexisting conditions. A significant goal of managed care is to provide consumers with quality healthcare. With managed care, guidelines are provided to help ensure predetermined protocols are followed, which may include specific diagnostics, medications, and treatment regimens based on the diagnosis of the consumer. The four major types of managed care plans are Health Maintenance Organization, Preferred Provider Organization, Exclusive Provider Organizations, and Point of Service plans. Individuals have the option to utilize in-network providers at a reduced cost or may use out of network providers at a higher price in specific managed care plans. Some managed care plans are more flexible and do not require referrals for specialist visits, while others are less flexible and may not pay any amount if a consumer does not get a referral before receiving services from a specialist and out of network provider. Workers' compensation insurance is a benefit to pay for medical treatment and loss of wages as a result of injury on the job.

6.12 REVIEW QUESTIONS

1. What are the major types of managed care organizations?
2. What were some problems associated with Fee-for-Services plans in the U.S.?
3. What are the differences between POS, HMO, PPO, and EPO managed care organizations?
4. How does managed care impact healthcare?
5. What are three general questions to ask before deciding on a healthcare plan?
6. Describe how worker's compensation insurance benefits employees who are injured on the job.

6.13 REFERENCES

Anderson, S. (2018, December 17). Private Insurance: The American way for nearly 100 years. Healthinsurance.org. https://www.healthinsurance.org/obamacare/private-health-insurance/

The Hartford. (2020). Workers' compensation history. Retrieved November 16, 2020, from https://www.thehartford.com/workers-compensation/history#:~:text=In%20 the%20late%2019th%20century,the%20Sickness%20and%20Accident%20 Laws.&text=Employers'%20Liability%20Law%20of%201871,a%20modern%20 workers'%20compensation%20system

Healthinsruance.org. (2020). What is medical underwriting? Retrieved from https:// www.healthinsurance.org/glossary/medical-underwriting/

Kiersz, A. & Hoff, M. (2020, June 3). The 34 deadliest jobs in America. Business Insider. Retrieved from https://www.businessinsider.com/the-most-dangerous-jobs-in-america-2018-7

Medical Mutual. (2020). What is a PPO? Understanding PPO health plans. Retrieved from https://www.medmutual.com/For-Individuals-and-Families/Health-Insurance-Education/Health-Insurance-Basics/Types-Health-Insurance/PPO-Health-Insurance-Plans.aspx

National Council on Disability. (n.d.) Appendix B. A brief history of managed care. Retrieved from https://ncd.gov/publications/2013/20130315/20130513_AppendixB#_ednref7

Norris, L. (2018). Individuals health insurance under Obamacare: What's changed since passage of Affordable Care Act? Healthinsurance.org. Retrieved from https://www.healthinsurance.org/obamacare/individual-health-insurance/

Silva. (2020). What is an exclusive provider organization? Policygenius. Retrieved from https://www.policygenius.com/health-insurance/epo-exclusive-provider-organization/

Small Business Majority. (2019). Point-of-service-plan (POS) Retrieved from https://healthcoverageguide.org/reference-guide/coverage-types/point-of-service-plan-pos/

Speights, K. (2018, October). What is managed care? The Motley Fool. Retrieved from https://www.fool.com/investing/general/2015/10/06/what-is-managed-care.aspx

U.S. Bureau of Labor Statistics. U.S. Department of Labor. (2020, November 4). Employer-reported workplace injuries and illnesses-2019. Retrieved November 16, 2020, from www.bls.gov › news.release › pdf › osh

U.S. Centers for Medicare & Medicaid. (n.d.). Health Maintenance Organization (HMO). Medicare.gov. Retrieved November 4, 2019, from https://www.medicare.gov/sign-up-change-plans/types-of-medicare-health-plans/medicare-advantage-plans/health-maintenance-organization-hmo

US Legal, Inc. (2019)."Managed care and HMOs." Health care, 2019, https://health care.uslegal.com/managed-care-and-hmos/

U.S. National library of medicine. (2018). Managed care. Medline Plus. https://medlineplus.gov/managedcare.html

7 Special Populations

7.1 LEARNING OBJECTIVES

By the end of this chapter, the student will be able to:
- Describe how healthcare programs for special populations fit into the U.S. healthcare system as a whole
- Define special populations in the U.S.
- Describe the importance of the Americans with Disabilities Act (ADA)
- Recall the role of Medicare, Medicaid, Social Security, correctional health programs, and the Veterans Administration in supporting the health needs of special populations

7.2 KEY TERMS

- adult disability
- Americans with Disabilities Act (ADA)
- childhood disability
- correctional health programs
- elderly
- incarcerated
- military veterans
- American Indians and Alaska Natives (AIAN)

7.3 INTRODUCTION

What is a special population, and why should the U.S. assist in care for these individuals? The U.S. government provides healthcare to special populations to reduce the burden of disability and illness. Achieving health equity for all Americans has remained a focus area of many government programs. The government has created programs to assist with costs for those unable to provide adequate healthcare coverage for themselves, whether through poverty, age, or disability.

How does the U.S. government fund programs for special populations? Medicare is funded through payroll taxes paid by employers and employees, general federal income tax revenue, income taxes paid on Social Security benefits, premiums paid by Medicare beneficiaries, interest earned on trust funds, Hospital Insurance (HI) and Supplementary Medical Insurance (SMI), and investments (Medicare.gov, n.d.). **Medicaid** is jointly funded through the federal government and individual states (Medicaid.gov, n.d.). This chapter will describe special populations in which the U.S. healthcare system provides healthcare benefits. Through a brief review, it will additionally highlight the federal and state programs which provide support to specific special groups. This chapter includes discussion of Native American and Alaska Natives, military veterans, children and adults with disabilities, elderly, and incarcerated individuals.

7.4 AMERICAN INDIANS AND ALASKA NATIVES

American Indians and Alaska Natives (AIAN) currently number 6.79 million or 2.09% of the U.S. population (World Population Review, 2020). This vulnerable population is disproportionately affected by many health conditions and have a higher rate of death than other Americans with these same conditions. Common conditions include diabetes, chronic lower respiratory diseases, chronic liver disease and cirrhosis, and mental health disorders that lead to intentional self-harm and suicide (Indian Health Services [IHS], 2019). In addition, American Indians and Alaska Natives suffer more unintentional injuries and assault/homicides. In 2017, the leading causes of death for AIAN were heart disease, cancer, and unintentional injuries (Centers for Disease Control and Prevention [CDC], 2020a). Sadly, this group of vulnerable citizens also has a life expectancy of 73 years of age, 5.5 years less than other Americans from any race (78.5 years of age) (IHS, 2019) (Figure 7.1).

The U.S. government and Indian tribes developed a "trust" relationship as far back as the eighteenth century, a relationship that has had an impact on and shaped the focus of health for the AIAN community (National Academy of Science, 2017). Indian Health Services (IHS), an agency within the Department of Health and Human Services (HHS), is the leading health provider for this vulnerable group of citizens. IHS has been federally recognized since 1954 with a transfer of health services from the Bureau of Indian Affairs to the Public Health Service. In addition, as a result of the 1975 Indian Self-Determination and Education Assistance Act (ISDEAA), tribes are able to have control and management of healthcare services. Over 60% of the IHS budget is appropriated and managed by tribes.

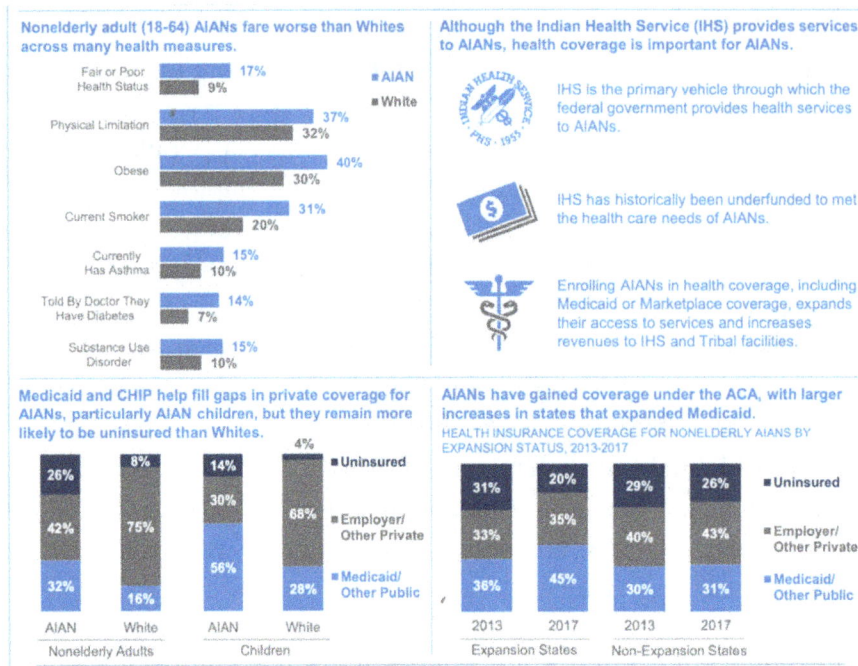

Figure 7.1: American Indians and Alaska Natives Health

Source: Kaiser Family Foundation

Attribution: Kaiser Family Foundation

License: © Kaiser Family Foundation. Used with permission.

American Indians and Alaska Natives are the only population in the U.S. who have a legal right to health services because of the current laws in place. Yet, there is inadequate funding to meet the health needs of this special population. A timeline of legislation regarding AIAN health appears in Figure 7.2. It is important to note that if there is a full repeal of the Affordable Care Act, the Indian Health Care Improvement Act (IHCIA) would be eliminated and IHS would have funding cuts and loss of services (Burrell Institute for Health Policy and Research, 2017).

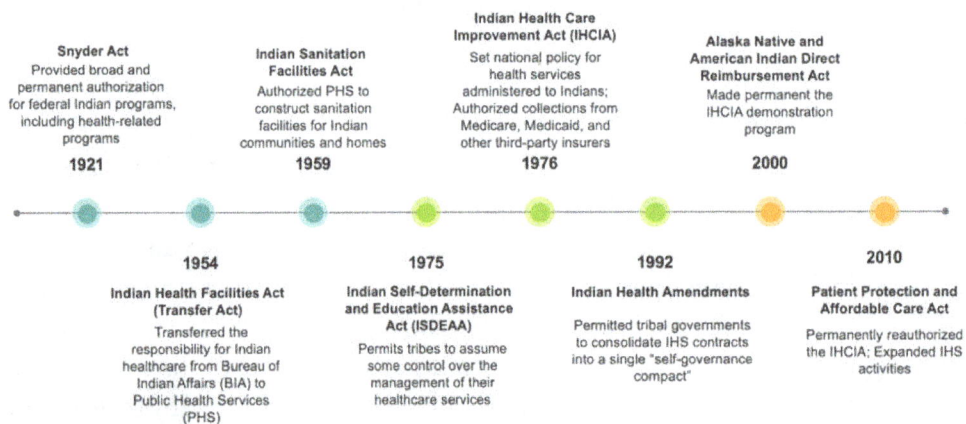

Figure 7.2: Timeline of Legislation Affecting AIAN Health

Source: Original Work

Attribution: Deanna Howe

License: CC BY-SA 4.0

Indian Health Services (IHS) works with American Indian and Alaska Native (AIAN) tribe governments to meet the complex needs of their people. Yet, only about 2.56 million are receiving comprehensive health services through the Indian Health Service organization. This in large part is because most IHS services occur in the rural tribal areas and abutting counties. A majority of AIAN's live outside of tribal areas in urban settings (70%) and may or may not have access to urban clinics (Office of Minority Health [OMH], 2018). Geographic inaccessibility and needed services that are not available could be reasons why AIAN do not seek care in urban areas. Lack of access to adequate healthcare is a common issue for AIAN's and results in poor health outcomes.

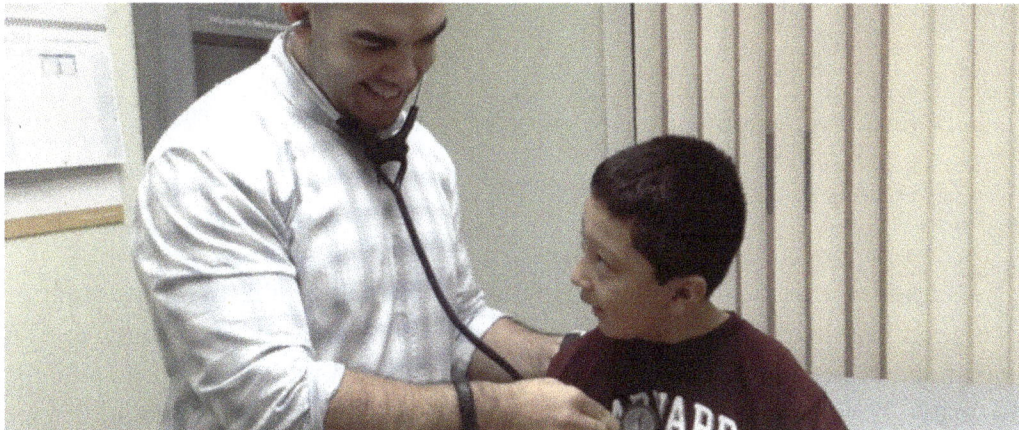

Figure 7.3: Child Receiving Care at an IHS Clinic

Source: Indian Health Service
Attribution: Indian Health Service
License: Public Domain

The Indian Health System is made up of direct care healthcare services, tribally operated healthcare services, and urban Indian healthcare services and resource centers. Funding is authorized by Congress annually, and IHS has received a small increase each year: $5.0 billion (b) for FY 2017, $5.5b for FY 2018, $5.8b for FY 2019, and $6.0b for FY 2020. However, IHS per user expenditure in FY2019 was only $4,078 compared to $9,726, U.S. National Health Expenditure per person in 2017 (IHS, 2020a). Clearly, more financial support is needed to increase this financial disparity and ensure American Indians and Alaska Natives have access to quality healthcare that can meet their health needs.

7.5 MILITARY VETERANS

The U.S. Armed Forces includes 1.3 million active duty, 1.1 million National Guard and Reserve, and over 20 million veterans (DMDC, 2019). Gulf War veterans—those serving from 1990 to the present—are now the largest group of **veterans** (Bialik, 2017). According to the U.S. Department of Veterans Association (VA) (2020a), the total veteran population is predicted to decline from 19.5 million in 2020 to 13.6 million in 2048. Figure 7.4 notes this predicted decline. This anticipated decline will likely result from aging veterans expected to die during the next twenty years: those from World War II, the Korean War, and the Vietnam War.

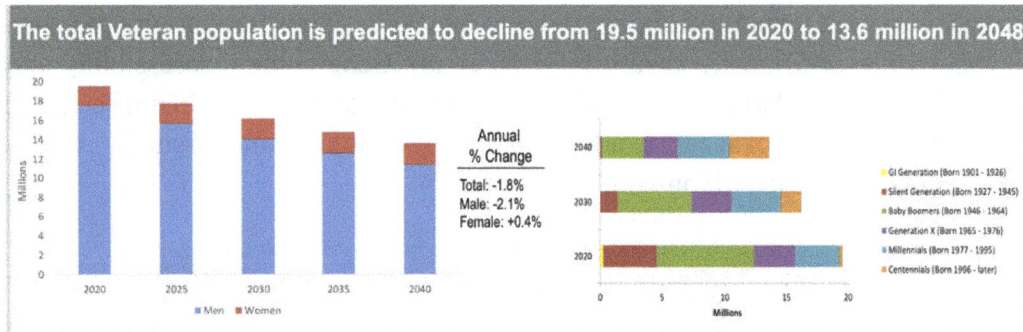

Figure 7.4: Total veteran population is predicted to decline

Source: US Department of Veterans Affairs
Attribution: US Department of Veterans Affairs
License: Public Domain

Men and women who have served in the military may be able to receive some or all of their healthcare benefits through the VA. Healthcare services through the VA are funded by the federal government. Each year, the VA requests funds to support the many programs for military veterans and their families. According to the VA (2020b), the VA has a proposed $243.3 billion budget for fiscal year 2021 which addresses veterans needs in areas of healthcare, benefits, national cemeteries, as well as compensation and pensions, housing and insurance. The house and senate must first vote on and approve this recommendation before funds are allocated.

As with all of the agencies discussed in this chapter, eligibility for VA healthcare must be determined by preset requirements. Limits in funding makes it impossible to serve all military veterans. Therefore, the VA has eight priority groups to make sure the most vulnerable and in-need groups of veterans are enrolled first. Priority group 1 (highest priority group) includes veterans with a service-connected disability rated 50% or higher, veterans determined by the VA to be unemployable as a result of a service-related condition, and those who have received the Medal of Honor. Two examples of service-related conditions causing disability are loss of limb or traumatic brain injury (TBI). Generally, eligible recipients with a 50% disability do not pay annual premiums, co-pays, or fees for services. Veterans with access to VA healthcare because of low-income may be required to assume a copay (NDNRC, 2019), that is, a set amount the veteran must pay at the time of service. Copay amounts may vary depending on the level of service (urgent care versus inpatient hospitalization) and frequency of service (once versus multiple times in one year). Copays, if required, are as low as $5 for prescription services and as high as $1,408 + $10/day for 90 days of inpatient care (VA, 2020c).

- -

First Person Perspective

Mr. B. is a retired U.S. Air Force veteran.

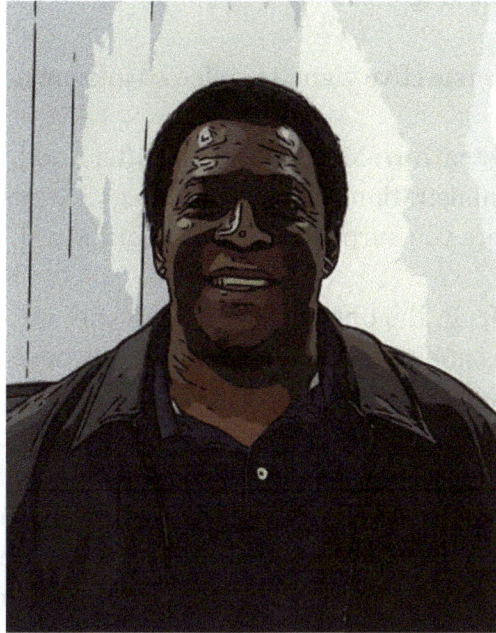

Figure 7.5: First Person Perspective

Source: Original Work
Attribution: Deanna Howe
License: CC BY-SA 4.0

I have experienced care with Veterans Affairs (VA) once I retired from the Air Force in 2004 and lived in Texas. After retirement, the VA diagnosed me with several conditions, acute and chronic. When I needed to see a doctor, the average wait time was three to four weeks to get an appointment. Once at the appointment, there could be long wait times in the lobby before I would see the doctor. Although the wait times were long, the doctors and staff were professional during most visits, with the exception of a few occasions.

Over time, I began to see improvements in many areas of the VA. They established a program to accelerate the appointment wait time and decrease the wait time in the VA lobby. My appointments to see a doctor decreased from a three-week wait to only a three to seven days wait. When the VA could not schedule an appointment for me within a few days, I was given an option to receive a referral to choose a doctor from town. This included all services, such as medical and dental. There was a $25.00 co-payment fee required for choosing a doctor in town. This extra fee was an issue for some folks, but I was okay with it in exchange for receiving quicker service. Due to all the changes and improvements made by the

VA, my experience with the VA changed to excellent from 2009–2016. I moved to Italy in 2016 and Germany from 2018 to the present. I haven't had any visits with VA clinics during this time. However, I would add, it would be great for the VA to have more facilities accessible for veterans to utilize while working overseas.

First person perspective vignette collected and created by D. Howe, 2020.

For your consideration: Mr. B. notes that after 2009, he had excellent care with the Veterans Administration. With so many negative stories in the media over the past few years, were you surprised to hear about Mr. B.'s positive experience with the VA?

The VA offered Mr. B. the opportunity to seek care outside of the VA health system to expedite his ability to see a doctor, but it would require a $25 copay. Once or twice, this fee may seem nominal, but for complicated health issues that require frequent medical visits, the copay fees can add up quickly. For veterans unable or unwilling to pay the $25 copay, their care may be delayed while waiting for an appointment with the VA. This scenario then becomes an access issue noting that those with money tend to receive quicker and better care.

In consideration of the many sacrifices our military members give in service, should all healthcare services be free to retired veterans? Should retired veterans have to pay copays to receive timely care? What solutions would you offer? Discuss and share your ideas.

━ ━ ━ ━ ━ ━ ━ ━ ━ ━ ━ ━ ━ ━ ━ ━ ━ ━ ━

Health issues affecting military veterans depends upon many unique factors, such as the era in which they served and their type of service (war or peacetime). The Veterans Administration (VA) has a specific site, "Veterans health issues related to service history," which covers all wars, from World War II (1939–1945) through Operation Enduring Freedom in Afghanistan (2001–2014). Each era has a link to specific health conditions, criteria for eligibility, and the steps needed to seek care. For example, World War II notes such conditions as noise, radiation, mustard gas, and extreme cold, and Operation Enduring Freedom (OEF) notes burn pit smoke, extreme cold, extreme heat, explosions, noise, and depleted uranium. In total, seven war time eras are presented for veterans to review. Other types of impact areas include mental health, military sexual trauma, substance abuse problems, exposure to hazardous materials, and women's healthcare needs (VA, 2019).

According to the United Health Foundation (2019), military returning from recent Gulf Wars have emerging health needs due to unusual combat-related circumstances. Our military members are experiencing more frequent and longer deployments exposing them to extreme stress in combat. As a result, extraordinary numbers of veterans are presenting with Post Traumatic Stress Disorder (PTSD) and Traumatic Brain Injury (TBI) (United Health Foundation, 2019). Less documented are the rates of depression because of the stigma associated with asking for help. Finally, there were 541 suicides of service members in 2018. This signals an increase in suicide rates from 21.9% in 2017 to 24.8% in 2018 (Lamothe, 2019). The projected VA 2021 budget, if passed by Congress, includes $10.2 billion for mental health services, of which $313 million is set aside for suicide-prevention outreach (VA, 2020b).

Pause and Reflect

Americans who serve voluntarily and in military conflicts or war may be hurt or physically injured in some way. Not all conditions are immediately evident, for instance, exposure cases or mental health. Some military members separate from the military after one or two tours of duty and may not be eligible to seek veteran's medical benefits in one of the higher priority groups. Does the U.S. government have a responsibility to provide care to these prior military who were injured during regular military duty? Funding is not always adequate, so how should we prioritize those prior military veterans injured or exposed to hazardous materials as noted above?

7.6 PERSONS WITH DISABILITIES

According to the CDC (2019a), "a disability is any condition of the body or mind (impairment) that makes it more difficult for the person with the condition to do certain activities (activity limitation) and interact with the world around them (participation restrictions)" (para. 1). Caring for a child or family member with physical or cognitive disability creates emotional, physical, and financial stress on the entire family. Healthcare costs for individuals with disabilities can be very high depending on the specific needs of those affected. The U.S. allocates publicly-funded health insurance to assist in the support and medical care of persons with disabilities from age birth to 18, and beyond in many cases. In 2017, there were an estimated 40+ million individuals with a disability in the U.S. (12.7% of the 320+ million individuals recorded in the U.S.) (NiDILRR, 2018).

7.6.1 Children with Disabilities

Treatments, therapies, equipment, medications, and time are all factors caregivers of disabled persons must manage. For example, a child born with cerebral palsy (CP), an incurable congenital disorder which affects muscle tone, movement, and motor skills, requires an extensive level of care to maximize quality of life (CDC, 2019b). Treatments for a child with CP will likely include physical, occupational, and speech therapies; surgery; braces; and medications. Another example is a child who is hit on the head by a line drive while playing baseball and suffers a traumatic brain injury. Depending on severity, emergency treatment including surgical intervention, medications, and rehabilitation therapies may be needed for years or a lifetime following the accident.

How does a family afford this care? One might think healthcare covers all of these needs for those with healthcare insurance. However, difficulties in obtaining coverage could include finding care providers "in network," ensuring the family deductible is met, and meeting the co-pay amount for each support service and medical appointment required. Families living in rural or low-care provider areas may have trouble meeting all health insurance coverage criteria, leading to added burdens and more out-of-pocket expenses. Costs can skyrocket if an insurance company's requirements for payment are inconsistent with a family's specific situation, leading to emotional and financial distress. Families with no health insurance may find it impossible to meet the many needs of a disabled child.

The definition of **childhood disability** changes depending on the specific funding source—state or federal—and current legislation. A strict definition used by the Social Security Administration (SSA) (2019a) is "the child must have a physical or mental condition(s) that very seriously limits his or her activities; and the condition(s) must have lasted, or be expected to last, at least 1 year or result in death" (para. 2). The example of the child born with cerebral palsy would meet this definition.

The Supplemental Security Income (SSI) program, administered by the SSA, provides monthly payments to a disabled child whose condition meets the above definition and whose family meets the criteria of low income (SSA, 2019a). The application process is complicated and requires supporting documentation of disability and evidence generation to support financial need; it also includes careful management with an SSA case manager. Additional funding sources include Medicaid and **Child Health Insurance Program (CHIP)**. According to Musumeci and Chidambaram (2019), "Medicaid and CHIP covered about half (47%) of the 13.3 million children with special healthcare needs in 2017" (para. 1). Medicaid/CHIP payments vary depending on the state of residence because some states provide more supplemental funds than others. Income eligibility for Medicaid is set at 138% of the Family Poverty Level (FPL). States have the option to expand eligibility above this percent. Musumeci and Chidambaram (2019) also write, "As of January 2019, the median financial eligibility level for Medicaid and CHIP children nationally is 255% FPL ($54,392/year for a family of three in 2019)" (para. 7). Figure 7.6 notes the 2017 health insurance status of children with special healthcare needs. However, of importance to consider is there being current legislation to cap Medicaid benefits, which in some states would include children with disabilities (Schubel, 2017).

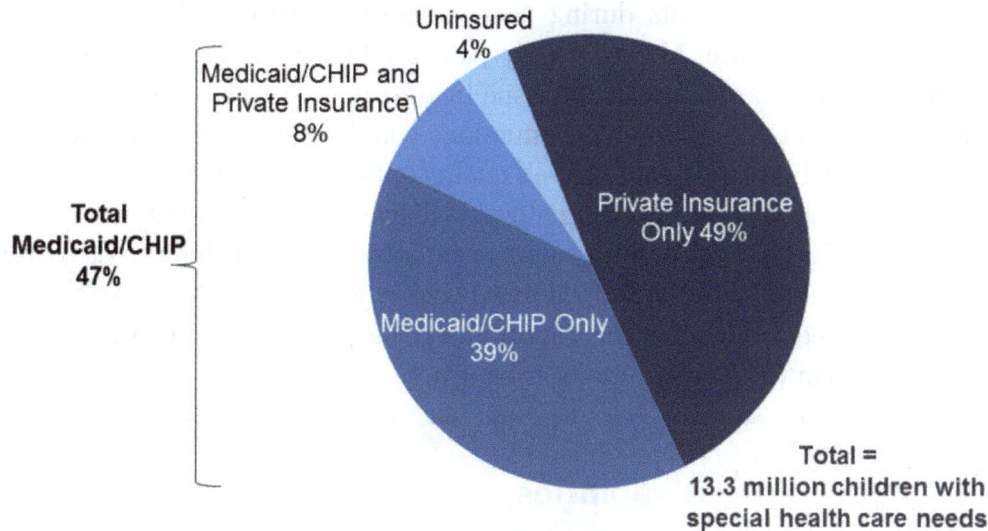

Figure 7.6: Health Insurance Status of Children With Special Healthcare Needs, 2017

Source: Kaiser Family Foundation
Attribution: Kaiser Family Foundation
License: © Kaiser Family Foundation. Used with permission.

The Tax Equity and Fiscal Responsibility Act (TEFRA)/Katie Beckett waiver offers another pathway for eligibility to the Medicaid program. Waiver programs, such as Katie Beckett, allows for Medicaid eligibility when a family's income is too high and focuses solely on the income of the child. This waiver for eligibility provides much-needed funds to families who have a higher (whole family) income but are still required to pay high-cost care to support their disabled child. Below is a brief description of the Katie Beckett story and how this legislation helps children today receive paid care at home rather than an institution. Continuation of benefits into adulthood is possible. Disabled children who turn 18 could qualify for the Social Security Disability Insurance (SSDI) benefits if they continue to meet the definition of the SSA for qualifying conditions and prove the low-income criteria (SSA, 2019b). In addition, adult children may use Social Security benefits if their parents paid into the fund through employment taxes.

- -

Katie Beckett

As a young five-month-old infant, Katie contracted viral encephalitis and went into a coma. She received ongoing inpatient care in a small hospital in Iowa for three years. Katie ultimately recovered from the infection but was left partially paralyzed and required a ventilator to assist with breathing. Medicaid paid for the hospitalization and treatments, but when Katie was cleared to return home she would do so without Medicaid financial support.

Although the treatments during hospitalization were considered six-times costlier than home care, Medicaid only paid for treatments within a hospital. President Reagan learned about the issue in 1981 and changed this rule so that Katie and other children in similar situations could return home for continued care rather than live in hospitals. Katie's quality of life improved through the years with home care and Katie was eventually able to live in her own apartment, where she relied on night care from nurses and a ventilator for fifteen-hours a day. After a series of illnesses, Katie succumbed unexpectedly and died at the age of 34. Her legacy has helped to highlight the importance of keeping disabled children in the home rather than within institutions. (Shapiro, 2012)

7.6.2 Adults with Disabilities

According to the CDC (2019c), one in four adults have some type of disability. And, according to the Social Security Administration (2019), "the sobering fact for 20-year-olds is that more than 1-in-4 will become disabled before reaching retirement age" (para. 5). Adults with disabilities also include those who became disabled prior to age 22 (consider our two child disability examples of cerebral palsy and traumatic brain injury). Disabilities could include back injuries occurring from work; physical or cognitive injuries from an accident; hearing loss from high-noise work environments; or decreased function resulting from disease processes, such as multiple sclerosis, chronic fatigue syndrome, or diabetes. In addition, many mental health conditions, such as severe depression, schizophrenia, or bipolar disorder, could create disability. Depending on the disability, adults affected may be unable to work. The need for financial support is tremendous in these cases. According to the National Council on Disability (2017):

- People with disabilities live in poverty at more than twice the rate of people without disabilities

- More than 65% of the 17.9 million working-age adults with disabilities participate in at least one safety net or income support program

- Only 32% of working-age people with disabilities are employed compared with 73% of those without disabilities

Table 7.1: Can You Spot Someone with a Disability?	
Which of the following disabilities can you visually identify in a person? Which disabilities are less apparent?	
cerebral palsy	visual deficit
hearing deficit	Down syndrome
speech impediment	autism
arthritis	depression
diabetes	HIV/AIDS
asthma	epilepsy

Source: Original Work
Attribution: Deanna Howe
License: CC BY-SA 4.0

The benefits of Social Security Income (SSI) and Social Security Disability Insurance (SSDI) assist adults who have disabilities to meet the needs of housing, food, and medical care. In addition, Medicare coverage is available for those under the age of 65 with some disability conditions such as end-stage kidney disease (ESRD) or amyotrophic lateral sclerosis (ALS). Forty-five states offer a buy-in Medicaid program for those ineligible for Medicaid through SSI eligibility (NCD, 2017).

Access to quality healthcare remains an issue for adults with disabilities. Figure 7.7 notes disability and health access barriers of adults with disabilities. According to the CDC (2019d), people with disabilities face many barriers and have poorer overall health; have less access to adequate healthcare; and engage in risky health behaviors, such as smoking and physical inactivity.

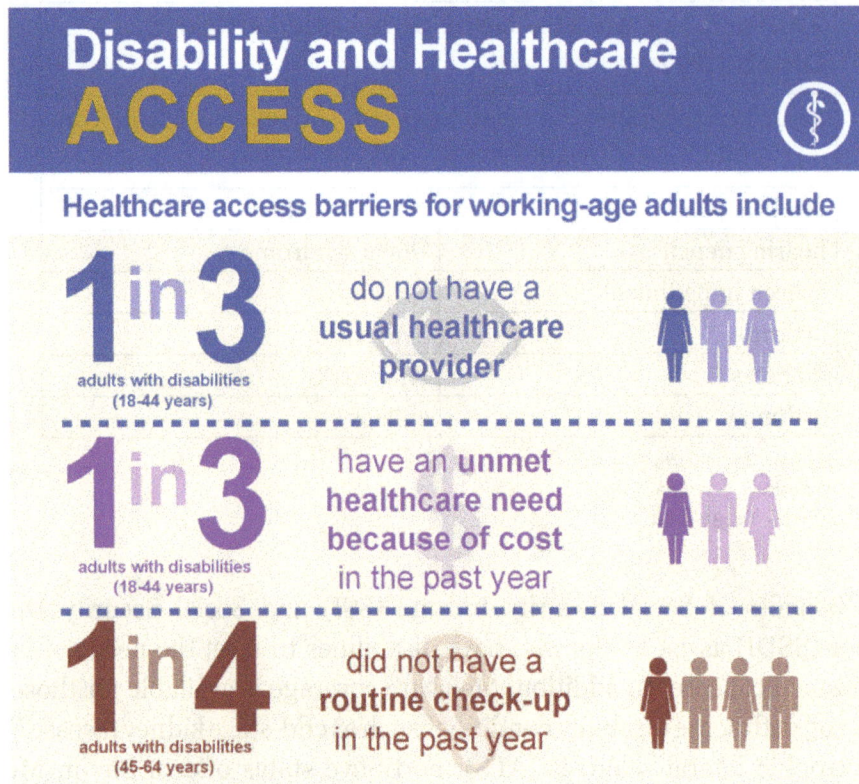

Figure 7.7: Disability and Healthcare Access

Source: Centers for Disease Control and Prevention
Attribution: Centers for Disease Control and Prevention
License: Public Domain

Of importance to note is that many adults with disabilities are able to work and earn a livable wage, thanks largely to the **Americans with Disabilities Act (ADA)**, signed into law by George H. W. Bush on July 26, 1990 (celebrating its 30-year anniversary in 2020). According to the Bureau of Labor Statistics (BLS) (2019a), persons with a disability accounted for 19.1% of the workforce compared with 65.9% of those without a disability in 2018. In the same year, the unemployment rate for persons with a disability was 8.0% compared to 3.7% for those without disability (BLS, 2019). This represents a decrease from the previous year for both groups.

7.7 ELDERLY

Thanks to advances in medicine and medical care, people are living much longer than those of generations past. Overall, **elderly** persons, those 65 and older, are expected to make up one-fifth of the population—approximately 77 million— by the year 2034 (U.S. Census Bureau, 2018). This statistic is significant because elderly persons are the fastest growing segment of our population. The aging of Baby Boomers, those born between 1946 and 1964, will create an immense strain upon the U.S. healthcare system to include expenditures, services, and workforce.

Disease and disability are not considered a normal part of aging. However, "in 2018, 49% of persons with a disability were age 65 and older" (Bureau of Labor Statistics (BLS), 2019b, para 4). Figure 7.8 notes the characteristics of the Medicare population.

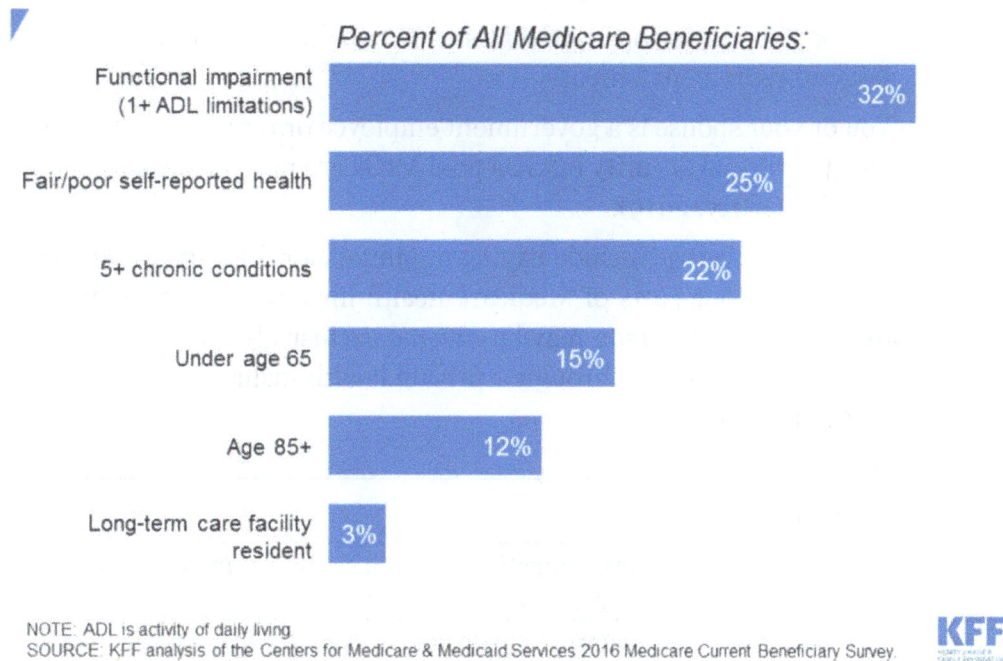

Percent of All Medicare Beneficiaries:

Functional impairment (1+ ADL limitations)	32%
Fair/poor self-reported health	25%
5+ chronic conditions	22%
Under age 65	15%
Age 85+	12%
Long-term care facility resident	3%

NOTE: ADL is activity of daily living.
SOURCE: KFF analysis of the Centers for Medicare & Medicaid Services 2016 Medicare Current Beneficiary Survey.

KFF

Figure 7.8: Characteristics of the Medicare Population

Source: Kaiser Family Foundation
Attribution: Kaiser Family Foundation
License: © Kaiser Family Foundation. Used with permission.

Pause and Reflect

According to the Center on Budget and Policy Priorities (2019), Medicare spending is projected to grow from 3.7% of GDP today to 5.9% in 2040. Consider the continued growth of the aging population. How will Medicare keep pace with the expected expenditures? Do you think there will be Medicare funds available for you at 65 years of age? Do you anticipate the government will increase the age of eligibility?

People are living longer, due in large part to improved medical care and positive behavioral changes (National Institutes of Health (NIH), 2018). Agencies, such as the CDC, and organizations, such as the Healthy People initiative, focus on population health, including but not limited to such areas as obesity, type 2 diabetes, high blood pressure, and stroke. Healthy People (2020) note that aging adults manage two or more chronic conditions that can lower quality of life and contribute to a leading cause of death.

The largest healthcare insurance for persons 65 and older is Medicare. Medicare was signed into law by President Lyndon B. Johnson, July 30, 1965. Before this time, only half of Americans had insurance to cover hospitalizations (Barry, 2019). The criteria to meet Medicare eligibility at age 65 includes the following:

- You are a U.S. citizen or permanent legal resident for at least five years

- You or your spouse has worked long enough for Social Security or railroad retirement benefits

- You or your spouse is a government employee or retiree who has not paid into Social Security but has paid Medicare payroll taxes while working (Barry, 2019).

Other ways to get coverage include paying premiums for the parts of Medicare (Table 7.2). There are four parts of Medicare health insurance: Parts A, B, C, D and Medicare Advantage. A person may be covered exclusively through Medicare or have some parts of the plans through a private health insurance approved by Medicare (see Chapter 5).

Table 7.2: Medicare Parts	
Part A	Hospital insurance: covers inpatient hospital stays, care in skilled nursing facility, hospice care, some home healthcare
Part B	Medical insurance: covers certain doctors' services, outpatient care, home healthcare, medical supplies, and preventive services
Part C	Medicare Advantage: an "all in one" option that bundles Parts A, B, and D
Part D	Prescription drug coverage: adds prescription drug coverage to original Medicare, some Medicare Cost plans, some Medicare Private Fee-for-Services plans, and Medicare Medical Savings Account Plans. (These plans are offered by insurance companies and other private companies approved by Medicare.)

Source: Medicare.gov
Attribution: Medicare.gov
License: Public Domain

7.8 INCARCERATED

The U.S. justice system houses approximately 2.3 million people throughout state prisons, federal prisons, juvenile correctional facilities, local jails, Indian Country jails, military prisons, immigration detention facilities, civil commitment centers, state psychiatric hospitals, and prisons in the U.S. territories (Sawyer & Wagner, 2019). The enormous burden of providing healthcare to an inmate is extremely important, not only for the overall health of the inmate but also to the health of the population once the inmate is released.

Incarcerated persons are more likely to have infectious diseases, such as tuberculosis, hepatitis C, and HIV (HealthyPeople.gov, 2019). If these infectious diseases are untreated, the released inmate could potentially spread the disease to others upon their return to society. Chronic conditions, such as arthritis, asthma, cancer, diabetes, heart disease, high blood pressure, and stroke, are most reported by prison inmates (CDC, 2019e). In addition, Healthy People (2019) note, "when compared to the general population, men and women with a history of incarceration are in worse mental and physical health" (para. 3.).

Individuals in prison, correctional facilities, and city or county jails receive medical care through **Correctional Health Programs** for minor aches and pains, medication regimens, or surgery if necessary. Generally speaking, persons incarcerated in a city jail have healthcare paid for the city. For those inmates in a county jail, the county pays for healthcare. Inmates residing in state penitentiaries have healthcare paid for by the state. And lastly, federal prisoner's healthcare is paid for by the federal government.

Many correctional health programs now assess a copay for services if an inmate requires medical care (Sawyer, 2017). In some states, inmates can earn a wage for work completed while in custody and bank this money for spending on commissary items or healthcare. However, some inmates earn less than a dollar an hour for work while incarcerated. This nominal wage would be depleted if a copay for healthcare were required because most inmates are "impoverished and earn little to no money for their work in prisons" (Bertram, 2019, para. 2.). For states in which no inmate wages are earned, copays could deter inmates from seeking healthcare altogether. Basically, inmates would have to prioritize healthcare, and the choice to not see a health provider could hurt not only the inmate but the public as well.

Pause and Reflect

Some will say healthcare is a right, yet incarcerated individuals may not receive ongoing preventative healthcare due to budget cuts or lack of services. The impact of low or no healthcare is the spread of communicable diseases, such as tuberculosis, through the inmate population and chronic diseases, such as diabetes, that may be poorly managed. These conditions could lead to disability upon release from the prison system, leading to an extended or lifetime use of Medicare or Medicaid services. In light of the impact on individuals, inmate population, and ultimately the community, is it a good idea to fully fund treatment for inmates while incarcerated? What are the pros and cons, as you see it?

7.9 COVID-19 VIRUS AND SPECIAL POPULATIONS

By now the entire world is familiar with the virus, COVID-19. An infection with the virus may include symptoms of fever, cough, and shortness of breath. The severity of symptoms from the virus depends on an individual's immune system. The virus spreads from person to person when an infected person coughs or sneezes. The tiny droplets fall and are inhaled by people close by and they become infected. The virus is very contagious and spreads quickly within a community. The COVID-19 virus has created tremendous risk to all Americans. However, special populations noted in this chapter are at increased risk for exposure and death.

The American Indian and Alaska Native (AIAN) population has been disproportionately affected by COVID-19. According to the CDC (2020c), the total amount of laboratory-confirmed cases is 3.5 times more in AIAN than non-Hispanic whites. The CDC also reports large data gaps for this population, which makes incidence, severity, and outcome analysis difficult (Hatcher et al., 2020). As discussed above, AIAN has a high prevalence of health conditions, such as respiratory diseases, diabetes, hypertension, and obesity. These conditions have been associated with more severe COVID-19 symptoms and a higher risk for death. The Indian Health Service has received more than $1 billion to provide enhanced services to AIAN's in response to the COVID-19 pandemic (IHS, 2020b). These funds were distributed to tribal health and urban Indian health programs to increase access to testing and the response to the virus pandemic.

Older adults often live with chronic diseases, which has been found to increase the risk for severe illness related to the virus. A lowered immune system may also contribute to the severe symptoms seen in older adults. According to the CDC (2020d), eight out of ten deaths in the U.S. are adults 65 years and older. Older adults have a higher risk for contracting the virus if they are reliant upon others for care or to assist in tasks related to daily living. Many nursing home residents are at high risk for infection related to living in a confined space and the inability to social distance. While the statistics are still emerging, one-third of all U.S. coronavirus deaths are nursing home residents or workers (Yourish et al., 2020). Additional risk factors include social isolation and an inability to access food and healthcare.

Adults and children with a disability are not inherently at risk for getting COVID-19. However, individuals with underlying chronic illnesses, such as chronic lung disease, severe heart disease, or a weakened immune system, are at higher risk for infection and severe illness (CDC, 2020e). According to the CDC (2020e), adults with disabilities are three times more likely than adults without disabilities to have chronic diseases, such as heart disease, diabetes, or stroke (para 1). Disability groups who are more at risk include people with limited mobility or those who cannot avoid close contact with others, those who have difficulty understanding information, and those who are unable to communicate symptoms of illness.

COVID-19 virus spreads quickly within communities, and the prison system is susceptible as well. Inmates are often housed in close quarters, which prevents social distancing and the ability to protect from infection. As noted above, many inmates have chronic diseases, which puts them at a higher risk of severe symptoms from COVID-19 infection. In response, the Federal Bureau of Prisons (BOP) (2020) has implemented modified operations by limiting social visits, decreasing inmate movement within and outside of a facility, and screening for the virus. According to the Marshall Project (2020), at least 25,239 cases and 373 deaths from COVID-19 are reported among prisoners. However, without wide testing in all facilities, it is unknown how many inmates may be infected. Figure 7.9 illustrates a six-week period of reporting of coronavirus cases cases between April and May 2020.. The large increase results from five states (Ohio, Tennessee, Arkansas, Michigan, and North Carolina) initiating aggressive testing of nearly all prisons in which people are becoming sick.

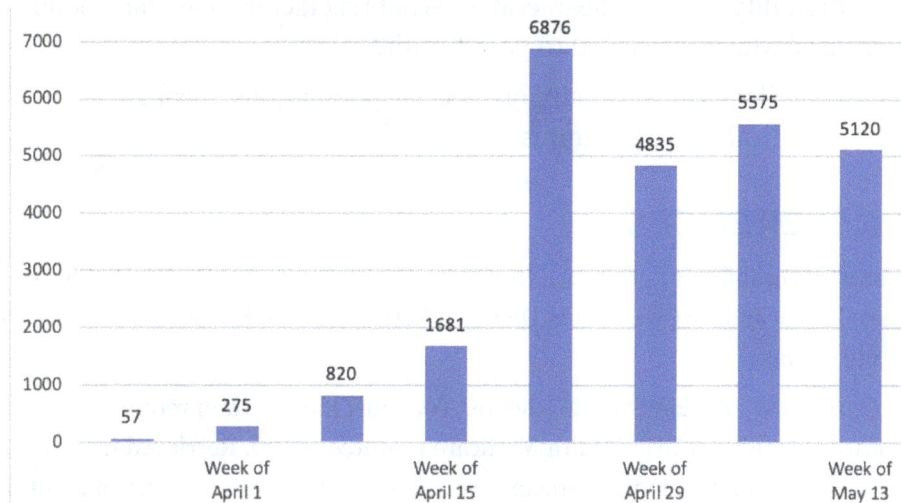

Figure 7.9: Corona Virus Cases Reported Among Prisoners

Source: The Marshall Project
Attribution: Corey Parson, Adapted from The Marshall Project
License: Fair Use

7.10 SUMMARY

The U.S. provides healthcare services and support to a few special populations. Military veterans, children and adults with disabilities, the elderly, and those incarcerated and living within our prisons all have specific health needs that are costly. The dynamics are complicated for each special group. This chapter included a discussion of available healthcare programs as well as how these programs are funded, some conditions of eligibility to receive assistance, and statistics of each special group. The programs discussed in this chapter provide many resources which help to contribute to the overall health of each individual. In addition, the chapter addresses the impact of the COVID-19 virus on special populations.

7.11 REVIEW QUESTIONS

1. How does legislation address American Indians and Alaska Natives receiving healthcare coverage?

2. How does policy, such as the Americans with Disabilities Act (ADA), support persons with disabilities?

3. What health services does the Veterans Administration provide to military veterans?

4. How did Katie Beckett's story ultimately benefit disabled children today?

5. How is correctional health funded? How do inmates pay for healthcare services?

6. Define the special populations addressed in this chapter: American Indian and Alaska Native, veterans, elderly, child and adults with disability, and the incarcerated. What risk factors does each population have which could lead to poor health?

7. How does the U.S. support special populations through federal and state healthcare programs?

7.12 REFERENCES

Americans with Disabilities Act (ADA). (n.d.). Introduction to the ADA. United States Department of Justice Civil Rights Division. Retrieved from https://www.ada.gov/ada_intro.htm

Barry, P. (2019). Do you qualify for Medicare? You must meet certain requirements for Medicare eligibility. AARP. Health Medicare resource center. Retrieved from https://www.aarp.org/health/medicare-insurance/info-04-2011/medicare-eligibility.html

Bertram, W. (2019, August 8). Momentum is building to end medical co-pays in prisons and jails. Prison Policy Initiative. Retrieved from https://www.prisonpolicy.org/blog/2019/08/08/copays-update/

Bialik, K. (2017). The changing face of America's veteran population. Pew research center. Retrieved from https://www.pewresearch.org/fact-tank/2017/11/10/the-changing-face-of-americas-veteran-population/

Bureau of Labor Statistics (BLS). (2019a). Economic new release. Persons with a disability: Labor force characteristics summary. Retrieved from https://www.bls.gov/news.release/disabl.nro.htm

Bureau of Labor Statistics (BLS). (2019b). Persons with a disability: Labor force characteristics summary. Retrieved from https://www.bls.gov/news.release/disabl.nro.htm

Centers for Disease Control and Prevention (CDC). (2020a). Health of American Indian or Alaska Native population: Data are for the U.S. Retrieved from https://www.cdc.gov/nchs/fastats/american-indian-health.htm

Centers for Disease Control and Prevention (CDC). (2020b). Coronavirus disease 2019 (COVID-19). Frequently asked questions. Retrieved from https://www.cdc.gov/coronavirus/2019-ncov/faq.html#Coronavirus-Disease-2019-Basics

Centers for Disease Control and Prevention (CDC). (2020c, August 19). CDC data show disproportionate COVID-19 impact in American Indian/Alaska Native populations. Retrieved from https://www.cdc.gov/media/releases/2020/p0819-covid-19-impact-american-indian-alaska-native.html

Centers for Disease Control and Prevention (CDC). (2020d). Coronavirus Disease 2019 (COVID-19). Older adults. Retrieved from https://www.cdc.gov/coronavirus/2019-ncov/need-extra-precautions/older-adults.html

Centers for Disease Control and Prevention (CDC). (2020e). Coronavirus disease 2019 (COVID-19). People with disabilities. Retrieved from https://www.cdc.gov/coronavirus/2019-ncov/need-extra-precautions/people-with-disabilities.html

Centers for Disease Control and Prevention (CDC). (2019a). Disability and health overview. Retrieved from https://www.cdc.gov/ncbddd/disabilityandhealth/disability.html

Centers for Disease Control and Prevention (CDC). (2019b). What is cerebral palsy? Retrieved from https://www.cdc.gov/ncbddd/cp/facts.html

Centers for Disease Control and Prevention (CDC). (2019c). Disability impacts all of us. Retrieved from https://www.cdc.gov/ncbddd/disabilityandhealth/infographic-disability-impacts-all.html

Centers for Disease Control and Prevention (CDC). (2019d). Disability and health information for health care providers. Retrieved from https://www.cdc.gov/ncbddd/disabilityandhealth/hcp.html

Centers for Disease Control and Prevention (CDC). (2019e). Correctional Health. Data on common health problems. Retrieved from https://www.cdc.gov/correctionalhealth/health-data.html

Defense Manpower Data Center (DMDC). (2019). DoD personnel, workforce reports & publications. Retrieved from https://www.dmdc.osd.mil/appj/dwp/dwp_reports.jsp

Federal Bureau of Prisons (BOP). (2020). BOP COVID-19 modified operations plan. Retrieved from https://www.bop.gov/coronavirus/

Hatcher, S. M., Agnew-Brune, C., Anderson, M., Zambrano, L. D., Rose, C. E., Jim, M. A., Baugher, A., Liu, G. S., Patel, S. V., Evans, M. E., Pindyck, T., Dubray, C. L., Rainey, J. J., Chen, J., Sadowski, C., Winglee, K., Penman-Aguilar, A., Dixit, A., Claw, E., & McCollum, J. (2020, August 28). COVID-19 among American Indian and Alaska Native persons- 23 states, January 31 – July 3, 2020. Morbidity and mortality weekly report (MMWR). 69(35); 1166–1169. Retrieved from https://www.cdc.gov/mmwr/volumes/69/wr/mm6934e1.htm

HealthyPeople.gov. (2020). Older adults. Retrieved from https://www.healthypeople.gov/2020/topics-objectives/topic/older-adults

HealthyPeople.gov. (2019). Incarceration. Retrieved from https://www.healthypeople.gov/2020/topics-objectives/topic/social-determinants-health/interventions-resources/incarceration

Indian Health Service (IHS). (2020a, August). IHS profile. Retrieved from https://www.ihs.gov/newsroom/factsheets/ihsprofile/

Indian Health Services (IHS). (2020b, April). IHS received more than &1 billion for coronavirus response. Retrieved from https://www.ihs.gov/newsroom/pressreleases/2020-press-releases/ihs-receives-more-than-1-billion-for-coronavirus-

response/#:~:text=The%20Indian%20Health%20Service%20has,respond%20to%20
the%20coronavirus%20pandemic

Indian Health Service (IHS). (2019, October). Disparities. Fact sheet. Retrieved from
https://www.ihs.gov/newsroom/factsheets/disparities/

Lamothe, D. (2019, September 27). U.S. military's suicide rate for active-duty troops up
over the past five years, Pentagon says. The Washington Post. Retrieved from https://
www.washingtonpost.com/national-security/2019/09/26/us-militarys-suicide-rate-
active-duty-troops-rises-fifth-consecutive-year-pentagon-says/

Medicaid.gov. (n.d.). Financial management. Retrieved from https://www.medicaid.gov/
medicaid/finance/

Medicare.gov. (n.d.). How is Medicare funded? Retrieved from https://www.medicare.
gov/about-us/how-is-medicare-funded

Musumeci, M. & Chidambaram, P. (2019, June 12). Medicaid's role for children with
special health care needs: A look at eligibility, services, and spending. Kaiser Family
Foundation. Retrieved from https://www.kff.org/medicaid/issue-brief/medicaids-
role-for-children-with-special-health-care-needs-a-look-at-eligibility-services-and-
spending/

National Academy of Sciences. (2017). Communities in action: Pathways to health equity.
Appendix A. Native American health: Historical and legal context. Retrieved from
https://www.ncbi.nlm.nih.gov/books/NBK425854/

National Council on Disability. (2017). Highlighting disability/poverty connection, NCD
urges congress to alter federal policies that disadvantage people with disabilities.
Retrieved from https://ncd.gov/newsroom/2017/disability-poverty-connection-
2017-progress-report-release

National Disability Navigator Resource Collaborative (NDNRC). (2019). Population
specific fact sheet - Veterans. Information for Veterans regarding Department of
Veterans Affairs health care. Retrieved from https://nationaldisabilitynavigator.org/
ndnrc-materials/fact-sheets/population-specific-fact-sheet-veterans/

National Institutes of Health (NIH). (2018). Disability in older adults. Retrieved from
https://report.nih.gov/nihfactsheets/viewfactsheet.aspx?csid=37

National Institute on Disability, Independent Living, and Rehabilitation Research
(NiDILRR). Retrieved from(2018). 2018 Annual disability statistics compendium.
https://disabilitycompendium.org/compendium/2018-annual-disability-statistics-
compendium?page=1

Office of Minority Health (OMH). (2018, March 28). Profile: American Indian/Alaska
Native. Retrieved October 6, 2020, https://www.minorityhealth.hhs.gov/omh/
browse.aspx?lvl=3&lvlid=62

Sawyer, W. (2017, April 19). The steep cost of medical co-pays in prison puts health
at risk. Prison policy initiative. Retrieved from https://www.prisonpolicy.org/
blog/2017/04/19/copays/

Sawyer, W. & Wagner, P. (2019, March 19). Mass Incarceration: The whole pie 2019. Prison policy initiative. Retrieved from https://www.prisonpolicy.org/reports/pie2019.html

Schubel, J. (2017, June 14). House ACA repeal bill puts children with disabilities and special health care needs at sever risk. Center on Budget and Policy Priorities. Retrieved from https://www.cbpp.org/research/health/house-aca-repeal-bill-puts-children-with-disabilities-and-special-health-care-needs

Shapiro, J. (2012, May 21). Katie Beckett defied the odds, helped other disabled kids live longer. Retrieved from https://www.npr.org/sections/health-shots/2012/05/21/153202340/katie-beckett-defied-the-odds-helped-other-disabled-kids-live-longer

Social Security Administration (SSA). (2019a). Child disability starter it- Fact sheet. Retrieved from https://www.ssa.gov/disability/disability_starter_kits_child_factsheet.htm

Social Security Administration (SSA). (2019b). Benefits for children with disabilities. Retrieved from https://www.ssa.gov/pubs/

Social Security Administration (SSA). (2019c). The faces and facts of disability. Retrieved from https://www.ssa.gov/disabilityfacts/facts.html

The Marshall Project. (2020). A state-by-state look at coronavirus in prisons. Retrieved from https://www.themarshallproject.org/2020/05/01/a-state-by-state-look-at-coronavirus-in-prisons

United States Census Bureau. (2018, March 13). Older people projected to outnumber children for first time in U.S. history. Retrieved from https://www.census.gov/newsroom/press-releases/2018/cb18-41-population-projections.html

U.S. Department of Veterans Association (VA) (2020a). Veteran Population Projections 2020-2040. Retrieved from https://www.va.gov/vetdata/docs/Demographics/New_Vetpop_Model/Vetpop_Infographic2020.pdf

U.S. Department of Veterans Association (VA) (2020b). VA strengthens care and benefits for Veterans with $243 billion budget request for fiscal year 2021. Retrieved from https://www.va.gov/opa/pressrel/pressrelease.cfm?id=5393

United States Department of Veterans Affairs. (2020c). VA health care copay rates. Retrieved from https://www.va.gov/health-care/copay-rates/

United States Department of Veterans Affairs. (2019). Veteran health issues related to service history. Retrieved from https://www.va.gov/health-care/health-needs-conditions/health-issues-related-to-service-era/

World Population Review. (2020). Native American population 2020. Retrieved from https://worldpopulationreview.com/state-rankings/native-american-population

Yourish, K., Lai, K. K. R., Ivory, D., & Smith, M. (2020, May 11). One-third of all U.S. coronavirus deaths are nursing home residents or workers. The New York Times. Retrieved from https://www.nytimes.com/interactive/2020/05/09/us/coronavirus-cases-nursing-homes-us.html

8 Access Issues in Healthcare

8.1 LEARNING OBJECTIVES

By the end of this chapter, the student will be able to:
- Define access to healthcare
- Discuss barriers to healthcare
- Define health literacy
- Explain initiatives to increase access to healthcare
- Describe possible improvements in the healthcare system

8.2 KEY TERMS

- access
- civilian
- equitable care
- health-seeking behaviors
- high deductible
- health disparities
- health literacy
- usual place of healthcare

8.3 INTRODUCTION

Having good health contributes to quality of life. Knowing that healthcare resources are available and easily accessible without depleting most of one's resources in times of need provides a sense of security. In this chapter, we explore the degree to which persons in the U.S. are without access to healthcare, barriers to healthcare access, consequences of inadequate access to healthcare, and possible measures to improve healthcare in the immediate future.

8.4 ACCESS TO HEALTHCARE

What does access to healthcare mean? Where is the U.S. regarding access to healthcare for the population? In 1993, the Institute of Medicine defined **access** to healthcare as "the timely use of personal health services to achieve the best possible health outcomes" (IOM, 1993, p. 31). The Office of Disease Prevention and Health Promotion (ODPHP, 2019a) uses this definition and lists three steps for obtaining access to needed healthcare services: (1) entrance into the system, usually through health insurance; (2) obtaining needed services within an accessible location; and (3) finding the right patient-provider relationship where communication, mutual trust, and respect are obtained. All three are essential in obtaining appropriate healthcare services.

8.4.1 Entrance into the System

Possessing health insurance may be considered as the gateway into the healthcare system. Without insurance coverage, most individuals are not willing to seek healthcare services unless faced with a life-threatening emergency—arguably, because of the expense. Hospital emergency departments are not allowed to turn anyone away because of the lack of health insurance. Conversely, physician offices can refuse to accept patients without insurance. Moreover, physician's offices may also turn patients away if they have only **Medicaid**; some also refuse **Medicare**.

Public health departments provide free or reduced-priced services to community members. Low-income pregnant women are eligible for Medicaid, and children of low-income families are eligible for Medicaid or state-sponsored insurance for children. Medicare is available to individuals with disability, who are on dialysis, or those age greater than 65 years. Of importance to note is that individuals' being eligible for insurance does not mean they are automatically enrolled or obtain insurance. However, without insurance, unless paying with cash, an individual will most likely have a difficult time accessing the healthcare system.

Pause and Reflect

Should physicians be able to turn patients away who have Medicaid? Should state or federal government require physicians to accept Medicaid patients? What sort of incentives might state or federal government provide to physicians so they will begin to or increase acceptance of Medicaid patients?

- -

First Person Perspective

Mr. J., M.A., is the Deputy Head for the Center for German-American Educational History

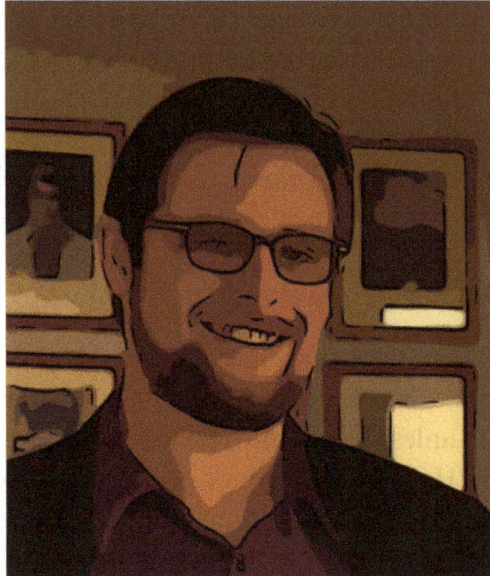

Figure 8.1: First Person Perspective

In college, I lost health insurance coverage through my parents—this was before the Obama-era mandate which allowed dependents to stay on their parent's health insurance coverage until they turned 26. Like a lot of college students, I gambled and went without health insurance, thinking that being young and healthy, I could spare the expense. I avoided going to the doctor and dentist for checkups, fearing the costs. I also would try to tough out illnesses, which ended up causing me to go to urgent care for a bronchial infection—something I could have avoided had I been able to go to the doctor without worry.

Still thinking I could manage on my own, life had other plans and I got in a serious car accident. My car was totaled and, because it had flipped over, paramedics forced me to take an ambulance ride to the nearest hospital. After running tests, the doctors determined that I was fine. Although I was very lucky to walk away from the accident with nothing more than a sore back, my lack of health insurance coverage impacted me negatively. Although my car insurance provider covered the hospital visit, it refused to cover my ambulance ride. This ended up costing me over $1,000, and I was soon dealing with aggressive debt collectors. The worst part about my story is knowing that this ambulance ride was relatively *cheap compared to what many young people in my situation have gone through.*

First person perspective vignette collected and created by D. Howe, 2020.

For your consideration: Mr. J. describes a time when he didn't have health insurance. Like many others without health insurance coverage, Mr. J. avoided going to the doctor or seeking routine care and also tried to "tough it out" in times of illness. Access issues to medical care are common when someone doesn't have health insurance. Are there any services available that Mr. J. could have used in order to get the healthcare he needed during times of illness? What about for yearly check-ups when he isn't sick? Have you ever known someone without health insurance? Did they also have access issues to healthcare services?

-- -- -- -- -- -- -- -- -- -- -- -- -- -- -- -- --

According to Cohen et al. (2019), 2018 National Health Interview Survey (NHIS) data from HHS and the CDC reveal that 30.4 million **civilian** individuals (9.4% of the noninstitutionalized population) were without health insurance coverage at the time of the interview, and this result shows a decrease in the uninsured over the last eight years. It is important to note that statistics may vary slightly depending on which data are used. Berchick et al. (2019) provide statistics from two U.S. Census Bureau surveys—data retrieved from a nationwide survey from the U.S. Department of Commerce, the Current Population Survey Annual Social and Economic Supplement (CPS ASEC); and a state-based survey, the American Community Survey (ACS). Berchick et al. report 27.5 million persons without health insurance, 8.5% of the total noninstitutionalized population in 2018 (compared to 9.4% from Cohen et al., 2019). Berchick et al. report this as a slight increase of uninsured persons from 2017. Over two-thirds of the insured population had private health insurance, while the rest of those insured were covered by public health insurance (Medicare or Medicaid) (Cohen et al., 2019). Other interesting and important data obtained in the NHIS 2018 survey among age groups are as follows:

- Ages 0-17 years: 5.2% were uninsured, 41.8% had Medicaid or Medicare, and 54.7% had private insurance
- Ages 18-64: 13.3% were uninsured; 19.4% had Medicaid or Medicare; and 68.9% (136.6 million) had private insurance
- Ages 25-34: the age group that lacked health insurance the most in 2018. Only 17% of individuals had a form of health insurance (Cohen et al., 2019).

At first glance, the number of children uninsured is alarming, when considering most children are eligible for insurance from federal or state funds. Berchick et al. (2019) found that the children without insurance were most likely to be from families with income categories of at or above 400% of poverty income level. Although findings were nonsignificant, the data thus indicates that most uninsured children live in high-income families, families possibly without any insurance for any family member. Two statistically-significant findings by Berchick et al. were that more uninsured children lived in the South and were of Hispanic descent. This is congruent with the NHIS 2018 findings that the racial characteristics of uninsured children reveal the least likely to be insured were Hispanic children (7.7%); followed by non-Hispanic whites (4.1%); non-Hispanic Blacks (4.0%); and non-Hispanic Asian (3.8%) children (NCHS, 2019) (Figure 8.2).

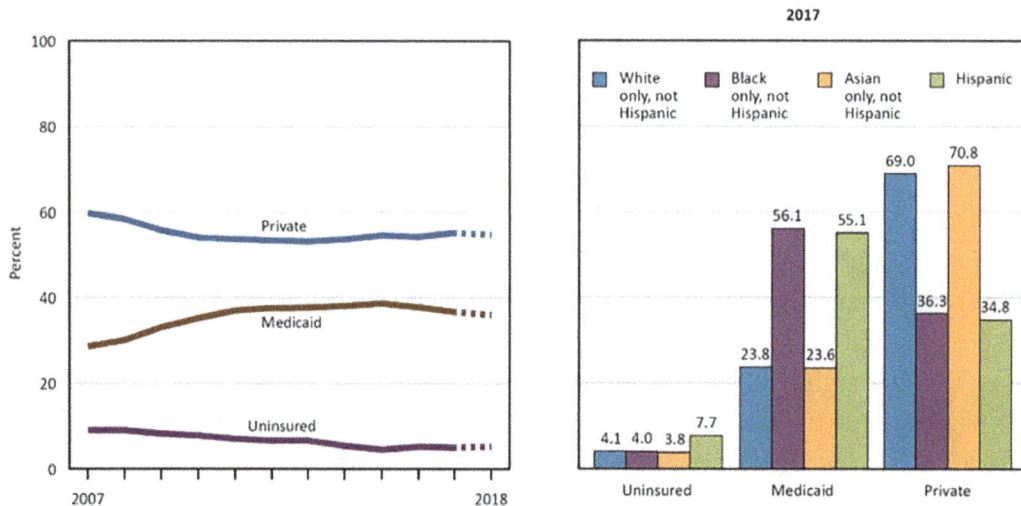

Figure 8.2: Health Insurance Coverage Among Children Under Age 18 Years, By Type of Coverage and Race and Hispanic Origin: United States, 2007–2018 (Preliminary Data).

NOTES: Estimates for 2018 are preliminary and are shown with a dashed line. Health insurance categories are mutually exclusive. A small percentage of children are covered by Medicare, military plans, or other plans. Estimates for this group are not presented.
Source: Health, United States 2018
Attribution: U.S. Department of Health and Human Services
License: Public Domain

Probably not surprisingly, the largest age group lacking health insurance in the U.S. is the age group 25-34 years, most of whom are no longer covered by their parent's insurance. This age group may be graduating from college and having difficulty finding full-time employment. Berchick et al. (2019) found that those working less than full-time and/or less than year-round were more likely to be uninsured.

For all adults, those of Hispanic origin were the most likely to be uninsured, followed by Blacks, Whites, and then Asians (NCHS, 2019). Data was not provided concerning legal citizenship. Importantly, health-wise, the NIHS (NCHS) discovered Hispanic persons had the highest rate of diabetes. See Figure 8.3 below for health insurance coverage for adults aged 18-64 and ethnicity.

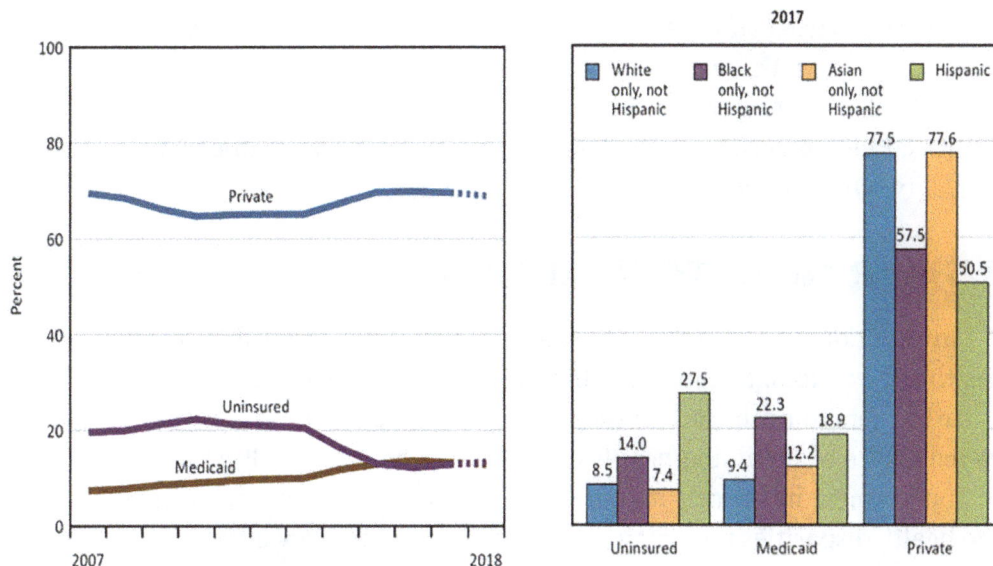

Figure 8.3: Health Insurance Coverage Among Adults Aged 18–64, By Type of Coverage and Race and Hispanic Origin: United States, 2007–2018 (Preliminary Data).

NOTES: Estimates for 2018 are preliminary and are shown with a dashed line. Health insurance categories are mutually exclusive. A small percentage of people are covered by Medicare, military plans, or other plans. Estimates for this group are not presented.
Source: Health, United States 2018
Attribution: U.S. Department of Health and Human Services
License: Public Domain

8.4.2 Obtaining Needed Services Within an Accessible Location

There is a shortage of primary care physicians throughout the U.S. Numbers of advanced practice professionals (best known as advanced practice providers, but sometimes also called physician extenders)—nurse practitioners and physician assistants—are increasing throughout the nation. Yet, at the present time, primary care services may not be available in many locations. Obtaining specialty services may not be available either. Important to note is that many locations offer public health departments or community health services. Having a healthcare provider or healthcare services in close proximity is essential for individuals to receive the appropriate care when healthcare is needed and in a timely manner. Moreover, **equitable care** with improved health outcomes and reduced healthcare costs occurs when individuals have healthcare services provided and utilized on a regular basis (Office of Disease Prevention and Health Promotion [ODPHP], 2019a).

8.4.3 Finding the Right Patient-Provider Relationship Where Communication, Mutual Trust and Respect are Obtained

Having a healthcare provider who demonstrates caring behaviors and attitudes is important in a healthcare provider-patient relationship. Caring is shown when there is respect and a non-judgmental attitude towards someone regardless of the individual's culture, race, religion, ethnicity, gender, age, or disability. Caring and respect lead to trust and open communication. Trust and open communication lead to increased **health-seeking behaviors** and eventually lower healthcare costs due to decreased emergency room and outpatient clinic visits (ODPHP, 2019a). Improved health-seeking behaviors also lead to a decrease in chronic illness and mortality (ODPHP, 2019a).

8.5 BARRIERS TO HEALTHCARE

In addition to lack of health insurance, lack of accessible and appropriate healthcare services, and inability to find the "right" healthcare provider, there are other barriers to healthcare in the U.S. Inadequate health insurance, not having a "usual" place of obtaining healthcare, the high costs of healthcare, not obtaining an appointment in a timely manner, having a language barrier, low health literacy, and health disparities for certain parts of the population are all barriers to receiving adequate healthcare and are discussed next. Factors that may influence these barriers are also discussed.

8.5.1 High Cost of Healthcare

As technology continues to evolve and improve, quicker and more reliable diagnostic tests are available, as well as more efficient medications with fewer side effects, all of which increases the costs of healthcare. Governmental health plans and many insurance plans are slow to approve and pay for new technology, including diagnostic tests, medications, and equipment. Physicians, however, order the most up-to-date diagnostic tests, medications, and equipment which they feel will help patients or improve their health. Often, patients need to take several medications to combat their disease processes. For example, it is not uncommon for persons with high blood pressure to be on three different medications to maintain a normal blood pressure. Kirzinger et al. (2019) found that individuals who have the most difficulty affording their prescription medications are taking four or more prescription medications; spending $100 or more per month on medications; are in the 50–64 year old age range; describe themselves in either fair or poor health; and have an income less than $40,000 annually. Obviously, having to pay exorbitant costs for medications may prevent individuals from receiving the healthcare they need. These findings may indicate that individuals who are aging— but not old enough for Medicare—and who are possibly in the lower income levels may be developing chronic illnesses in their younger years of age.

Examining similar information as the Kirzinger report, the federal government's latest data concerning delay or nonreceipt of healthcare are found in the 2017 National Health Interview Survey (NHIS) (NCHS, 2019, Trend Table 29) where 320,182 individuals (adults or an adult speaking for a child in the home) were interviewed concerning delay or nonreceipt of needed medical care due to cost, nonreceipt of needed prescription drugs due to cost, and nonreceipt of needed dental care due to cost. Results from the 2017 survey were compared to results from 1997, 2005, and 2010. In 2017, 7.4% of respondents stated they delayed or did not receive needed medical care due to costs. This percentage was the lowest percentage in the 10- year recorded period. Of those responding to the question about not receiving needed prescription drugs due to cost, 5.1% stated they had not received medications as needed. Only the year 1997 was lowest, with 4.8% not receiving medications due to cost. Of those responding that they didn't receive needed dental care due to cost, 9.5% agreed that they had not received dental care. Again, this was the second lowest percentage, with 8.6% responding in 1997 that this was a problem. Although these are relatively small percentages, the goal is that no one delays or doesn't receive medical care when needed.

8.5.2 Health Insurance Costs and the Relationship to Access

Costs associated with health insurance, such as high deductibles, copays, and out-of-pocket expenses, can be a barrier to healthcare. Many individuals have private insurance with **high deductibles**, some employer-based and some individually purchased. The U.S. Centers for Medicare and Medicaid Services (U.S. CMS, n.d.) define a high deductible health plan as "a plan with a higher deductible than a traditional insurance plan" (para. 1). With a high deductible plan, the monthly premiums are lower, but the beneficiary pays a large amount of the healthcare costs before the insurance company pays for any of the healthcare costs. "For 2020, the IRS defines a high deductible health plan as any plan with a deductible of at least $1400 for an individual or $2800 for a family" and limits "total yearly out-of- pocket expenses (deductibles, copayments, and coinsurance) to $6,900 for an individual or $13,800 for a family," if using in-network services only (receiving services outside of the insurance's approved providers would result in higher costs to the individual and/or family) (U.S. CMS, n.d., para 3).

The 2018 National Health Interview Survey (NHIS) indicated that the numbers of individuals with high deductible health plans increased from 43.7% in 2017 to 45.8% in 2018 for persons under the age of 65 (Cohen et al., 2019). Moreover, according to Kirzinger et al. (2019), surmising the results of several Kaiser Family Foundation (KFF) healthcare tracking polls suggested that about one-fourth of insured workers were required to pay an increased deductible averaging 212% over the last decade, resulting in an approximate deductible of $2000 or more for a single person.

Having a high deductible where out of pocket costs must be paid prior to the insurance covering prescription drugs or medical costs may deter individuals from seeking healthcare. Kirzinger et al. (2019) described one KFF 2018 poll where results indicated that 34% of insured adults found it difficult to pay health insurance deductibles, 28% found it difficult to pay monthly premiums for health insurance, and 24% found it difficult to pay the co-pays for health-related costs, such as visits to a physician's office and prescription medications. Another KFF poll, performed in 2017, (Kirzinger et al., 2019), presented a scenario to those with employee-sponsored insurance (ESI) asking them if they had to pay $500 of an unexpected healthcare bill, would they be able to pay the bill. Fifty-nine percent said they would be able to pay the bill at the time of service, whereas 34% said they would not and would need to use a credit card, borrow money, or not be able to pay it at all. The results of this 2017 poll is depicted in Figure 8.4.

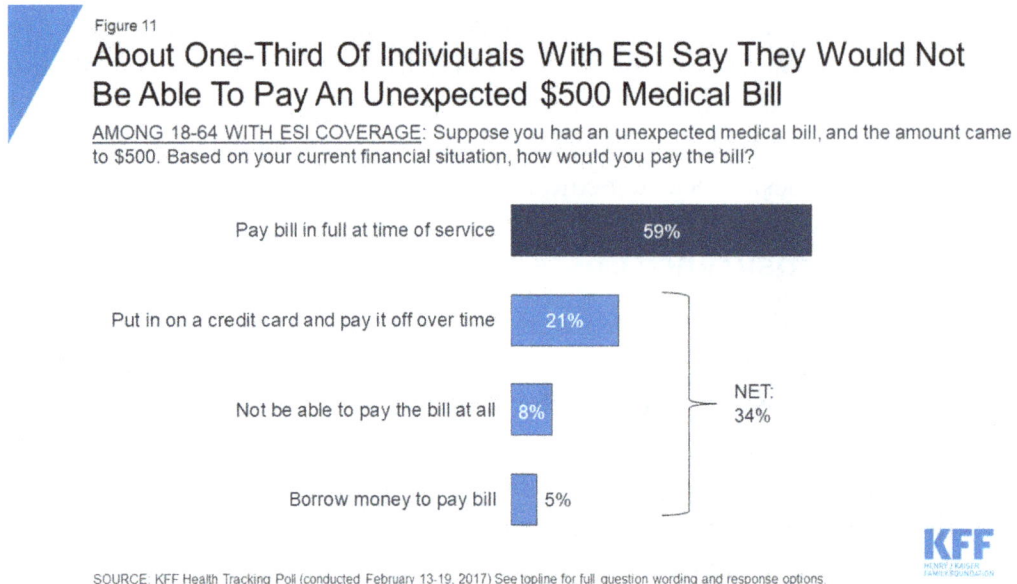

Figure 11

About One-Third Of Individuals With ESI Say They Would Not Be Able To Pay An Unexpected $500 Medical Bill

AMONG 18-64 WITH ESI COVERAGE: Suppose you had an unexpected medical bill, and the amount came to $500. Based on your current financial situation, how would you pay the bill?

Pay bill in full at time of service	59%
Put in on a credit card and pay it off over time	21%
Not be able to pay the bill at all	8%
Borrow money to pay bill	5%

NET: 34%

KFF
HENRY J KAISER
FAMILY FOUNDATION

SOURCE: KFF Health Tracking Poll (conducted February 13-19, 2017) See topline for full question wording and response options.

Figure 8.4: About One-Third of Individuals with ESI say They Would Not be Able to Pay an Unexpected $500 Medical Bill

Source: Kaiser Family Foundation
Attribution: Kaiser Family Foundation
License: © Kaiser Family Foundation. Used with permission.

For those with public health insurance (Medicare or Medicaid), Medicaid does not pay hospitals or physicians the same rate as Medicare. Medicare does not pay the same as most private health insurance plans. Original Medicare does not provide the supplemental benefits that Medicare Advantage does. Medicare Part D has cost limits for medications. Therefore, one may have insurance, but the insurance may not be enough to obtain needed services or may not pay sufficiently to prevent exorbitant costs to the individual. Moreover, healthcare providers cannot depend on third parties to reliably provide any, or even some, form of payments (Elrod & Fortenberry, 2017).

8.5.3 Not Having a "Usual" Place to Obtain Healthcare

One of the questions on the 2018 National Health Interview Survey (NHIS) asked whether interviewees (249,456 individuals 18 years and older) had a usual place of healthcare (Cohen et al., 2019). Having a **usual place of obtaining healthcare** often involves having an easily accessible location with appropriate services provided and development of a rapport with caregivers. Interview results indicate that among adults aged 18 and over, 85% have a usual place of healthcare. The most often-cited place for healthcare was a doctor's office or HMO (69.7%), followed by clinic or health center (26.1%), hospital outpatient department (1.5%), hospital emergency room (1.4%), and some other place (1.3%). Specific variables that may affect having a usual place of healthcare identified in the 2018 NHIS are gender, race and ethnicity, education, employment, poverty level, and not having insurance. See results of these variables from the 2018 NHIS (CDC, n.d.) in Table 8.1.

Table 8.1: CDC Summary Health Statistics: National Health Interview Survey, 2018, Adults 18 and Over	
Do you have a usual place of obtaining healthcare: Yes or No?	
Yes	85%
No	15%
Race/ethnicity and gender combined	**Percentage having a usual place of healthcare**
White females	90.8%
Black female	88.8%
Hispanic or Latino female	84.9%
White male	83.6%
Black male	81.9%
Hispanic or Latino males	73.9%
Education level	**Percentage having a usual place of healthcare**
Bachelor's degree or higher	90.1%
No high school diploma	79.1%
Current Employment	**Percentage having a usual place of healthcare**
Have worked full-time; may be unemployed at this time	85.6%
Work part-time	83.8%
Poverty status	**Percentage having a usual place of healthcare**
Below poverty threshold	79.6%
Near poor (income 100% to less than 200% of poverty level)	79.7%
Not poor (incomes higher than 200% of poverty threshold or greater)	87.8%

Uninsured	Percentage having a usual place of healthcare
Yes	51.5%
No	48.5%

8.5.4 Timeliness of Obtaining an Appointment or Treatment

Sometimes individuals cannot receive an appointment with a healthcare provider as quickly as needed or desired. This causes a delay in treatment and possible worsening of symptoms. Many individuals end up in the emergency department or outpatient clinic, and higher costs may be incurred or poorer health outcomes may result from delays. Long waits in physician's offices or in emergency departments is another barrier to healthcare (Office of Disease Prevention and Health Promotion [IDPHP], 2019a). Patients may leave without being seen if the wait is long, thus delaying care further. Patient dissatisfaction may occur also. Often, tests are ordered and there is a delay in obtaining those services. The delay may lead to distraught feelings, development or extension of complications requiring hospitalization and possible poor health outcomes, and likely increased costs (ODPHP, 2019a).

8.5.5 Language Barrier

The number of individuals in the U.S. with English as a second language is increasing (Meuter et al. 2015), posing a language barrier issue between non-English speaking patients and healthcare workers. A language barrier prevents ideal communication between the patient and the healthcare provider, with possible errors in assessment of problems, services rendered, and in care instructions. A lack of culturally-competent care may also be present if the healthcare provider is not aware of, or chooses not to be aware of, cultural differences that affect the communication between patient and healthcare provider. A lack of culturally-competent care may lead to inequitable care for those who cannot speak English fluently (Meuter et al., 2015).

Pause and Reflect

How might a language barrier affect seeking healthcare? Consider if you were visiting a different country whose people speak a different language. What if you become ill? How would you find healthcare? How would you communicate the problem?

8.5.6 Health Literacy

The official definition of **health literacy** from the HHS (2020b) is "the degree to which individuals have the capacity to obtain, process, and understand basic health information needed to make appropriate health decisions" (para. 1). Navigating the healthcare system may be difficult if an individual is not aware of what steps need to be taken and where to go for assistance. Without health literacy skills, individuals do not have the knowledge of where and how to obtain healthcare services or navigate the complex U.S. healthcare system. Reading and comprehending health resources may be a challenge.

The World Health Organization (WHO) (1998) characterizes health literacy as overall encompassing of what is needed for healthcare services to be accessed and utilized by an individual: health literacy implies the achievement of a level of knowledge, personal skills and confidence to take action to improve personal and community health by changing personal lifestyles and living conditions. Thus, health literacy means more than being able to read pamphlets and make appointments. By improving people's access to health information—and their capacity to use it effectively—health literacy is critical to empowerment.

Health literacy itself depends upon more general levels of literacy. Poor literacy can affect people's health directly by limiting their personal, social, and cultural development, as well as hindering the development of health literacy (p. 10). In addition, making healthcare decisions and taking responsibility for self-care are also concerns for those who have low health literacy skills (CDC, 2019j).

According to Hickey et al. (2018), characteristics associated with low health literacy are those with lower income levels, limited education, chronic diseases, older age, and non-native English speakers (p. 49). Significantly, however, healthcare providers may not be able to tell from looking at a person which level health literacy they have. Therefore, it is important to assume every patient needs careful instruction and an assessment of understanding because lower health literacy levels can adversely affect healthcare-seeking behaviors, such as understanding of instructions, importance of following directions, and follow-up care.

The Agency for Healthcare Research and Quality (2015) encourages healthcare organizations to develop quality improvement measures to make information simple to comprehend and healthcare systems easy to maneuver. Hickey et al. (2018), recommend incorporating health literacy into the standard clinical care for all patients. Some easy suggestions include the following:

- Use *plain language*—organize the information, break up complex information, define technical or medical terms with simple language

- Use *visual aids*—illustrations, simple drawings, clear labels

- Use *technology*—patient portals, telemedicine, mobile apps

- Use *effective teaching methods*—open-ended questions, "teach-back" communication method, "show back" to demonstrate skills (ACP, 2019)

> **Pause and Reflect**
>
> A non-native English speaker is about to be discharged from the hospital following surgical removal of the appendix. The nurse comes into the room and discusses the need for proper care of the surgical wound, to continue taking all the antibiotic medications provided, and to call the primary doctor if there are any complications (excess pain, fever, draining from surgical site). The nurse asks if the patient understands the directions and they nod their head in the affirmative. The patient is asked to sign the form, given the written discharge instructions, and discharged to home. In this scenario, how do we know the patient understood the instructions?

8.5.7 Health Disparities

Orgera and Artiga (2018) define health and **healthcare disparities** as "differences in health and healthcare between population groups" (para. 1). Various factors, such socioeconomic status, race, ethnicity, gender, sexual orientation, age, disability status, and regions of the nation, may affect the care individuals receive. We have already discussed reasons an individual may not seek healthcare and/or delay care and the costs associated with health insurance. Arguably, some variables consistently indicate there are some groups who receive less healthcare. The U.S. Office of Disease Prevention and Health Promotion (ODPHP, 2019a) states that those in a lower socioeconomic status receive less healthcare. And many persons in the poor and near-poor categories, according to the research presented here, delay healthcare or have difficulty with the costs of healthcare. One should note that many poor do receive Medicaid. However, as stated previously, Medicaid may not be accepted by all physicians.

Delving deeper into the unmet healthcare needs of persons based on poverty levels, the NCHS (2019) compared unmet (delayed or received) healthcare needs due to costs in persons based on national poverty levels from 2017 to results obtained in 2007 (based on data from the 2017 NHIS previously discussed). The poverty levels compared were the same as previously discussed elsewhere (below poverty level; nearly poor: 100–199% of poverty level) except two groups of not-poor were established: the first group of not-poor lived at 200–399% of the poverty level, and the next group of not-poor lived at or above 400% of the poverty level. Results indicated that although there has been improvement in meeting the medical needs in all groups since 2007, a divide remains between the percentage of unmet medical needs of the poor and those in the not-poor groups because of costs. Thus, those in the poor groups have unmet healthcare needs, and, as greater levels of poverty were identified, the discrepancy increased incrementally.

The NCHS (2019) also interviewed these same individuals in the 18–64 age group to determine if they received needed prescription medications. Again, despite the vast improvements in the last decade, there remains a difference in the poor, near-poor, and not-poor categories (Figure 8.5).

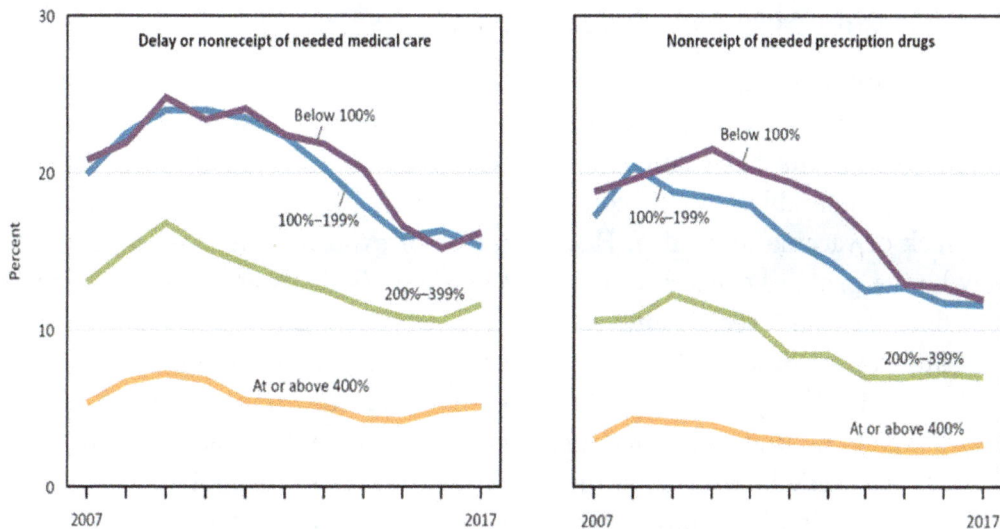

Figure 8.5: Delay or Nonreceipt of Needed Medical Care and Nonreceipt of Needed Prescription Drugs in the Past 12 Months Due to Cost Among Adults Aged 18–64, By Percent of Poverty Level: United States, 2007–2017

Source: Health, United States 2018
Attribution: U.S. Department of Health and Human Services
License: Public Domain

8.5.8 Geographic Location

Geographic location is another factor that may affect whether individuals receive healthcare (NCHS, 2019). Individuals in rural areas receive less healthcare access and utilization than those in urban areas. Of all children aged 19–35 months in the U.S. in 2017, 29.6% did not receive adequate vaccination coverage. Children living in rural areas received the appropriate vaccination less than their urban counterparts (66.8% compared to 71.9%, respectively) (NCHS) (Figure 8.6).

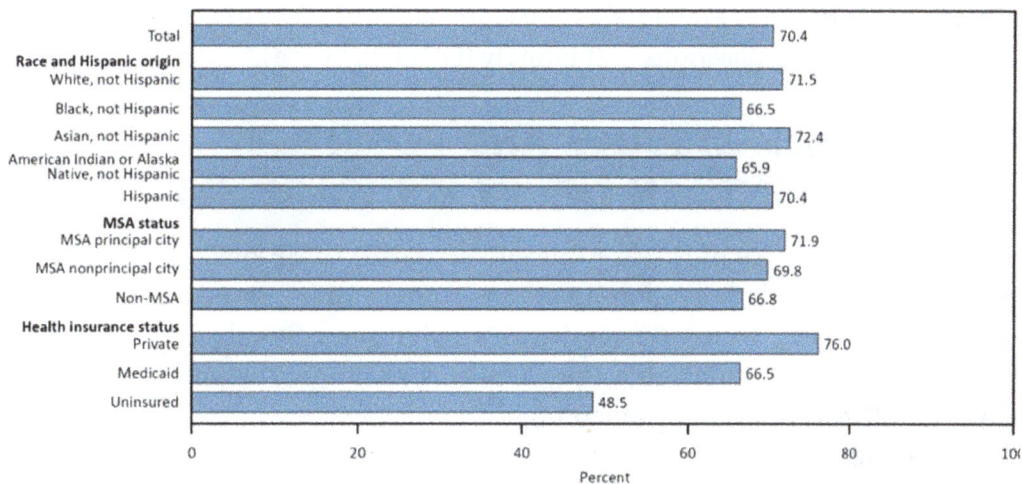

Figure 8.6: Vaccination Coverage for Combined Series Among Children Aged 19–35 Months, By Selected Characteristics: United States, 2017.

NOTES: MSA is a metropolitan statistical area.
Source: Health, United States 2018
Attribution: U.S. Department of Health and Human Services
License: Public Domain

8.5.9 Health Access for Illegal Immigrants

Many variables have already been discussed about why different persons or populations delay seeking healthcare or possibly receive inadequate healthcare. Illegal immigrants have unique health concerns as they may be mentally and physically vulnerable. Specific concerns for this population may be sex trafficking and lack of vaccinations, also. However, fear of exposing their residency status may be the primary concern of undocumented individuals and may explain why they delay or do not seek healthcare.

Language or other cultural barriers may be an issue when receiving needed healthcare for this population. Only some communities have clinics to address health needs of undocumented persons seeking care and include translation services as needed. Also, some health departments are available that provide childhood vaccinations and other health education services to undocumented families. For emergency situations, individuals could seek care in emergency rooms. Regardless of the legality of citizenship, no person is turned down in the U.S. emergency departments for healthcare.

8.6 CONSEQUENCES OF INADEQUATE ACCESS TO HEALTHCARE

Individuals without access to healthcare overall, are likely to have poorer health and quality of life (Office of Disease Prevention and Health Promotion, 2019a). Individuals without access to healthcare are more likely to encounter increased healthcare costs to self and family and to society (ODPHP, 2019a). They are less likely to participate in preventive health measures and obtain needed healthcare services in a timely manner (ODPHP, 2019a). They are more likely to seek healthcare in emergency departments and outpatient clinics and be hospitalized for avoidable illnesses (ODPHP, 2019a). And, they are more likely to live with chronic conditions and succumb to complications prematurely (ODPHP, 2019a).

8.7 EMERGING ISSUES AND POSSIBLE IMPROVEMENTS IN THE HEALTHCARE SYSTEM

Through the Office of Disease Prevention and Health Promotion, the federal government each decade develops initiatives striving for improved health for every American (ODPHP, 2020). Currently, Healthy People 2030 objectives are being formulated, while the 2020 objectives are being analyzed. The public may attend any committee meeting. Other emerging noteworthy issues are the COVID-19 virus, illegal immigration, numbers and availability of healthcare providers and work models used, telehealth, and lack of use of evidence-based preventive services.

8.7.1 Healthy People 2020

The Healthy People 2020 objectives (ODPHP, 2019b) and corresponding findings are as follows:

- Increase the proportion of persons with health insurance.

    ◇ 2020 Goal: 100% (83.2% in 2008) (90.6% in 2018 [Cohen et al., 2019])

- Increase the number of persons with a usual primary care provider.

    ◇ 2020 Goal: 83.9% (76.3% in 2007) (85.4% in 2018 [Cohen et al., 2019])

- (Developmental) Increase the number of practicing primary care providers.

- Increase the proportion of persons who have a specific source of ongoing care.

    ◇ 2020 Goal: 95% (86.4% in 2008)

- Reduce the proportion of persons who are unable to obtain or who delay in obtaining necessary medical care, dental care, or prescription medicines.

    ◇ 2020 Goal: 4.2% (4.7% in 2007) (4.4% did not receive medical care due to cost, and 6.3% delayed seeking medical care in 2018 [Cohen et al.); 11.9% did not receive their prescription medicines in 2017 (NCHS, 2019)

- (Developmental) Increase the proportion of persons who receive appropriate evidence-based clinical preventive services.

- (Developmental) Increase the proportion of persons who have access to rapidly-responding prehospital emergency medical services.

- Reduce the proportion of hospital emergency department visits in which the wait time to see an emergency department clinician exceeds the recommended time frame.

8.7.2 Numbers and Availability of Healthcare Providers and Work Models Used

Shortages of healthcare providers, specifically primary care providers, will continue (Institute of Medicine, 2015). New methods of scheduling patients and utilizing resources may need to be addressed. Better utilization of resources might meet the access needs and reduce delays in care. The Institute of Medicine (IOM) describes one issue with access due to a supply-demand mismatch: scheduling and wait times. Any imbalance, or mismatch, with what is needed in terms of healthcare services and what is available in terms of those services results in delays in receiving care and may cause patients to not seek healthcare services or seek services elsewhere. Other issues may be office culture, operational inefficiencies and inadequate or underuse of resources (IOM, 2015).

All healthcare providers need to switch to a patient-centered approach to care as opposed to the provider-centered method of the past (IOM, 2015). A patient-centered approach may mean having providers available for walk-in appointments—where the patients don't have to have an appointment—as done in retail clinics. Providers scheduling later office hours and weekends so that individuals might be able to see their regular healthcare provider also promotes a patient-centered approach.

National benchmarks should be evaluated by practitioners to help identify factors that would more closely align their practice with patient-centered care and respect for patients' time. One benchmark offered by the IOM (2015) is evaluating wait times for all healthcare provider's office visits. The IOM also suggests evaluating driving times for patients to doctor's visits.

8.7.3 Telehealth Increasing Access to Care

Telehealth (communication through phone or video), also known as **telemedicine**, may be a useful resource in a physician practice. According to the IOM (2015), up to 25% of patients call the physician's office on any given day, and the use of telehealth could curtail an office visit. Utilizing nurses and advanced-practice professionals to help with providing care, health teaching and preventive management, informatics managers, and coordinators of care should be evaluated.

The COVID-19 outbreak may have changed telehealth forever. The Centers for Medicare and Medicaid (CMS) have relaxed the rules for payment to healthcare providers during the COVID-19 pandemic. Telehealth waivers (for both video and phone) from CMS during this national crisis include allowing healthcare providers to perform telehealth visits in rural and non-rural areas, cross state lines, care for established and non-established patients, and bill the same as if the visit were in person (HHS, 2020). Also covered are emergency department visits, initial nursing facility and discharge visits, home visits, and therapy visits. Federally Qualified Health Centers and Rural Health Clinics have also been added to provide telehealth sites at a distance or to arrange telehealth services for those unable to travel (HHS, 2020), thereby possibly reaching those who are disadvantaged. With the use of telehealth expansion, especially for Federally Qualified Health Centers and Rural Health Clinics during COVID-19, hopefully payment for these services can continue so that all persons can easily access a healthcare provider and in a timely manner.

8.8 SUMMARY

This chapter discussed variables and statistics related to access to healthcare, barriers of access and utilization of healthcare services, problems associated with lack of access, and possible measures going forward. Considering the statistics provided, the factors associated with increased access to healthcare, seeking care when needed, and not delaying seeking healthcare are: higher educational levels, higher family income levels, and having healthcare insurance. Whether other variables affect health and better outcomes is debatable, considering the statistics provided, and should continue to be evaluated. Perhaps healthcare providers need education and training to identify their own biases to ensure equitable care for all racial and ethnic cultures.

8.9 REVIEW QUESTIONS

1. What does access to healthcare mean?
2. Discuss three barriers to adequate healthcare.
3. What does it mean to be health literate?
4. Describe two specific ways to improve access to healthcare.

8.10 REFERENCES

Advance Care Planning (ACP). (2019, September). Four simple strategies for improving your patient's health literacy. Retrieved from https://acpdecisions.org/four-simple-strategies-for-improving-your-patients-health-literacy/#:~:text=An%20important%20strategy%20for%20improving,find%20to%20meet%20their%20needs

Agency for Healthcare Research and Quality. (2015). Create a health improvement literacy plan: Tool #2. Retrieved from https://www.ahrq.gov/health-literacy/quality-resources/tools/literacy-toolkit/healthlittoolkit2-tool2.html

Berchick, E. R., Barnett, J. C., & Upton, R. D. (2019, November). Health insurance coverage in the United States: 2018, Current population report, P60-267 (RV). U.S Department of Commerce, U.S. Census Bureau. Retrieved from census.gov.

Casida, J. M. (2018). Low health literacy. Implications for managing cardiac patients in practice. Nurse Practitioner, 43(8); 49-55. DOI: 10.1097/01.NPR.0000541468.54290.49

Centers for Disease Control and Prevention (CDC). (2020a). Coronavirus disease 2019 (COVID-19). https://www.cdc.gov/coronavirus/2019-ncov/cases-updates/cases-in-us.html

Centers for Disease Control and Prevention (CDC). (2020b). CDC COVID data tracker. United States forecasting. Retrieved from https://covid.cdc.gov/covid-data-tracker/?CDC_AA_refVal=https%3A%2F%2Fwww.cdc.gov%2Fcoronavirus%2F2019-ncov%2Fcases-updates%2Fcases-in-us.html#forecasting

Centers for Disease Control and Prevention (CDC). (2020b). Coronavirus disease 2019 (COVID-19): People who are at higher risk for severe illness. Retrieved from https://www.cdc.gov/coronavirus/2019-ncov/need-extra-precautions/index.html

Centers for Disease Control and Prevention (CDC). (2020c, October). Provisional death counts for Coronavirus disease (COVID-19): Distribution of deaths by race and Hispanic origin. Retrieved from https://data.cdc.gov/NCHS/Provisional-Death-Counts-for-Coronavirus-Disease-C/pj7m-y5uh

Centers for Disease Control and Prevention (CDC). (2020d, May). Provisional death counts for Coronavirus disease (COVID-19): Weekly state-specific data updates. Retrieved from https://data.cdc.gov/d/pj7m-y5uh/visualization

Centers for Disease Control and Prevention (CDC). (2020e). Weekly updates by select demographic and geographic characteristics: Co-morbidities Retrieved from https://www.cdc.gov/nchs/nvss/vsrr/covid_weekly/index.htm#Comorbidities

Centers for Disease Control and Prevention (CDC) (n.d.). Summary health statistics: National health interview survey, 2018. Retrieved from https://ftp.cdc.gov/pub/Health_Statistics/NCHS/NHIS/SHS/2018_SHS_Table_A-16.pdf

Cohen, R. A., Terlizzi, E. P., & Martinex, M. E. (2019). Health insurance coverage: Early release of estimates from the National Health Interview Survey, 2018. National Center for Health Statistics. Retrieved from https://www.cdc.gov/nchs/nhis/releases.htm

Ducharme, J. (2020, March 11). World Health Organization declares COVID-19 a 'Pandemic': Here's what that means. Times. Retrieved from https://time.com/5791661/who-coronavirus-pandemic-declaration/

Elrod, J. K., & Fortenberry, J. L., Jr. (2017). Bridging access gaps experienced by the underserved: The need for health care providers to look within for answers. BioMed Central Health Services Research, 17(Suppl 4):791, pp 37–41. DOI 10.1186/s12913-017-2756-4.

Hickey, K. T., Creber, R. M., Reading, M., Sciacca, R. R., Riga, T. C., Frulla, A. P., & Institute of Medicine (IOM). (2015). Transforming health care scheduling and access. Washington, DC: The national academies press. https://doi.org/10.17226/20220

Institute of Medicine (IOM). (1993). Access to health care in America. Washington, D.C.: National academies press. https://doi.org/10.17226/2009

Johns Hopkins University. (2020, October 8). COVID-19 dashboard by the Center for Systems Science and Engineering (CSSE) at Johns Hopkins University (JHU). Retrieved from https://coronavirus.jhu.edu/map.html

Kirzinger, A., Munana, C., Wu, B., & Brodie, M. (2019, June 11). Data note: Americans' challenges with health care costs. Kaiser Family Foundation. Retrieved from https://www.kff.org/health-costs/issue-brief/data-note-americans-challenges-health-care-costs/

Mayo Clinic. (2020, October 8). Coronavirus disease 2019 (COVID-19): Overview. Retrieved from https://www.mayoclinic.org/diseases-conditions/coronavirus/symptoms-causes/syc-20479963

Meuter, R. F., Gallois, C., Segalowitz, N. S., Ryder, A. G., & Hocking, J. (2015). Overcoming language barriers in health care: A protocol for investigating safe and effective communication when patients or clinicians use a second language. BioMed Central Health Services Research, 15 (371). DOI: 10.1186/s12913-015-1024-8.

National Center for Health Statistics (NCHS). (2019). Health, United States, 2018. Hyattsville, MD. Retrieved from https://www.cdc.gov/nchs/data/hus/hus18.pdf

Office of Disease Prevention and Health Promotion (ODPHP). (2020). Development of the national health promotion and disease prevention objectives for 2030. Retrieved from https://www.healthypeople.gov/2020/About-Healthy-People/Development-Healthy-People-2030

Office of Disease Prevention and Health Promotion (ODPHP). (2019a). Access to health services. Retrieved from https://www.healthypeople.gov/2020/topics-objectives/topic/Access-to-Health-Services

Office of Disease Prevention and Health Promotion (ODPHP). (2019b). Access to health services: Objectives. Retrieved from https://www.healthypeople.gov/2020/topics-objectives/topic/Access-to-Health-Services/objectives

Orgera, K. & Artig, S. (2018, August 8). Disparities in health and health care: Five key questions and answers. Kaiser Family Foundation. Retrieved from https://www.kff.org/disparities-policy/issue-brief/disparities-in-health-and-health-care-five-key-questions-and-answers/

Pew Research Center. (2019). U.S. unauthorized immigrant population estimates by state, 2016. Retrieved from https://www.pewresearch.org/hispanic/interactives/u-s-unauthorized-immigrants-by-state/

U.S. Center for Medicare and Medicaid Services (CMS). (n.d.). High deductible health plan. Retrieved from https://www.health care.gov/glossary/high-deductible-health-plan/

U.S. Department of Health & Human Services (HHS). (2020). Telehealth: Delivering care safely during COVID-19. Retrieved from https://www.hhs.gov/coronavirus/telehealth/index.html. Retrieved May 26, 2020.

U.S. Department of Homeland Security. (n.d.). Table 13. Refugee arrivals: Fiscal years 1980 to 2018. Yearbook of immigration statistics, 2018. Retrieved from https://www.dhs.gov/immigration-statistics/yearbook/2018/table13

World Health Organization (1998). Health promotion glossary. Retrieved from https://www.who.int/healthpromotion/about/HPR%20Glossary%201998.pdf?ua=1

9 Cost of Healthcare

9.1 LEARNING OBJECTIVES

By the end of this chapter, the student will be able to:

- Explain the five main factors associated with healthcare costs and their impact on the healthcare system
- Compare the cost of U.S. healthcare with other developed nations
- Compare physician salaries in the U.S. with physician salaries in other countries
- Explain possible ways pharmaceutical consumers can help decrease the cost of prescription drug costs
- Summarize how National Health Expenditure Accounts influence the cost of U.S. healthcare

9.2 KEY TERMS

- Choosing Wisely Campaign
- defensive medicine
- gross domestic product
- National Health Expenditure Accounts (NHEA)
- overutilization
- service price and intensity
- service utilization

9.3 INTRODUCTION

Much time and attention has been devoted to understanding healthcare and the impact on the U.S. economy. Healthcare spending, quality, and affordability are quite complex and can be difficult for many to understand. Americans typically pay much more for healthcare services than other developed countries, yet health outcomes are nearly the worst in all measured categories (Peter G. Peterson Foundation, 2020). Not surprisingly, healthcare costs in the U.S. can put a heavy financial burden on consumers. Even with healthcare coverage, many consumers are left wondering why the cost of healthcare is so high. According to Centers for Medicare & Medicaid Services (2020), national healthcare spending is expected to increase in the future. By 2028, projections are that national health spending will reach approximately $6.2 trillion (Centers for Medicare & Medicaid Services, 2020). This chapter will present information on the costs of healthcare in the U.S., and factors influencing these costs. Projected healthcare costs for the future are presented as well.

9.4 GROSS DOMESTIC PRODUCT AND HEALTHCARE

Gross domestic product (GDP) is defined as the comprehensive value of goods and services generated in a country (Bureau of Economic Analysis, 2020). The GDP is an indicator of the financial status of a country. GDP is usually reported in yearly increments and the healthcare costs as a percentage of the GDP have more than tripled from 1960 to today (Figure 9.1). In 2019, the U.S. gross domestic product was approximately 21,200 billion dollars (Trading Economics, 2020).

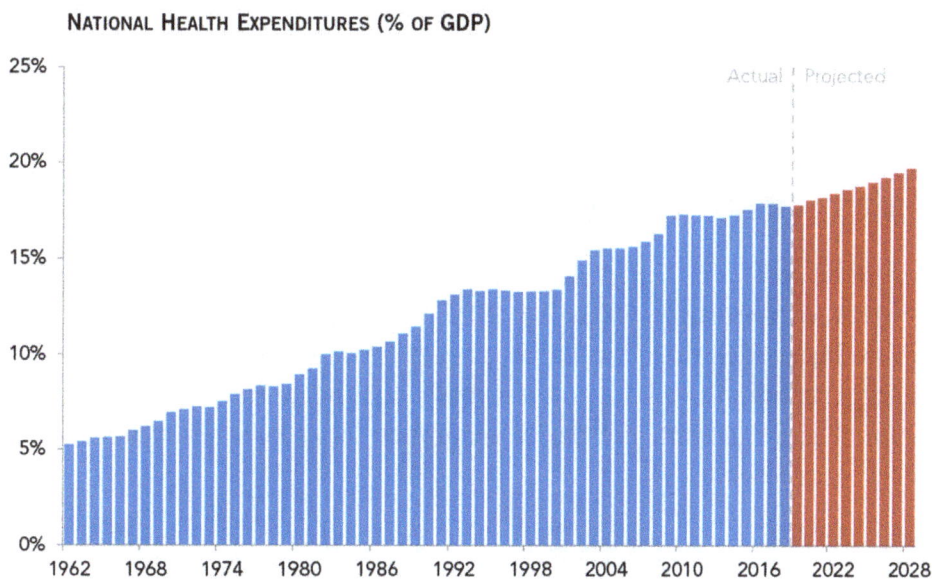

PETER G. PETERSON FOUNDATION — Healthcare costs in the United States have increased drastically over the past several decades

NATIONAL HEALTH EXPENDITURES (% OF GDP)

SOURCE: Centers for Medicare and Medicaid Services, *National Health Expenditure Data*, March 2020.
© 2020 Peter G. Peterson Foundation   PGPF.ORG

Figure 9.1: Healthcare Cost Increases and Projections

Source: Peter G. Peterson Foundation
Attribution: Peter G. Peterson Foundation
License: © Peter G. Peterson Foundation. Used with permission.

In 2019, the U.S. spent 18% of its gross domestic product (GDP) on healthcare (USAFacts, 2020). Moreover, the health share of the GDP is projected to increase to 19.4% by the year 2027 (Centers for Medicare & Medicaid Services, 2020). Although the U.S. healthcare spending is highest among ten other countries (Switzerland, Sweden, France, Germany, Netherlands, Canada, United Kingdom, New Zealand, Norway, and Australia), the overall health, access, and life expectancy in the U.S. are not reflective of the amount of healthcare spending (OECD, 2019). See Figure 9.2 for a comparison on healthcare spending in 2017 between top developed countries. According to Nunn et al. (2020), public spending by the U.S. is similar to percentages in other countries; it is the private spending in the U.S. which exceeds other countries.

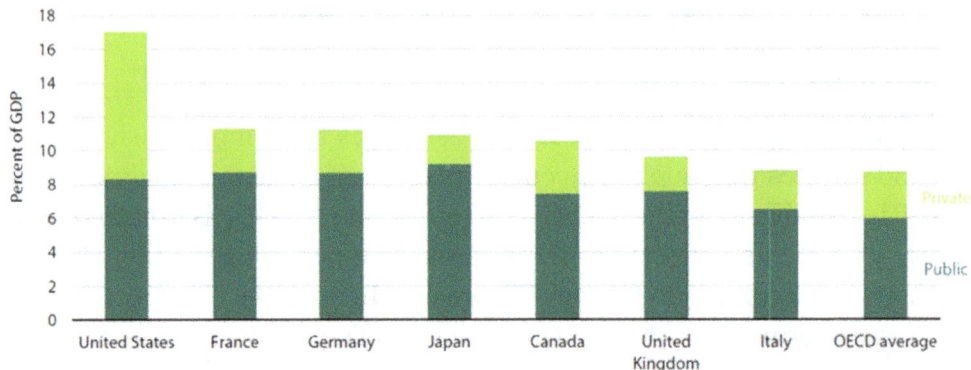

Source: World Health Organization (WHO) 2019a.
Note: Data are for 2017. Figure shows selected Organisation for Economic Co-operation and Development (OECD) countries; OECD average includes all OECD member countries as of February 2020. Public expenditures include: expenditures on government schemes and social health insurance schemes. Private expenditures include: compulsory private insurance schemes, voluntary health-care payment schemes, household out-of-pocket payments, and rest of the world financing schemes (non-resident). See WHO (2019b) for details.

Figure 9.2: Public and Private Healthcare Expenditures as a Share of the Gross Domestic Product by Country (2017 Data)

Source: The Brookings Institution
Attribution: The Brookings Institution
License: Fair Use

9.5 NATIONAL HEALTH EXPENDITURE ACCOUNTS

The total cost of U.S. healthcare is estimated by **National Health Expenditure Accounts (NHEA)**. NHEA has been providing estimates for healthcare in the U.S. since the 1960s (Center for Medicare & Medicaid Services, 2019). Reports from the NHEA contain yearly healthcare rates for goods, services, government management, net health insurance fees, community health events, and healthcare reserves.

9.6 U.S. HEALTHCARE SPENDING

The economy of the U.S. is the largest in the world (Bajpai, 2020). It is estimated that healthcare spending accounts for one-sixth of the U.S. economy (American Hospital Association [AHA], 2020). There has been an overall 80% increase in healthcare spending between 1996 and 2013 (Dieleman et al., 2017). Healthcare cost is a complicated subject and encompasses many variables to include the patient, type and level of service, healthcare setting, and the payer source. There is no set cost structure across all sectors of the healthcare system in the U.S. which has led to inconsistencies in healthcare spending. Dieleman et al. (2017) note five factors associated with increases in healthcare spending: population growth, population aging, disease prevalence or incidence, service utilization, and service price and intensity.

9.7 POPULATION GROWTH

According to the U.S. Census Bureau (2020), a preview of the 2020 census count will show a slow growth in our population. While our population does continue to grow, from 311+ million people in 2011 to 328+ million people in 2019, the overall percentage of population growth has slowed significantly since 2015. Some states see a higher growth rate than others (Texas, Florida, and Utah) while others are experiencing a negative growth rate (Illinois and West Virginia) (U.S. Census Bureau, 2020). Although the overall population growth is slowing, the U.S. has hundreds of millions of citizens who impact the healthcare system daily which ultimately effects the cost for services. Population growth is associated with a 23.1% or $269.5 billion in spending increases in areas of inpatient, ambulatory, retail pharmaceutical, nursing facility, emergency department, and dental care (Masterson, 2017). Medicine has advanced tremendously through the years and even unhealthy persons or those living with chronic diseases can live long lives. However, healthcare spending will increase as a result of chronic disease maintenance and longer living.

9.8 POPULATION AGING

The U.S. population is living longer and soon persons 65 and older will reach more than 20% of the population (Peter G. Peterson Foundation, 2020) (Figure 9.3). The sentiment "50 is the new 40" or "70 is the new 60" is common. Our perceptions of aging are changing as people are living longer. What was considered old age in the 1970's is not what is considered old today. According to the World Health Organization (WHO) (2018), for those over 60 years of age, the proportion of the world's population is expected to almost double from 12% to 22% between the years of 2015 and 2050. This growth has resulted in more people 60 years and older than children 5 years and younger, expected in the year 2020 (WHO, 2018).

According to Dieleman et al. (2017), between 1996 and 2013 there was an 11.6% increase in healthcare spending associated with our aging population. Common health conditions associated with aging include hearing loss, osteoarthritis, cataracts, and some chronic diseases such as diabetes, chronic obstructive pulmonary disease (COPD), depression, and dementia (WHO, 2018). Healthcare services commonly needed are related to doctor's visits and medications for disease management. There may be equipment needs to assist with mobility such as wheelchairs, walkers, canes and adjustable seats. Sensory functioning is enhancement with eye-glasses and hearing aids. Lastly, quality of life drivers such as affordable senior housing and home maintenance with cooking and cleaning assistance may be needed. When taken as a whole, it is easy to see how elderly are a driving force in healthcare spending.

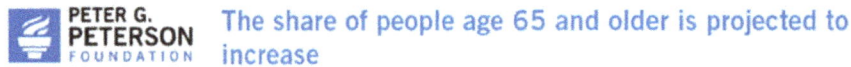

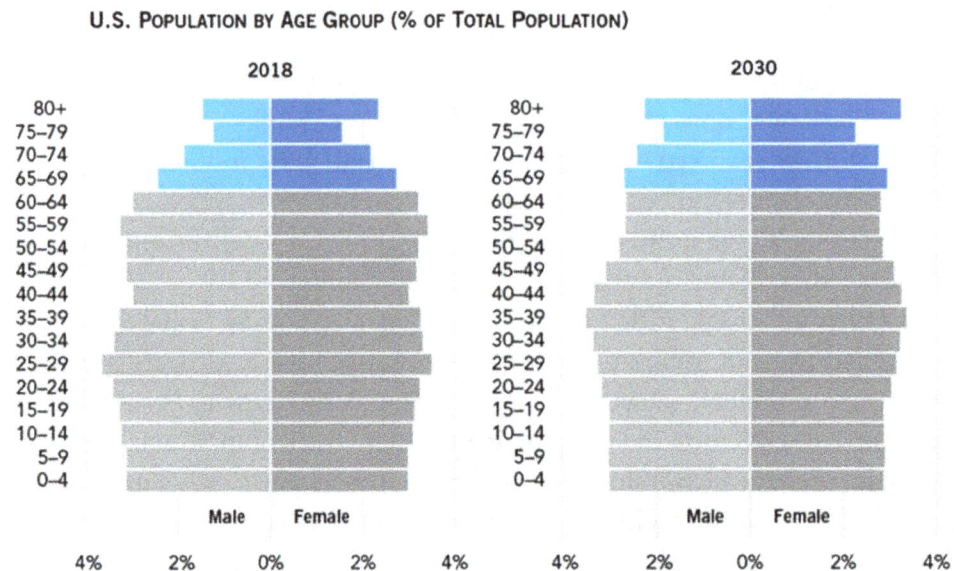

Figure 9.3: Aging Population, Age 65 and Older

Source: Peter G. Peterson Foundation
Attribution: Peter G. Peterson Foundation
License: © Peter G. Peterson Foundation. Used with permission.

With the population of citizens over 65 years of age growing, healthcare needs and spending will increase. Medicare insurance is a primary source of health insurance for those 65 and older. According to Cubanski et al. (2019), the next ten years are expected to see a projected increase in Medicare spending from $605 billion in 2018 to $1,278 billion in 2029. Increases in the aging population and subsequent increases in healthcare spending has a potential negative impact on the healthcare system related to availability of caregivers, services, and financial support. Important to note here is that actuaries for the Medicare program project that **Part A** trust fund will be depleted by 2026 (Figure 9.4). This is in part due to spending levels being higher than asset levels and more people being without health insurance as a result of the ACA repeal of the individual mandate (Cubanski et al., 2019). For more on Medicare specifics, refer back to Chapter 5.

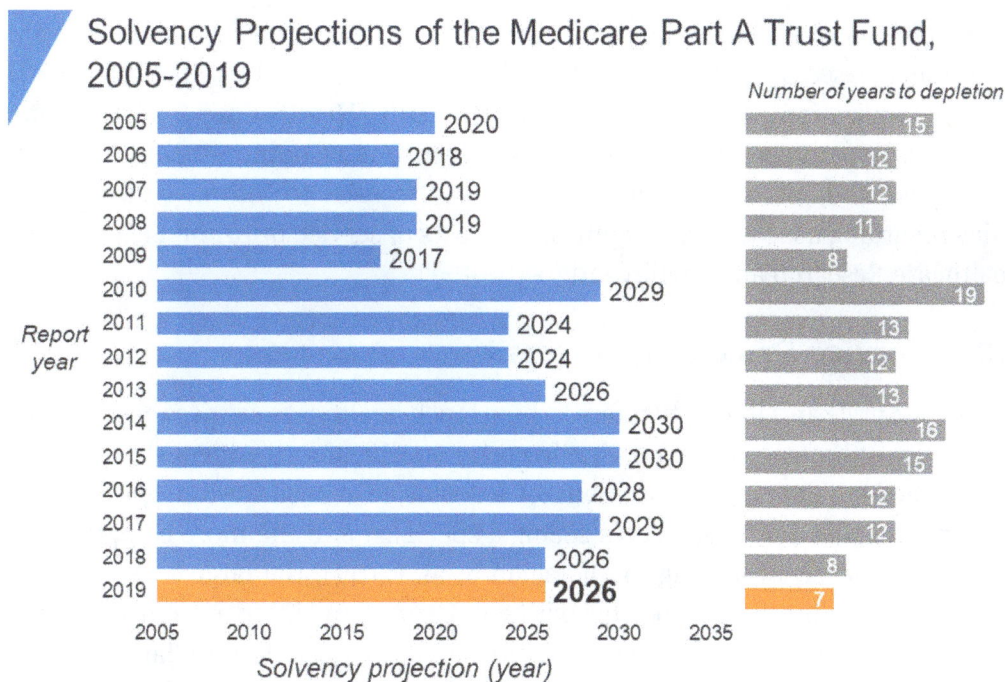

Solvency Projections of the Medicare Part A Trust Fund, 2005-2019

Number of years to depletion

Report year	Solvency projection	Years to depletion
2005	2020	15
2006	2018	12
2007	2019	12
2008	2019	11
2009	2017	8
2010	2029	19
2011	2024	13
2012	2024	12
2013	2026	13
2014	2030	16
2015	2030	15
2016	2028	12
2017	2029	12
2018	2026	8
2019	**2026**	7

Solvency projection (year)

SOURCE: Intermediate projections from 2005-2019 Annual Reports of the Boards of Trustees of the Federal Hospital Insurance and Federal Supplementary Medical Insurance Trust Funds.

KFF

Figure 9.4: Medicare Part A Projections

Source: Kaiser Family Foundation
Attribution: Kaiser Family Foundation
License: © Kaiser Family Foundation. Used with permission.

9.8.1 Disease Prevalence or Incidence

As noted in Chapter 2, the U.S. has a high incidence of chronic disease conditions such as diabetes, hypertension, depression, osteoarthritis, and more. The many risk factors of smoking, sedentary lifestyle, and obesity have contributed to chronic disease which requires ongoing medical follow-up and medications to manage symptoms. However, Dieleman et al. (2017) note that overall disease prevalence or incidence impact on healthcare spending, although variable depending on the specific condition, has decreased. Some specific conditions do show variability when analyzing spending. For example, between 1996 and 2013, diabetes was a condition in which disease prevalence were associated with increases in spending and heart disease and cerebrovascular disease prevalence had decreased spending (Dieleman et al., 2017).

9.8.2 Service Utilization

Service utilization refers to "use of services by persons for the purpose of preventing and curing health problems, promoting maintenance of health and well-being, or obtaining information about one's health status and prognosis" (Carrasquillo, 2013). These services are often sought through in-patient admissions, out-patient procedures and visits, professional services, and prescription drugs and medical devices. For persons younger than 65, the overall use of healthcare services decreased 0.2% between 2013 and 2017 (Health Care Cost Institute, 2018) however, utilization grew 1.8% from 2017 to 2018 (Health Care Cost Institute, 2019). Service utilization data is collected from many points, including forty-eight states and the District of Columbia, and is used to inform research and policy regarding use, access, outcomes, and costs of service utilization (Agency for Healthcare Research and Quality, 2020).

9.8.3 Service Price and Intensity

Service price and intensity refers to how much healthcare services cost and the complexity of the care received. Service price specifically considers the cost of a hospital bed per day, hip replacement, or a doctor office visit for example. Service intensity includes services such as seeing a specialist and the more complex care given at this level. According to Dieleman et al. (2017), the largest increases in healthcare spending were associated with service price and intensity and accounted for an overall 50% increase, accounting for nearly $450 billion dollars, between 1996 and 2013. Interestingly, the price paid for services will vary depending on the funding source. For example, the cost of an inpatient stay is higher for private insurance payers than for both Medicare and Medicaid payers (Figure 9.5). According to Claxton et al. (2018), after analyzing trends in prices over time, prices for healthcare services have risen more rapidly than general economic inflation, and there is a wide geographic variance in price for services across the U.S.

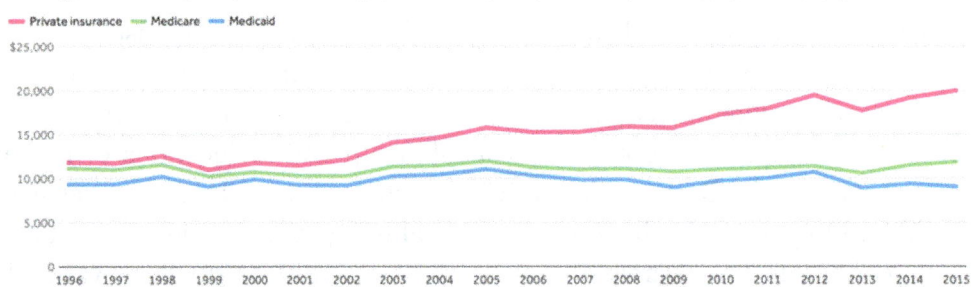

Average inflation-adjusted, standardized payment rates per inpatient hospital stay, by primary payer, 1997-2015

— Private insurance — Medicare — Medicaid

The average payment rates were computed as if each primary payer paid for all non-maternity adult stays in a given year. Payments were adjusted for inflation and standardized across payers in terms of patient's age, sex, race/ethnicity, geography, household income as a percentage of the federal poverty level, conditions, charges, length-of-stay, and whether or not a surgical procedure was performed. They were not standardized for changes over time in the bundles of treatments and services provided during inpatient stays.

Source: Thomas M. Selden analysis of AHRQ's Medical Expenditure Panel Survey for the Kaiser Family Foundation. Update of earlier analysis, available here: https://www.healthaffairs.org/doi/abs/10.1377/hlthaff.2015.0706
• Get the data • PNG

Peterson-KFF
Health System Tracker

Figure 9.5: Prices for Inpatient Hospital Growth Higher and Faster for Private Insurance

Source: Green Imaging
Attribution: Kaiser Family Foundation
License: © Kaiser Family Foundation. Used with permission.

Administrative cost

Administrative insufficiency contributes to the cost of healthcare. An investigation conducted by Shrank et al. (2019) estimated healthcare administrative cost to be approximately 265.6 billion. In fact, when compared to other areas of the healthcare system as identified by the Institute of Medicine (IOM), administrative complexities are the highest area of healthcare waste. And, when compared to other countries, the U.S. expenditures on administrative costs is extraordinarily high as a percentage of the GDP (Nunn et al., 2020) (Figure 9.6). Tasks such as billing, coding, scheduling, and payroll contribute to administrative costs. Insurance offices, hospitals, doctors' offices, and clinics are examples of healthcare entities utilizing numerous administrative personnel. Additionally, the amount of time spent on administrative duties by healthcare personnel such as physicians, nurses, and allied health personnel also contributes to administrative costs.

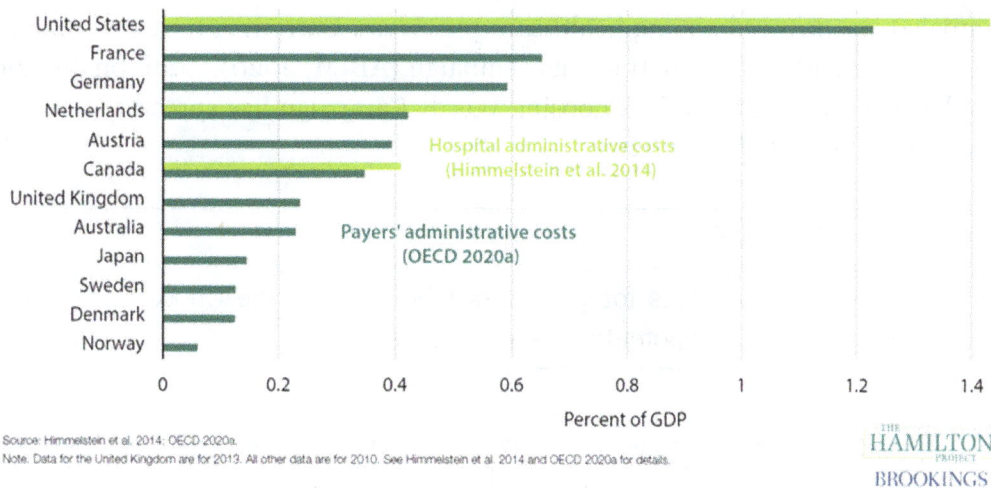

Source: Himmelstein et al. 2014; OECD 2020a.
Note: Data for the United Kingdom are for 2013. All other data are for 2010. See Himmelstein et al. 2014 and OECD 2020a for details.

Figure 9.6: Selected Administrative Costs as a Share of the Gross Domestic Product, by Country

Source: The Brookings Institution
Attribution: The Brookings Institution
License: Fair Use

Overutilization

The overutilization of healthcare services is another problem influencing the cost of healthcare in the U.S. Overutilization occurs when patients undergo numerous healthcare exams and procedures that are not necessary. Fortunately, around 2012, the American Board of Internal Medicine (ABIM) began collaborating with physicians and organizations to help decrease the overutilization of healthcare services to reduce associated costs. One such example of this collaboration is seen with initiatives started by Dr. Howard Brody.

Dr. Brody proposed that healthcare providers begin to assess ways to reduce healthcare costs (Brody, 2009). He requested that healthcare specialties collaborate with a specialist within their area to seek out the *Top Five* commonly prescribed, most expensive diagnostics that yielded few benefits to patients. Once the list was generated, he proposed that specialties devise methods to educate other physicians in their specialty areas regarding the unnecessary usage of these diagnostics and thereby discouraging needless ordering for patients. The National Physicians Alliance (NPA) worked concurrently with Dr. Brody to stimulate plans to decrease spending among internal medicine, family medicine, and pediatric medical practices. These specialty areas created three lists outlining steps for those in the identified practices to follow to help decrease cost (ABIM, 2020).

The **Choosing Wisely Campaign** is a follow-up campaign stemming from the work of Dr. Brody. An essential goal of the Choosing Wisely Campaign is to encourage discussion among healthcare providers and patients to help decrease costs. The mission of the campaign includes discussions to help provide evidence-based care, eliminate duplication of diagnostic testing, and to provide safe and essential care to patients (ABIM, 2020). The advent of the Choosing Wisely Campaign was favored among healthcare providers. Currently, over one million healthcare providers are a part of this campaign (ABIM, 2020). Additionally, the popularity associated with the Choosing Wisely Campaign has spread to another nineteen countries (ABIM, 2020).

Pause and Reflect

What are some advantages for providers who support the Choosing Wisely Campaign? What are the potential disadvantages

---

First Person Perspective

Dr. H has a Doctorate in Health Sciences (DHSc), MSN, RN. She is a dual citizen of the United Kingdom (U.K.) and the U.S. She lives full time in the U.S. and works as nurse faculty teaching at a university.

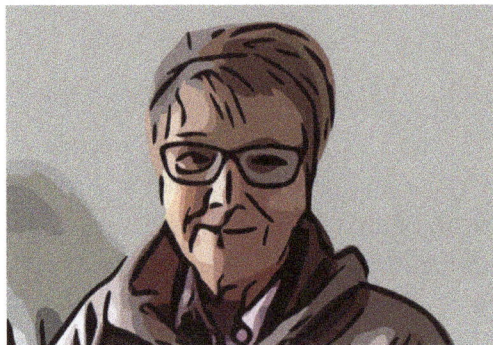

Figure 9.7: First Person Perspective

Source: Original Work
Attribution: Deanna Howe
License: CC BY-SA 4.0

While visiting family in the U.K., I became unwell with severe abdominal pain and vomiting. I went to the emergency room, completed diagnostic tests, and was seen by a surgeon before being admitted to the hospital for care and treatment. It was decided I needed surgery to have my gallbladder removed. I was given the option to have the surgery in the U.K or wait until I went home to the U.S. I decided to have the surgery at home and after five days I was well enough to be discharged from the hospital. I received copies of my medical chart, physician notes, diagnostic testing results, C.T. and other scan reports, lab work, and a baggy with all medications needed until I saw a U.S. surgeon.

Back home in the U.S. (ten days later), I tried to make an appointment with a surgeon. The surgeon would not see me unless I was referred from my primary care physician. My primary care physician would not make a referral without an appointment with him directly. I had to wait another ten days to see my primary physician. At this appointment, my doctor insisted I repeat every diagnostic test (which was another delay in getting to the surgeon).

Once I was seen by the surgeon, he agreed I needed the surgery immediately but required I pay a $2,000 deposit to cover his fee. The surgery was completed approximately two months after my return back to the U.S. and out of pocket costs were $5,000 with deductibles and copays. My cost in the U.K. for the emergency room, five days in the hospital, diagnostic tests, and medications were nothing, even though I had not lived in the U.K. for decades. No one in the U.K. ever asked how I was going to pay for my care.

First person perspectives collected and created by D. Howe, 2020.

For your consideration: Dr. H required surgery and decided to get the procedure done at home in the U.S. rather than in the United Kingdom. The U.K. hospital sent all of the documentation and diagnostic test results to support the diagnosis and need for surgery. Why do you think the surgeon would not accept these documents directly and required Dr. H to get a referral? Dr. H.'s primary care physician insisted she come in for a visit before he would send a referral to the surgeon. He would not accept the documentation from the U.K. and insisted on a repeat of all tests. Would you consider this a good use of resources or an unnecessary waste?

The costs Dr. H. incurred as a result of these repeated tests is a testament to overuse of services. In addition, Dr. H. notes the delays she had before finally getting the surgery two months from her initial diagnosis. How could this situation have improved with greater coordination of care between physicians? What are your thoughts about Dr. H. having to pay $2,000 to the surgeon before he would perform her surgery? What if she didn't have the money? How many of your friends or relatives have $2,000 readily available to pay a doctor for necessary care prior to receiving the care? Even if you have insurance, sometimes hospitals and doctors ask for payment in advance.

What are your thoughts about prepayment for healthcare services? Discuss and share your ideas.

— —

Physician salaries

Physician salaries are influential to the cost of U.S. healthcare (Mikulic, 2019). For instance, physicians in the U.S. have salaries far surpassing physicians in other countries (Mikulic, 2019). According to Mortensen (2020) the average yearly income for a specialist in the U.S. is $350,000 and the average pay for a general practice doctor in the U.S. is $242,400. In comparison with doctors' salaries in ten other countries, the U.S. is second only to Luxembourg in highest physician salaries. Australia, Netherlands, Austria, Ireland, Switzerland, Canada, Germany, and Belgium all have physician salaries lower than the U.S. (Mortensen, 2020).

Defensive medicine

According to Torrey (2019), another issue influencing the cost of healthcare in the U.S. is **defensive medicine**. Defensive medicine accounts for 2.4% of healthcare spending in the U.S. (Sullivan, 2018). The practice of defensive medicine is two-fold. The first aspect of defensive medicine is the practice of physicians ordering excessive diagnostics for clients in hopes of preventing litigation. When this occurs, clients often have tests or procedures ordered at their request or because the physician is being overly cautious. Physicians often decide to go above and beyond what is considered normal to keep the clients appeased as well.

While clients may feel more at ease with the over-testing, it should be noted that there are disadvantages to this type of regime. A client's sense of false security is a severe disadvantage to over-testing (Torrey, 2019). Over testing may seem like you are experiencing optimal health when the over-testing may not have investigated other underlying health problems (Torrey, 2019) (Box 9.1).

Often, the cost of over-testing as in defensive medicine is passed along to the client through increased healthcare insurance premiums (Torrey, 2019). Unfortunately, when this occurs, strategies to address the increase in insurance premiums are often implemented, which may ultimately trickle down as the taxpayers' burden and serve as a prelude to increased healthcare costs (Torrey, 2019). Clients may wish to contact their healthcare insurance providers to get pre-approval before undergoing diagnostic testing. If this happens, clients are then able to gain knowledge on the type of diagnostic testing that the insurance company will approve and are then able to make informed decisions as to whether they wish to have the prescribed diagnostic testing.

The second aspect of defensive medicine is when physicians refuse to treat what they consider to be high-risk clients. This is in part due to the fear of malpractice litigations. When this occurs, those clients who are expected to achieve favorable healthcare outcomes are desired and accepted by the physicians rather than those clients who are more than likely to experience less than optimal outcomes (Torrey, 2019). This practice may result in high-risk clients not having the option to be treated by top-ranking physicians (Torrey, 2019).

Defensive medicine alludes to physicians and healthcare centers receiving additional money for over-testing and procedures (Torrey, 2019). The practice of defensive medicine is more likely to be seen by physicians who practice in high-risk specialty areas (Torrey, 2019).

Example of Over-Testing Based on Client Apprehensions

Client Jane Doe comes into her primary physician's office to have the results of her previously administered Mantoux tuberculin skin test read. Her physician notes no induration and records her results as negative meaning she has had no exposure to the disease. However, the physician orders a chest x-ray to further confirm the results of the negative tuberculosis (TB) skin test. Although Jane has no signs or symptoms of TB and is considered to a be low risk client for TB, she feels elated after her doctor agrees to order a chest x-ray and TB blood test to further address her apprehension about any possible TB exposure.

Medications

When attempting to view a more comprehensive cost estimate of medications, it is vital to include prescription medications, over the counter medications, and medical non-durable products. *Prescription* **medications** are those medications requiring a physician or advanced healthcare provider to prescribe. *Over-the-counter medications (OTC)* are those medications that can be purchased without a healthcare provider's permission. Over-the-counter medications include medications such as Tylenol, Benadryl, and Aspirin. Also included in over-the-counter drugs are many homeopathic medicines such as St. John's wort, ginkgo, and fish oil. *Medical-nondurables* include non-prescription items such as medical supplies and equipment, such as syringes, and Band-Aids. Medical non-durables comprise roughly 5% of the cost of prescription medications (Organisation for Economic Cooperation and Development [OECD], 2019).

Prescription drug cost. When calculating the cost of healthcare, it is essential to include the cost of medications. It is estimated that 17% of overall personal healthcare service is attributed to prescription medications (Kesselheim et., 2016). In 2016, approximately 448.2 billion dollars was spent on prescription drug sales (Schumock et al., 2017). Prescription medications comprise about 75% of retail medication costs. The amount of money spent per capita in the U.S. on prescription medications is more significant than any other industrialized country (Kesselheim et al., 2016) (Figure 9.8).

10.2. Expenditure on retail pharmaceuticals per capita, 2017 (or nearest year)

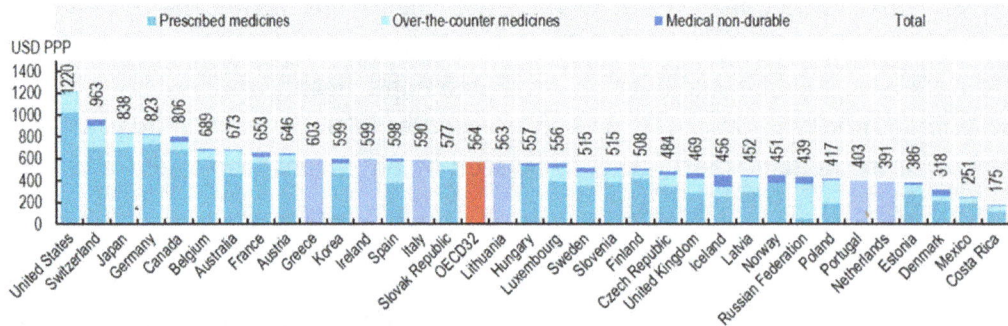

Source: OECD Health Statistics 2019.

Figure 9.8: Expenditure on Retail Pharmaceuticals Per Capita, 2017 (or nearest year).

Source: OECD Health Statistics
Attribution: OECD Health Statistics
License: Fair Use

The cost of prescription medication coverage is expected to increase (Campbell, 2019). One possible solution to help decrease this cost is the use of generic medications whenever possible. This use should help due to a significant cost difference between generic and brand prescription drug costs. According to Franki (2019), the average cost of brand-name medication was 18.6 times higher than the generic medication equivalent (Figure 9.9). For instance, the cost of generic medications can be 80 to 85% less than brand name medications (Wagener, 2019). Perhaps unsurprisingly, the use of generic drugs has increased from 66% in 2010 to 82% in 2016 (Blue Cross Blue Shield Association, 2017).

Average annual cost of therapy: Generics vs. brand-name drugs

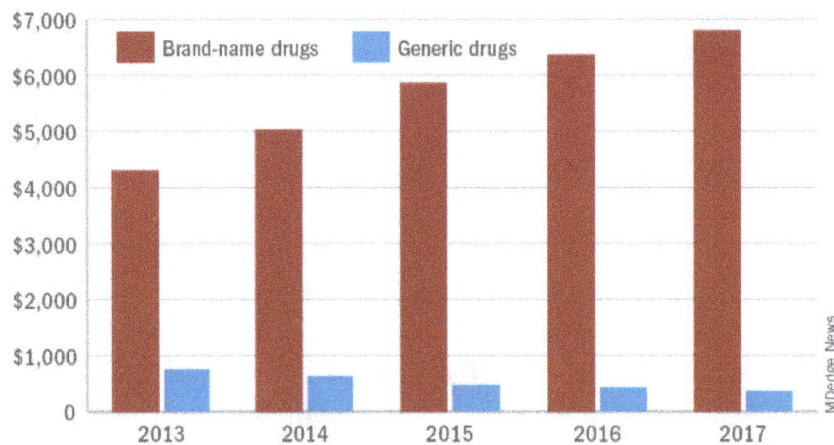

Note: Based on a market basket of 260 drugs widely used by older adults for chronic conditions.

Source: AARP Public Policy Institute and the PRIME Institute, University of Minnesota

Figure 9.9: Generic vs. Brand-Name Medication Prices

Source: The Hospitalist
Attribution: The Hospitalist
License: Fair Use

One reason provided for expensive medications in the U.S. is because the cost is decided by drug manufacturing companies (Taube, 2019). There is much political conversation about how to regulate the cost of medications in our country. Unfortunately, legal ramifications often prevent interference with lowering the drug medication cost. For example, the Centers for Medicaid and Medicare (CMS) are not currently able to legally negotiate drug prices. Although, the Medicare Drug Price Negotiation Act of 2017 was introduced on January 4, 2017, it has yet to be enacted (GovTrack.us, 2020). If passed, this bill would allow the CMS to work with pharmaceutical companies to try and reduce drug costs.

Over-the-counter medications (OTC) and non-durable supplies. Four attributes are associated with the value of over-the-counter medications in the U.S. healthcare system: accessibility, affordability, trust, and empowerment (Consumer Healthcare Products Association [CHPA], 2019a). The movement of medications from a prescription-required status to OTC allows consumers considerable flexibility and access to medications in treating common ailments. Consumers are able to address many acute health problems with OTC rather than go to a doctor. For example, if you wake up with a fever and stuffed nose, you may try an OTC fever reducer and decongestant medication to see if you can resolve the problem before calling the doctor for an appointment. CHPA (2019a) note that consumers make about twenty-six trips a year to purchase OTC medications while they visit a doctor on average only about three times a year.

According to CHPA (2019b), approximately 19% of retail spending is from OTC medications. CHPA notes that households spend on average $442 a year for OTCs. Cost savings include a decrease in doctor/clinic visits and prescription drug costs along with increased productivity.

Hospitalization

Approximately 32% of total health spending in the U.S. is attributed to hospital spending (Kamal & Cox, 2018). Hospitalization can be required in emergent situations, such as traumatic injury or acute disease conditions, and also for non-emergent cases, such as joint replacement or cataract removal. Costs resulting from hospitalization will depend on the cause, depth of treatment, skilled care required, and the length of stay. Worldwide, the cost of hospitalization in the U.S. far surpasses the cost in other countries (Elflein, 2019). Although the average hospital stay in the U.S. is shorter than in other countries, such as Switzerland and Australia, the costs of these stays are higher (Kamal & Cox, 2018). In 2017, the average cost of a hospital stay was $15,734 (Debt.org, 2019). The five most expensive conditions requiring in-patient hospitalization were septicemia, osteoarthritis, liveborn (newborn) infants, acute myocardial infarction, and heart failure (Liang et al., 2020).

9.9 IMPACT OF COVID-19 ON HEALTHCARE COSTS

As a result of the COVID-19 virus pandemic and efforts to reduce the spread from person to person, many economies have shut down or severely restricted access to services. This has impacted many individuals through job loss and subsequent loss of health insurance. Such a loss of health insurance may lead persons who are sick to skip the doctor visit or, if they must see a doctor, to worry about an inability to pay for services. For those who become infected with COVID-19 and require hospitalization, the costs can be financially devastating.

9.10 SUMMARY

This chapter discussed the cost of healthcare in the U.S., National Health Expenditure Accounts (NHEA), and the impact of healthcare on the GDP. It compared healthcare costs between the U.S. and other developed countries. And it presented factors influential to healthcare costs, such as population growth, population aging, disease prevalence or incidence, service utilization, service price and intensity, physician salaries, prescription drugs, administrative costs, overutilization, hospital stays, and defensive medicine.

9.11 REVIEW QUESTIONS

1. What are National Health Expenditure Accounts?
2. How does the U.S. rank among other industrialized countries in terms of healthcare costs?
3. Explain how prescription drug cost influences the overall cost of consumer healthcare.
4. Describe three factors that influence the cost of healthcare in the U.S.
5. How do physician salaries in the U.S. compare with physician salaries in other countries?

9.12 REFERENCES

Agency for Healthcare Research and Quality. (2020, March 25). Health care cost and utilization project fact sheet. Retrieved November 15, 2020, from https://www.hcup-us.ahrq.gov/news/exhibit_booth/hcup_fact_sheet.jsp

American Board of Internal Medicine. (2020). Facts and figures. Retrieved from http://www.choosingwisely.org/our-mission/facts-and-figures/

American Hospital Association (2020). Health care: The big picture. Retrieved from https://www.aha.org/data-insights/health-care-big-picture

Bajpai, P. (2020, January 22). The 5 largest economies in the world and their growth in 2020 Retrieved from https://www.nasdaq.com/articles/the-5-largest-economies-in-the-world-and-their-growth-in-2020-2020-01-22

Blue Cross Blue Shield Association. (2020). Why does health care cost so much? Retrieved from https://www.bcbs.com/issues-indepth/why-does-health care-cost-so-much

Blue Cross Blue Shield Association. (2017). Rising cost of patented drugs drive growth of pharmaceutical spending in the U.S. Retrieved from https://www.bcbs.com/the-health-of-america/reports/rising-costs-patented-drugs-drive-growth-pharmaceutical-spending-us

Brody, H. (2009). Medicine's ethical responsibility for health care reform-The Top Five List. New England Journal of Medicine, 362, 283–285. DOI: 10.1056/NEJMp0911423

Bureau of Economic Analysis. (2020). Gross domestic product. May 18, 2020 Retrieved from https://www.bea.gov/resources/learning-center/what-to-know-gdp

Campbell, K. (2019). Why are prescription drug prices rising? And what can be done? Retrieved from https://health.usnews.com/health-care/for-better/articles/2019-02-06/why-are-prescription-drug-prices-rising

Carrasquillo, O. (2013) Health care utilization. In: Gellman M.D., Turner J.R. (eds) Encyclopedia of Behavioral Medicine. Springer, New York, NY. https://doi.org/10.1007/978-1-4419-1005-9_885

Centers for Medicare and Medicaid Services. (2020). National health expenditure projections 2019-29. Retrieved from https://www.cms.gov/files/document/national-health-expenditure-projections-2019-28.pdf

Centers for Medicare & Medicaid Services. (2019). National health expenditure data. Retrieved from https://www.cms.gov/research-statistics-data-and-systems/statistics-trends-and-reports/nationalhealthexpenddata/nationalhealthaccountshistorical

Claxton, G., Rae, M., Levitt, L. & Cox, C. (2018, May 8). How have health care prices grown in the U.S. over time? Peterson-KFF Health System Tracker. Retrieved from https://www.healthsystemtracker.org/chart-collection/how-have-health care-prices-grown-in-the-u-s-over-time/#item-start

Consumer Health care Products Association. (2019a). Statistics on OTC use. Retrieved from https://chpa.org/MarketStats.aspx

Consumer Health care Products Association. (2019b). White paper: Value of OTC medicines to the U.S. health care system. Retrieved from http://overthecountervalue.org/white-paper/

Cubanski, J., Neuman, T., & Freed, M. (2019, August 20). The facts on Medicare spending and financing. Kaiser Family Foundation. Retrieved from https://www.kff.org/medicare/issue-brief/the-facts-on-medicare-spending-and-financing/#:~:text=Medicare%20is%20funded%20primarily%20from,percent)%20(Figure%207).&text=Part%20A%20is%20financed%20primarily,percent%20of%20Part%20A%20revenue)

Debt.org. (2020). Hospital and surgery cost. Retrieved from https://www.debt.org/

medical/hospital-surgery-costs/

Dieleman, J. L., Squires, E., Bui, A. L., Campbell, M., Chapin, A., Hamavid, H., Horst, C., Li, Z., Matyasz, T., Reynolds, Al, Sadat, N., Schneider, M. T. & Murray, C. J. L. (2017). Factors associated with increases in US health care spending, 1996-2013. JAMA, 318 (17); 1668–1678. DOI: 10.1001/jama.2017.15927

Elflein, J., (2019, September 17). U.S. hospital care expenditure 1960-2019. Stratista. Retrieved from https://www.statista.com/statistics/184772/us-hospital-care-expenditures-since-1960/

Frank, R. (2019). Cost gap widens between brand-name, generic drugs. The Hospitalist. Retrieved from https://www.the-hospitalist.org/hospitalist/article/198828/business-medicine/cost-gap-widens-between-brand-name-generic-drugs

GovTrack.us. (2020). H.R. 242 — 115th Congress: Medicare Prescription Drug Price Negotiation Act of 2017. Retrieved from https://www.govtrack.us/congress/bills/115/hr242

Health Care Cost Institute. (2019). 2018 Health care cost and utilization report. Retrieved from https://healthcostinstitute.org/health-care-cost-and-utilization-report/annual-reports

Health Care Cost Institute. (2018). 2017 Health care cost and utilization report. Retrieved from https://healthcostinstitute.org/health-care-cost-and-utilization-report/annual-reports

Kesselheim, A., Avorn, J., & Sarpatwari, A. (2016). The high cost of prescription drugs in the United States: Origins and prospects for reform. JAMA 316(8), 858-71. DOI: 10.1001/jama.2016.11237

Lankford, K. (2017). 50 ways to save on health care. Kiplinger's personal finance. Retrieved from https://www.kiplinger.com/slideshow/spending/T027-S001-30-ways-to-cut-your-health-care-costs/index.html

Lian, L., Moore, B., & Soni, A. (2020, July). National inpatient hospital costs: the most expensive conditions by payer, 2017. Agency for Healthcare Research and Quality. Retrieved from https://www.hcup-us.ahrq.gov/reports/statbriefs/sb261-Most-Expensive-Hospital-Conditions-2017.jsp#:~:text=The%20 average%20cost%20per%20hospital,expensive%20types%20of%20health care%20utilization.&text=Higher%20costs%20are%20documented%20 for,(%2413%2C600%20for%20Medicare%20vs

Masterson, L. (2017, November 8). Price increases, population growth drive majority of rising health care spending. Healthcaredive. Retrieved from https://www.health caredive.com/news/health-care-costs-rising-prices/510434/

Medicare Interactive. (2020). Introduction to Medicare. Retrieved from https://www.medicareinteractive.org/get-answers/medicare-basics/medicare-overview/introduction-to-medicare

Medicare Rights Center. (2017, August 11). What is Medicare? [YouTube video]. Retrieved from https://www.youtube.com/watch?v=Bcs6se5ONY4&feature=youtu.be

Mikulic, M. (2019, August 9). U.S. health expenditure as percent of GDP 1960-2019. Retrieved from https://www.statista.com/statistics/184968/us-health-expenditure-as-percent-of-gdp-since-1960/

Mortensen, R. (2020). 10 highest paying countries for doctors. Medic Footprints. Retrieved from https://medicfootprints.org/10-highest-paid-countries-world-doctors/

Nunn, R., Parsons, J., & Shambaugh, J. (2020, March 10). A dozen facts about the economic of the US health-care system. Brookings. Retrieved from https://www.brookings.edu/research/a-dozen-facts-about-the-economics-of-the-u-s-health-care-system/

Organisation for Economic Cooperation and Development. (2020). Pharmaceutical expenditure. Retrieved from https://www.oecd-ilibrary.org/sites/4dd50c09-en/1/2/10/1/index.html?itemId=/content/publication/4dd50c09-en&_csp_=8258 7932df7c06a6a3f9dab95304095d&itemIGO=oecd&itemContentType=book#indicator-d1e26642

Organisation for Economic Cooperation and Development. (2019). Health care quality framework. Retrieved from http://www.oecd.org/health/health-care-quality-framework.htm

Peter G. Peterson Foundation (2020, April 20). Why are Americans paying more for health care? Retrieved November 11, 2020, from https://www.pgpf.org/blog/2020/04/why-are-americans-paying-more-for-health care

Schumock, G., Li, E., Wiest, M., Suda, K., Stubbings, J., Matusiak, L., Hunkler, R., Vermeulen, L. (2017). National trends in prescription drug expenditures and projections for 2017. American Journal of Health-System Pharmacy, 74(15), 1158–1173. DOI: 10.2146/ajhp170164

Shrank, W., Rogstad, T., & Parekh, N. (2019). Waste in the US health care system. JAMA, 322 (15):1505–1509. DOI:10.1001/jama.2019.13978

Sullivan, T. (2018, May 5). Defensive medicine adds $45 billion to the cost of health care. Policy & Medicine. Retrieved from https://www.policymed.com/2010/09/defensive-medicine-adds-45-billion-to-the-cost-of-health care.html

Taube, S., (2019, April 14). Who profits from high prescription drug prices? Wealth Daily. Retrieved from https://www.wealthdaily.com/articles/who-profits-from-high-prescription-drug-prices-/92030

Torrey, T. (2020, February 27). Defensive medicine and how it affects health care cost. Verywellhealth. Retrieved from https://www.verywellhealth.com/defensive-medicine-2615160

Torrey, T. (2020, Jan 15). How to avoid unnecessary medical test. Verywellhealth. Retrieved from https://www.verywellhealth.com/why-does-my-doctor-send-me-for-so-many-medical-tests-2615097

United States Census Bureau. (2020). Nation's population growth slowed this decade. Retrieved November 13, 2020, from https://www.census.gov/library/stories/2020/04/nations-population-growth-slowed-this-decade.html

USAFacts. (2020). Health care. Retrieved from https://usafacts.org/issues/health care/?utm_source=bing&utm_medium=cpc&utm_campaign=ND-Health care&msclkid=a75323a7f35f1f0c3d3b7d6389de7ccf

Wagener, D. (2019). What's the difference between a brand-name drug and a generic drug? GoodRx. Retrieved from https://www.goodrx.com/blog/brand-vs-generic-drugs-whats-the-difference/

World Health Organization (WHO). (2018, February 5). Ageing and health. Retrieved from https://www.who.int/news-room/fact-sheets/detail/ageing-and-health

10 Quality in Healthcare

10.1 LEARNING OBJECTIVES

By the end of this chapter, the student will be able to:

- Explain how healthcare is regulated in the U.S.
- Name three accreditation agencies
- State the advantages of accreditation
- Explain the importance of quality improvement programs
- Differentiate between the Merit-Based Incentive Payment System and the Advanced Alternative Payment Models
- List the five principles of Lean
- Define health disparities

10.2 KEY TERMS

- accreditation
- Advanced Alternative Payment Models (APMs)
- healthcare quality
- health disparities
- Merit-Based Incentive Payment System
- quality improvement
- Quality Payment Program
- Sustainable Growth Rate Formula

10.3 INTRODUCTION

A vital aspect of healthcare in the U.S. is the quality of services rendered. According to the Institute of Medicine (as cited in Peerpoint, 2019, para. 1), healthcare quality "is the extent to which health services provided to individuals and patient populations improve desired health outcomes." Improvement of health outcomes should be the goal of all healthcare services. When desired health outcomes are met, the cost of healthcare decreases. Although the cost of healthcare in the U.S. is rising, much needs to be done to help improve the quality of overall healthcare and health within our country. This chapter will discuss the quality of the U.S. healthcare system, various programs, and initiatives geared towards rendering the best healthcare possible to U.S. constituents.

10.4 QUALITY IN HEALTHCARE

According to the Organisation for Economic Co-operation and Developments (OCED) (2019), quality in healthcare should be effective, safe, and patient-centered. When healthcare is effective, needed healthcare services produce desired outcomes and unnecessary healthcare services are avoided. Healthcare is considered safe when it is delivered in a manner that is of little harm to the client. The patients are the focus in patient-centered care, hence the designation.

Blue Shield of California, the California Health Care Foundation, the Robert Wood Johnson Foundation, and the Institute of Medicine have worked to create a four-domain framework for classifying main measures for health and healthcare. The purpose of this framework was to help provide a clear, focused means to assess the quality of health and healthcare for individuals in the U.S. and establish standards (Institute of Medicine [IOM], 2015). This four-domain framework is presented in *Vital Signs: Core Metrics for Health and Health Care Progress*. Healthy people, care quality, lower cost, and engaged people are the four identified domains (Institute of Medicine, 2015). These domains were used to create fifteen comprehensive core measures (see Table 10.1). These in turn were used to provide standards to measure health and ultimately help improve health and decrease healthcare costs for individuals in the U.S. (IOM, 2015). See below for an outline of these core measures.

Table 10.1: Core Measures Set with Related Priority Measures		
1. Life expectancy • Infant mortality • Maternal mortality • Violence and injury mortality	2. Well-being • Multiple chronic conditions • Depression	3. Overweight and obesity • Activity levels • Healthy eating patterns
4. Addictive behavior • Tobacco use • Drug dependence/ illicit use • Alcohol dependence/ misuse	5. Unintended pregnancy • Contraceptive use	6. Healthy communities • Childhood poverty rate • Childhood asthma • Air quality index • Drinking water quality index

7. Preventive services	8. Care access	9. Patient safety
• Influenza immunization • Colorectal cancer screening • Breast cancer screening	• Usual source of care • Delay of needed care	• Wrong-site surgery • Pressure ulcers • Medication reconciliation
10. Evidence-based care	11. Care match with patient goals	12. Personal spending burden
• Cardiovascular risk reduction • Hypertension control • Diabetes control composite • Heart attach therapy protocol • Stroke therapy protocol • Unnecessary care composite	• Patient experience • Shared decision making • End-of-life/ Advanced care planning	• Healthcare-related bankruptcies
13. Population spending burden	14. Individual engagement	15. Community engagement
• Total cost of care • Healthcare spending growth	• Involvement in health initiatives	• Availability of healthy food • Walkability • Community health benefit agenda

Source: Original Work

Attribution: Deanna Howe, adapted from National Academy of Sciences, 2015

License: CC BY-SA 4.0

10.5 REGULATORY AGENCIES FOR HEALTHCARE

The regulation of quality healthcare in the U.S. involves numerous organizations with somewhat different focuses. Some of the organizations are influenced by congressional input, while others are regulated and funded by the government. A list of the Department of Health and Human Services (HHS) agencies and offices are listed below. HHS provides general oversight about the healthcare of U.S. citizens. Patient outcomes and affordable healthcare services have been at the forefront of HHS for several years. Its mission is "to enhance and protect the health and well-being of all Americans. We fulfill that mission by providing for effective health and human services and fostering advances in medicine, public health, and social services" (U.S. Department of Health & Human Services [HHS], 2019, para 1).

HHS Agencies & Offices

Administration for Children and Families (ACF)	Food and Drug Administration (FDA)
Administration for Community Living (ACL)	Health Resources and Services Administration (HRSA)
Agency for Healthcare Research and Quality (AHRQ)	Immediate Office of the Secretary (IOS)
Agency for Toxic Substances and Disease Registry (ATSDR)	Indian Health Service (IHS)
Assistant Secretary for Administration (ASA)	National Institutes of Health (NIH)
Assistant Secretary for Financial Resources (ASFR)	Office for Civil Rights (OCR)
Assistant Secretary for Health (ASH)	Office of Global Affairs (OGA)
Assistant Secretary for Legislation (ASL)	Office of Inspector General (OIG)
Assistant Secretary for Planning and Evaluation (ASPE)	Office of Intergovernmental and External Affairs (IEA)
Assistant Secretary for Preparedness and Response (ASPR)	Office of Medicare Hearings and Appeals (OMHA)
Assistant Secretary for Public Affairs (ASPA)	Office of National Security (ONS)
Center for Faith-Based and Neighborhood Partnerships (CFBNP)	Office of the Chief Technology Officer (CTO)
Centers for Disease Control and Prevention (CDC)	Office of the General Counsel (OGC)
Centers for Medicare & Medicaid Services (CMS)	Office of the National Coordinator for Health Information Technology (ONC)
Departmental Appeals Board (DAB)	Substance Abuse and Mental Health Services Administration (SAMHSA)

10.6 COMPARING THE U.S. WITH OTHER COUNTRIES

The quality of healthcare in the U.S. differs from that of other industrialized countries (Schneider et al., 2017). Schneider et al. (2017), in conjunction with the Commonwealth Fund (2017), collected data about healthcare from the following countries: Australia, Canada, France, Germany, Netherlands, New Zealand, Norway, Sweden, Switzerland, United Kingdom, and the U.S. The results of this study revealed that, unfortunately, adults in the U.S. are less likely to obtain healthcare due to the cost of healthcare services than those in other countries. Additionally, the participants in this study considered themselves to be in poorer health than did those in other comparable countries. These countries were compared in the areas of the care process, access, administrative efficiency, equity, and healthcare outcomes (See Table 10.2). The U.S. ranking was the lowest overall on a scale of 1 (best) to11(worst). This should be very alarming, given that the U.S. spends more on healthcare than other comparable countries.

Table 10.2: Healthcare System Performance Ratings										
	AUS	CAN	FRA	GER	NETH	NZ	NOR	SWE	SWIZ	UK	US
Overall ranking	2	9	10	8	3	4	4	6	6	1	11
Care Process	2	6	9	8	4	3	10	11	7	1	5
Access	4	10	9	2	1	7	5	6	8	3	11
Administrative Efficiency	1	6	11	6	9	2	4	5	8	3	10
Equity	7	9	10	6	2	8	5	3	4	1	11
Healthcare Outcomes	1	9	5	8	6	7	3	2	4	10	11

Source: The Commonwealth Fund
Attribution: The Commonwealth Fund
License: Fair Use

10.6.1 Hospital Admissions

People are admitted to the hospital with preventable diseases more often in the U.S. than comparable countries (Peterson Center on Healthcare, 2019). As indicated by Figure 10.1, the U.S. has more hospital admissions with congestive heart failure, asthma, hypertension, and diabetes than comparable countries. One contributing factor to this problem is lack of access to prevention, health promotion, and maintenance services to those most in need (Blumenthal et al., 2015). Efforts geared towards making healthcare services affordable and more accessible could decrease rates of many preventable diseases and help limit possible complications to already-diagnosed illnesses. This could improve the quality of healthcare for individuals living in the U.S.

Age standardized hospital admission rate per 100,000 population for asthma, congestive heart failure, hypertension, and diabetes, ages 15 and over, 2015 or nearest year

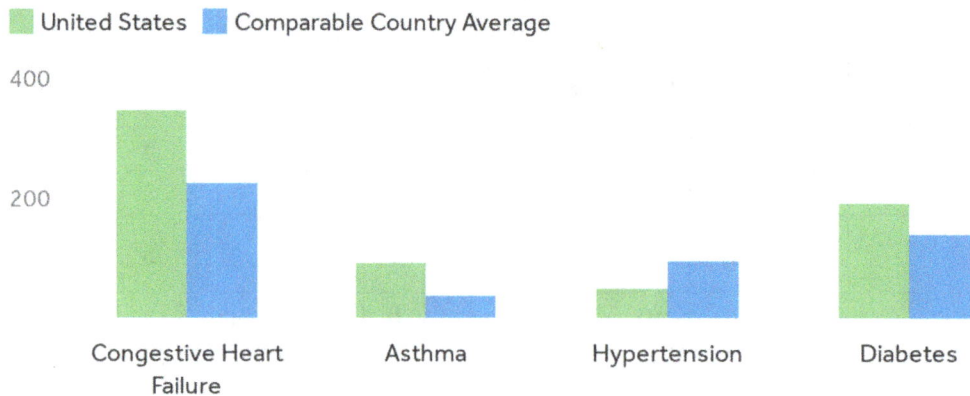

Data for Australia, Belgium, and the US are from 2014. Diabetes admission rates for Austria are also from 2014.

Source: KFF analysis of OECD data

Peterson-KFF
Health System Tracker

Figure 10.1: Hospitalizations in the U.S. Per Disease Compared to Other Countries

Source: Kaiser Family Foundation
Attribution: Kaiser Family Foundation
License: © Kaiser Family Foundation. Used with permission.

10.6.2 Healthcare Errors

Medical errors in healthcare negatively influence the quality of healthcare rendered. Many factors can contribute to medical errors, including human error, understaffing, increased patient acuity, and miscommunication. More medical, medication, and laboratory mistakes occur in the U.S. than other comparable countries. See Figure 10.2 for an indication of how the U.S. ranks in this area compared to other countries.

Percent of adults who have experienced medical, medication, or lab errors or delays in past two years, 2016

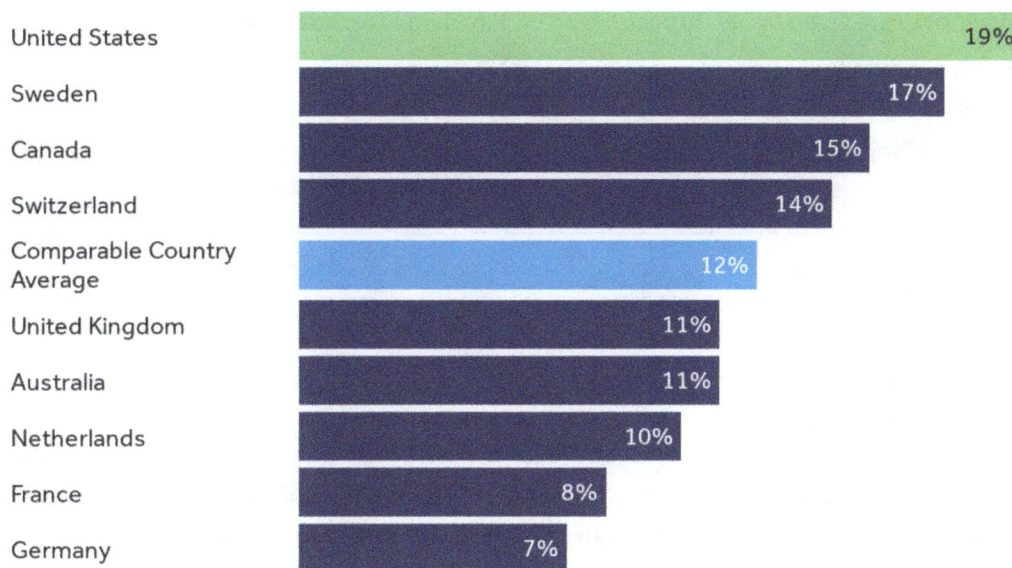

Country	Percent
United States	19%
Sweden	17%
Canada	15%
Switzerland	14%
Comparable Country Average	12%
United Kingdom	11%
Australia	11%
Netherlands	10%
France	8%
Germany	7%

Source: Unpublished data from 2016 Commonwealth Fund
International Health Policy Survey

Peterson-KFF
Health System Tracker

Figure 10.2: Medical Errors in the U.S. Compared to Other Countries

Source: Kaiser Family Foundation
Attribution: Kaiser Family Foundation
License: © Kaiser Family Foundation. Used with permission.

10.7 VALUE-BASED CARE

To value something is to treasure and attempt to protect it. In **value-based healthcare**, the focus is on providing coordinated care among healthcare workers to ensure patients are receiving the focused attention and care needed. According to the Centers for Medicare & Medicaid Services (2019), with value-based healthcare, healthcare providers are given incentives to render quality care. When this occurs, healthcare cost is decreased (Rouse, 2019).

Value-based care helps to prevent duplicate healthcare services or oversights in care (Rouse, 2019). This result differs from tradition-based healthcare where the healthcare providers are paid based on the number of services a patient receives (CMS, 2019). Many value-based care programs are associated with the Centers for Medicare & Medicaid Services (CMS). Some examples of value-based programs are as follows: End-Stage Renal Disease Quality Incentive Program, Hospital Value-Based Purchasing, Hospital Readmission Reduction Program, Value Modifier Program, Hospital-Acquired Conditions, Skilled Nursing Facility Value-Based program, and Home Health Based Program (CMS, 2019). See the Value-Based versus Fee-for-Service comparison chart below.

Table 10.3: Comparison of Value-Based Versus Fee-for-Service	
Value-Based	**Fee-for-Service**
Incentives are given for quality care: • Incentives for improved patient outcomes • Bundling of services is an option	Payment is received for the quantity of care: • Physicians are paid for services completed • No bundling of services

Source: Original Work
Attribution: Andrea Dozier
License: CC BY-SA 4.0

10.8 ACCREDITATION

Many healthcare agencies in the U.S. are accredited by certain organizations. According to BHM HealthCare Solutions (n.d.), "accreditation is a process by which an impartial organization will review a company's operations to ensure that the company is conducting business in a manner that is consistent with national standards." Much planning and effort are necessary for a healthcare agency to become accredited. Accreditation helps signify quality in health agencies (BHM, n.d.).

There are five major healthcare accreditation organizations (BMH):

- Utilization Review Accreditation Commission
- National Committee for Quality Assurance
- The Joint Commission
- Commission on Accreditation of Rehabilitation Facilities
- Council on Accreditation

Agencies that are accredited receive national recognition and repayment services from certain insurance companies (BMH). There is usually a cost that agencies must pay to become accredited. Once granted, the accreditation has a limited time frame and should be renewed accordingly. Accredited agencies help maintain performance improvement standards and are often notably recognized within the community and perhaps even nationwide. The accreditation certification also helps recruit top-notch healthcare workers to become members of the healthcare team.

First Person Perspective

Nurse C., FNP-C, RN, has a Master of Science in Education (MSN) and Master of Healthcare Administration (MHA). She has twenty-eight years of experience as a nurse, five years certified in Healthcare Accreditation, and works as Accreditation Coordinator in the Quality Department at her local hospital.

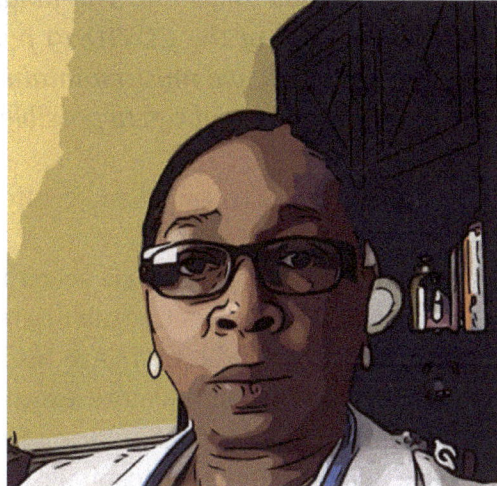

Figure 10.3: First Person Perspective

Source: Original Work
Attribution: Deanna Howe
License: CC BY-SA 4.0

Quality in healthcare seeks to create an environment which increases the likelihood of desired health outcomes, consistent with current professional knowledge and standards. Today's world challenges us in ways we have not experienced before related to quality and safety. Quality, safety, and infection prevention are amplified and at the forefront of our current practice because of the novel coronavirus known as COVID-19. In 2020, hospitals were met with many required changes related to infection prevention and control due to the virus. To stay compliant with guidance from organizations like the CDC, hospitals were making many changes to already-implemented practices. My hospital's systematic and previously hardwired process for distribution of organizational information sharing supported us in maintaining quality care delivery and safety. This is in part due to organizational accreditation standardization practices. I love my position as an Accreditation Coordinator; it affords me the opportunity to impact safety and quality for all of our patients, staff and visitors.

As Accreditation Coordinator, I view healthcare accreditation as a stamp of approval that says to our consumers (patients) and peers that we have met all required regulatory standards set forth by recognized professional organizations. The standard set forth reinforces the requirement to provide the safest and highest quality in our delivery of healthcare. Compliance is achieved by consistently monitoring, measuring, and analyzing the processes in our organization. This is a job that I enjoy immensely. When we fall out of those requirements, action must take place for correction immediately; this is how we achieve optimal healthcare quality. We are challenged daily to remember our individual roles in quality. We must keep quality at the forefront of every patient encounter for the best possible outcome. The landscape of healthcare is forever changed as a result of the COVID-19 pandemic. Due to this unprecedented healthcare crisis, we must maintain an intense focus on the delivery of the highest quality and safety possible.

First person perspectives collected and created by D. Howe, 2020.

For your consideration: Nurse C notes that accreditation is a stamp of approval that shows the organization has met regulatory standards. What are the advantages for hospitals to seek accreditation? Are healthcare agencies who are accredited more trustworthy? Considered more excellent? Have you ever investigated if your local hospital is accredited? Would you feel safer if the hospital was accredited? If you had a choice between two hospitals, one accredited and one not accredited, which would you choose for care? What type of challenges might a non-accredited healthcare agency experience? How does Nurse C's experience and certification in accreditation benefit her organization?

10.9 MEDICARE ACCESS AND CHILDREN'S HEALTH INSURANCE PROGRAM REAUTHORIZATION ACT OF 2015 (MACRA)

On April 16, 2015, the Medicare Access and Children's Health Insurance Program Reauthorization Act of 2015 (MACRA) legislation went into effect. The Quality Payment Program was developed by MACRA (CMS, 2019). The Quality Payment Program was created to provide incentives for healthcare providers offering value-based care. This program was also created to help eradicate a Fee-for-Service system (Rouse, 2019). In a Fee-for-Service payment system, healthcare providers are paid per service or procedure rendered to patients. Fee-for-Service payment programs often result in unnecessary exams and procedures for patients and yet more payments received by healthcare providers.

Pause and Reflect

How has the Medicare Access and Children's Health Insurance Program impacted healthcare services? List two benefits and two challenges.

Before the enactment of MACRA, Medicare payments for physicians were based on a sustainable-growth rate. MACRA annulled the **Sustainable Growth Rate Formula**, which provided a formula by which Medicare would pay physicians. The Sustainable Growth Rate Formula was evaluated and modified as needed yearly.

Healthcare providers can use two options to participate in the Quality Payment Program. The optimal selection is based on certain characteristics of the healthcare providers' client types, geographical area, area of practice, and size of practice (CMS, 2019). Healthcare providers may choose from the **Merit-based Incentive Payment System (MIPS)** or the **Advanced Alternative Payment Models**.

10.9.1 Merit-based Incentive Payment System (MIPS)

According to Practice Fusion (2020), the MIPS allowed for the reorganization of the following Medicare programs:

- Physician Quality Reporting System

- Value-Based Payment Modifier (VM)

- Medicare Electronic Health Record (HER) Incentive Program (Meaningful Use)

The MIPS performance-based system provides Medicare Part B payment adjustments for qualified healthcare providers based on a MIPS Composite Performance Score, as seen in Figure 10.4. There are four categories of the MIPS: Cost, Clinical Practice Improvement Activities (CPIA), Advancing Care Information (ACI), and Quality (PQRS). Participating providers receive a composite performance score (MIPS) that is used to determine their Medicare Part B reimbursements. The healthcare providers' scores can range from 0-100.

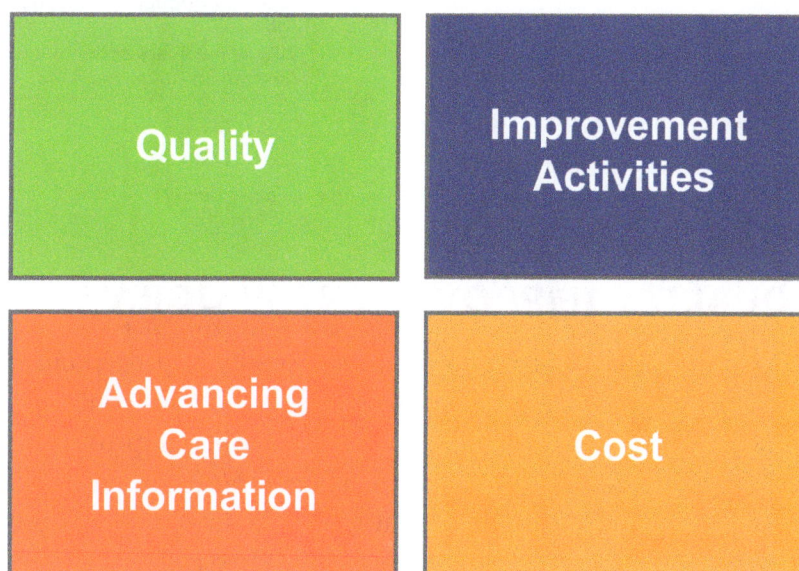

Figure 10.4: Merit-Based Incentive Payment System (MIPS) Categories

Source: Original Work
Attribution: Corey Parson
License: CC BY-SA 4.0

10.9.2 Advanced Alternative Payment Models

Like MIPS, **Advanced Alternative Payment Models (APMs)** are an option of the Quality Payment Program. APMs also reward healthcare providers for providing high-quality, more affordable care (Practice Fusion, 2019). Eligible healthcare providers receive a 5% incentive when predetermined patient payment thresholds are met (See Figure 10.5) (Quality Payment Program, n.d.). In addition to the 5% bonus, some benefits of Advanced APM include exclusion from MIPS and additional APM rewards (Quality Payment Program).

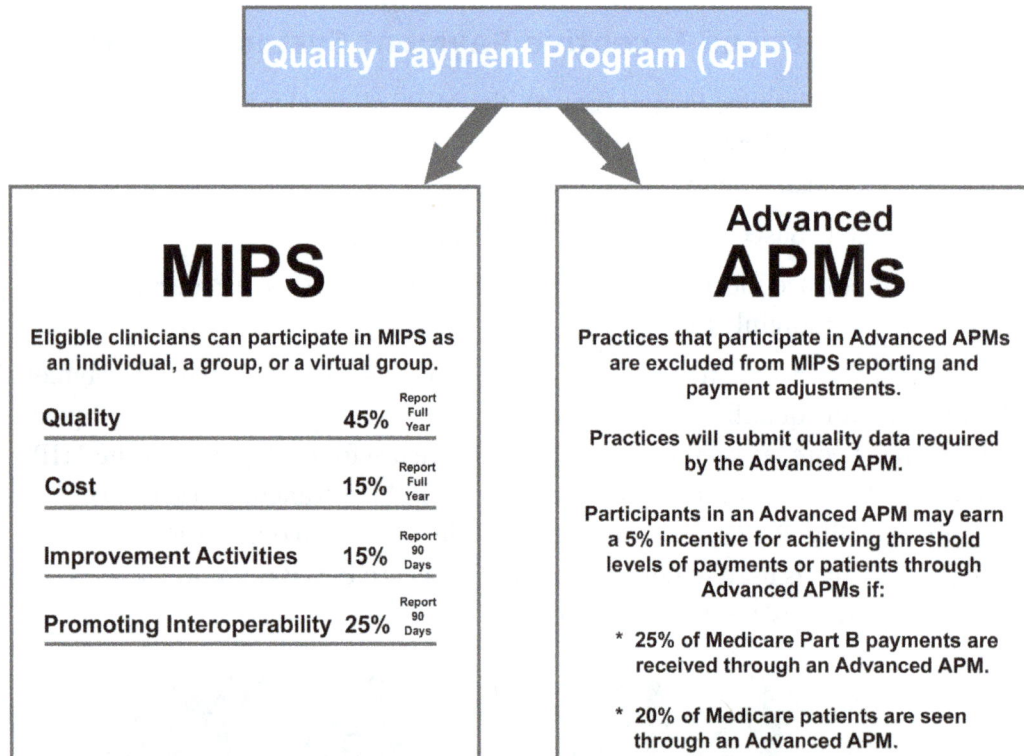

Figure 10.5: Comparison of MIPS and APMs

Source: Medical Group Management Association
Attribution: Corey Parson, Adapted from Medical Group Management Association
License: Fair Use

10.10 QUALITY IMPROVEMENT PROGRAMS

Associated with the healthcare spectrum are quality improvement programs. Quality improvement is continuous and is often referred to as continuous quality improvement (CQI). Individuals involved in the quality improvement process include many members of the healthcare team. There are many definitions for quality improvement, but the end goal of quality improvement programs is improved patient outcomes, cost-efficiency, and effective care.

At the forefront of an organization's quality improvement initiatives is an assessment of the organizations' systems and protocols (Health Catalyst, 2017). In other words, quality improvement initiatives should first begin with the discovery of *What is the process or protocol? How can we make this process better?* and *How can we prevent this from happening again in the future?* According to Health Catalyst, quality improvement programs must have the following components:

- A comprehended problem
- Defined improvement
- A created aim statement
- Quantifiable improvement

Quality improvement members evaluate the processes involved in patient care, its effectiveness, and how its processes can be improved. Members of the quality improvement process often collect analytics about patient care and services. These help to outline baselines and provide guidelines to measure. If any improvements occur, analytics help determine how much of an improvement has occurred (Health Catalyst, 2017).

According to Serino (2019), quality improvement programs are essential to healthcare because they help decrease waste by improving processes, thereby increasing the proficiency of healthcare staff and improving patient outcomes. The Institute for Healthcare Improvement (2019) outlines six goals for quality improvement:

- **Safe**: avoid harm to patients from the care that is intended to help them
- **Effective**: provide services based on scientific knowledge to all who could benefit and refrain from providing services to those not likely to benefit (avoid underuse and misuse, respectively)
- **Patient-centered**: provide care that is respectful of and responsive to individual patient preferences, needs, and values and ensure that patient values guide all clinical decisions
- **Timely**: reduce waits and sometimes harmful delays for those who receive and give care
- **Efficient**: decrease wastefulness
- **Equitable**: provide care that does not vary in quality because of personal characteristics, such as gender, ethnicity, geographic location, and socioeconomic status

Key components of an effective quality improvement program comprise the *problem, goal, aim,* and *measures* (Health Catalyst, 2019). The problem component is the process that needs to be investigated. The goal component is the desired result. The aim is a more systematically-organized plan for achieving the goal. And the measures component allows evaluation of the effectiveness of the intervention based on the initial problem. An example of these key components is illustrated in Table 10.4 below:

Table 10.4: Example of Problem Viewed Through Quality Improvement

Problem	Increase in reported medication errors in hospital-inpatients
Goal	Decrease the number of medication errors by 75% within 3 months
Aim	Conduct one-hour weekly mandatory professional development training for nursing and pharmacy staff
Measures	Investigate the number of reported medication errors after three months of intervention

Source: Original Work
Attribution: Andrea Dozier
License: CC BY-SA 4.0

10.11 QUALITY IMPROVEMENT EXAMPLES

Healthcare entities may choose to use a quality improvement framework to formulate an individualized framework. What follows is a brief discussion of a few common frameworks often adopted in healthcare when referring to quality improvement.

10.11.1 The Institute for Healthcare Improvement

The Institute for Healthcare Improvement (IHI) began working towards quality in healthcare in the late 1980s but was formally founded in 1991 (Institute for Healthcare Improvement, 2019). First, it is the goal of restructuring healthcare into a safer, more cost-efficient, time-sensitive entity for clients. The mission of the IHI helps promote quality in healthcare, as can be noted in these vision and mission statements:

> IHI vision: "Everyone has the best care and health possible."
> IHI mission: "Improve health and healthcare worldwide."

The delivery of quality healthcare requires continuous evaluation. When required to do so, healthcare leaders need to be flexible in order to implement changes to improve healthcare quality. The IHI suggests a Plan-Do-Study-Act cycle (PDSA) to evaluate changes. The following three questions are a part of the PDSA cycle with questions to help foster continuous quality improvement

1. What are we trying to accomplish?
2. How will we know that a change is an improvement?
3. What change can we make that will result in improvement?

10.11.2 Lean

Quality increases client health and safety. Poor quality may negatively affect patient outcomes, while high-quality healthcare may positively influence patient outcomes. Lean, a program originally developed and used in manufacturing, was created to eradicate waste and increase quality in production. Please refer to Figure 10.6 for the five Lean principles.

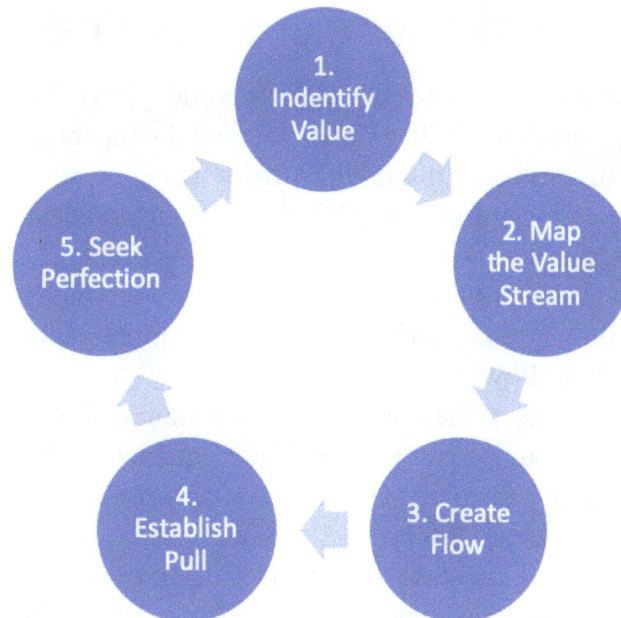

Figure 10.6: Principles of Lean

Source: Lean Enterprise Institute
Attribution: Corey Parson, Adapted from the Lean Enterprise Institute
License: Fair Use

More often, the principles of Lean production have been adopted in non-manufacturing areas, such as healthcare (Lean Enterprise Institute, 2019). One reason for this introduction of Lean into healthcare is because it offers diversity to customary quality improvement programs. When utilized in healthcare, Lean principles help improve patient outcomes, increase the effectiveness of medical services rendered, and decrease costs (Health Catalyst, 2020).

10.11.3 Six Sigma

Another framework used to improve quality is Six Sigma. Although Six Sigma is sometimes used along with Lean production, Six Sigma incorporates more statistical analyses. A major focus of Six Sigma is to reduce cost and increase productivity (American Society for Quality, [ASQ] 2019). Additionally, Six Sigma uses the DMAIC approach: Define, measure, analyze, improve, and control. It focuses on providing a framework for the improvement of performance and the decrease of process variations (ASQ, 2019).

10.11.4 Lean Six Sigma

The Lean Six Sigma approach combines the Lean production and Six Sigma framework. Lean Six Sigma in healthcare can decrease patient wait times, medication errors, and falls (Purdue, 2020). Additionally, using Lean Six Sigma in healthcare is beneficial because it can increase revenue, patient satisfaction, and turnaround time for laboratory results (Purdue, 2020).

10.12 HEALTHCARE WORKERS AND QUALITY

The delivery of quality healthcare requires several types of healthcare workers. Each member of the multidisciplinary team serves a distinct purpose and function. Some members of this multidisciplinary team may include these healthcare professionals: registered nurses, physicians, licensed practical nurses, certified nursing assistants, social workers, and therapists (speech, respiratory, physical, and occupational). To provide the best, most efficient care possible requires the team members having among them such skills as good communication, collaboration, organization, and flexibility.

Oftentimes, members of the multidisciplinary team will participate in regular meetings to help plan and organize care. The frequency of these meetings may be contingent upon such factors as the type of healthcare facility, client acuity, or healthcare facility protocol. This type of coordinated patient care helps improve healthcare services and increase the quality of those services. Collaborated meetings help foster open dialog between members of the healthcare team, avoid duplication of healthcare procedures, and promote improved patient outcomes.

10.13 HEALTH DISPARITIES

A serious problem affecting the quality of healthcare in the U.S. is health disparities. According to Potter et al. (2018), health disparities are "preventable differences in the burden of disease, injury, violence, or opportunities to achieve optimal health that are experienced by socially disadvantaged populations" (p. 33). The unequal dispersal of resources to disadvantaged persons contributes to health disparities (Potter et al., 2018). For example, the availability of healthcare facilities may be limited in some geographical areas, which may make health screenings and routine appointments difficult for some individuals without transportation. The Centers for Disease Control have sponsored numerous programs by various agencies to try and reduce health disparities. Some of these programs include early colorectal cancer screening, HIV prevention for high-risk individuals, health promotion, and diabetes prevention in high affected ethnic groups (U.S. Department of Health & Human Services, 2019b).

10.14 SUMMARY

There continues to be much discussion regarding the best way to ensure quality healthcare services for individuals in the U.S. The delivery of quality healthcare is of utmost importance. While the U.S. spends a great deal of money on healthcare as compared to other countries, much improvement is needed. Organizations, such as the Centers for Medicare & Medicaid Services, are now offering tangible incentives for healthcare providers based on the quality of care rendered and patient outcomes. This chapter included discussion on accreditation agencies for healthcare facilities and how they influence healthcare services. It also presented information regarding the Quality Payment Programs and Quality Improvement Programs.

10.15 REVIEW QUESTIONS

1. In what areas of healthcare does the U.S. rank lower than other countries?
2. What are the five principles of LEAN? How are they being integrated into healthcare?
3. What are the goals of quality improvement programs?
4. What is accreditation?
5. Why was the Quality Payment Program created?

10.16 REFERENCES

American Society for Quality. (2019). What is Six Sigma? Retrieved from https://asq.org/quality-resources/six-sigma

BHM Health care Solutions. (n.d.). The big five health care accreditation organizations: A side by side comparison. Retrieved from https://bhmpc.com/calltoaction/accreditation-comparison-cta/Accreditation-Comparison-Tool.pdf

Blumenthal, D., Abrams, M., & Nuzum, R., (2015). The Affordable Care Act at 5 years. New England Journal Medicine, 372, 2451–2458. DOI: 10.1056/NEJMhpr1503614

Centers for Medicare & Medicaid Services. (2019). Value-based programs. Retrieved from https://www.cms.gov/Medicare/Quality-Initiatives-Patient-Assessment

Health Catalyst. (2018). Lean health care: 6 methodologies for improvement from Dr. Brent James. Retrieved from https://downloads.healthcatalyst.com/wp-content/uploads/2018/10/Lean-Health care-6-Methodologies-for-Improvement-from-Dr.-Brent-James.pdf

Institute for Health care Improvement. (2019). Vision, mission, and values. Retrieved from http://www.ihi.org/

Institute of Medicine. (2015). Vital signs: Core metrics for health and health care progress. Washington, D.C.: The National Academies Press. https://doi.org/10.17226/19402

Instruments/Value-Based-Programs/Value-Based-Programs Health Catalyst. (2017). The top five essentials for quality improvement in health care. Retrieved from https://www.healthcatalyst.com/wp-content/uploads/2016/06/Top-Five-Essentials-for-Quality-Improvement.pdf

Lean Enterprise Institute. (2019). Principles of Lean. Retrieved from https://www.lean. org/whatslean/principles.cfm

Lehmann, C. (2019, July). Addressing social determinants of health. PT in Motion, 11(6), 28–39. Retrieved from http://www.apta.org/PTinMotion/2019/7/Feature/ SocialDeterminants/

McGill, N. (2016). Education attainment linked to health throughout lifespan: Exploring social determinants of health. The Nation's Health August, 46(6), 1–19. Retrieved from http://thenationshealth.aphapublications.org/content/46/6/1.3.full

Organisation for Economic C-Operation and Development. (2019). Health care quality framework. Retrieved from http://www.oecd.org/health/health-care-quality-framework.htm

PeerpointMedical Education Institute. (2019). The definition of health care quality and the institute of medicine. Retrieved from http://www.peerpt.com/ performancequality-

Peterson Center on Health care. (n.d.). Appropriate treatment: Preventable hospital admissions. Retrieved from https://www.healthsystemtracker.org/indicator/quality/ preventable-hospital-admissions/improvement/the-definition-of-health care-quality-and-the-institute-of-medicine/

Practice Fusion. (2020). Value-Based reimbursement and quality initiatives. Retrieved from https://www.practicefusion.com/value-based-reimbursement/

Potter, P., Perry, A., Stockert, P. & Hall, A. (2018). Community-based nursing practice. In: Fundamentals of Nursing, 9th ed. Elsevier

Purdue University. (2020). Advance in health care with Lean Six Stigma. Retrieved from https://www.purdue.edu/leansixsigmaonline/blog/health care-advancement-with-lean-six-sigma/

Rouse, M. (2019). MACRA (Medicare Access and CHIP Reauthorization Act of 2015) Retrieved from https://searchhealthit.techtarget.com/definition/MACRA-Medicare-Access-and-CHIP-Reauthorization-Act-of-2015

Schneider, E., Sarnak, D., Squires, D. Shah, A., & Doty, M. (2017). Mirror, mirror 2017: International comparison reflects flaws and opportunities for better U.S. health care. The Commonwealth Fund. Retrieved from https://interactives.commonwealthfund. org/2017/july/mirror-mirror/

Serino, A. (2020). Five examples of quality improvement in health care & hospitals. Ascendant Strategy Management Group. Retrieved from https://www. clearpointstrategy.com/examples-of-quality-improvement-in-health care/

U.S. Department of Health & Human Services. (n.d.) HHS agencies & offices. Retrieved from https://www.hhs.gov/about/agencies/hhs-agencies-and-offices/index.html

U.S. Department of Health and Human Services. (2016). Strategies for reducing health disparities: Selected CDC-sponsored interventions, United States, 2016. Retrieved from https://www.cdc.gov/minorityhealth/strategies2016/

U.S. Department of Health and Human Services, Office of Disease Prevention and
Health promotion. (2019). Social determinants of health. In Healthy People 2020.
Retrieved from https://www.healthypeople.gov/2020/topics-objectives/topic/social-
determinants-of-health

11 Technology Use in Healthcare

11.1 LEARNING OBJECTIVES

By the end of this chapter, the student will be able to:
- Describe benefits of technology use in healthcare
- Discuss activities that threaten security of personal health information (PHI)
- Explain importance of HIPAA rules and regulations
- Discuss the impact of telehealth on patients with access issues or patients in rural communities
- Describe the importance of interoperability of electronic health record systems

11.2 KEY TERMS

- artificial intelligence
- Clinical Decision Support Systems
- data analytics
- electronic health record
- HIPAA
- interoperability
- patient portal
- personal or protected health information
- point of care
- telehealth
- wearable health technology

11.3 INTRODUCTION

Healthcare technology is a vital component in providing advancements in diagnostics and assessments of patients as well as creating processes that allow us to record and retain records in digital format: "Health technologies encompass all the devices, medicines, vaccines, procedures and systems designed to streamline healthcare operations, lower costs and enhance quality of care" (Reddy, 2019, para. 1). Because so much technology is flooding the market, it is necessary to make smart choices. *Healthcare Weekly* (2019) noted 20 billion dollars of technology is available to create solutions that assist in improving efficiency and cutting operating costs. There are five criteria for selecting technology assets: functionality, usability, security, interoperability, and cost (Bailey et al., 2017).

Examples of technology that help streamline processes include automation of administrative duties, ease of workflow, use of scheduling apps, claims processing, and supply chain management technology. Examples of patient care technology that enhances quality and safety include bed alarms for the elderly; video monitoring (virtual sitter) for the elderly; medication administration; robotics for surgery; electronic health records; electronic pharmacy records; telemedicine for chronic disease management; implantable devices to manage diabetes, arrhythmias, and seizure disorders; and laser surgery to improve eyesight.

Emerging technologies include artificial intelligence (AI), 3D printing, telehealth, augmented and virtual reality, wearable health monitors, and next generation sequencing. Technology is available in every aspect of healthcare at this time. Yet, we have only scratched the surface of what is to come. This chapter looks at the health information technology support people who help healthcare technology run efficiently and meet the needs of stakeholders. It also offers a snapshot of technology used in today's healthcare system and discusses the benefits of technology, safety and quality through technology use, and emerging technologies. And it explores important concepts related to interoperability of systems, privacy, security, and legislation.

11.4 HEALTH INFORMATION TECHNOLOGY SUPPORT

Technology use in healthcare is booming, and the need for specialists to create, guide, and troubleshoot technology is vital. A number of growing health information technology professionals are essential to the operating processes throughout healthcare. Of note are analytics consultants, chief security officers, clinical informaticists, health information technicians, and medical and health services managers. A brief description of each can be found in Table 11.1.

Table 11.1: Health Information Technology Professionals

Title	Role Description	Key Skills
Analytics Consultant	• Lead the development team and implement data analytics solutions • Develop methodologies to inform best strategies • Work with teams to determine proper business process changes	• programming • data processing • problem solving • time management
Chief Security Officer (CSO) *or* Chief Information Security Officer (CISO)	• Lead information security efforts in the organization • Work with IT and Engineering departments to implement strategies for compliance • Support information security best practices • May provide physical security for employees	• written and oral communications • business management comprehension • problem-solving • research
Clinical Informaticist	• Work with clinical data and technology to streamline workflow and improve patient experiences • Ensure health data collected is used to support existing standards and best practices • Support implementation of information systems (EHR's)	• data analysis • data mining • software programming • communications • project management
Health Information Technician	• Manage and organize health information and data while meeting quality, security, and accessibility standards • Track patient outcomes for quality assessments • Categorize patient information for insurance reimbursement, updates to databases, and patient records	• software • data analysis • coding • customer service
Medical and Health Services Manager	• Plan and direct healthcare services • Oversee compliance of healthcare laws and regulations • Direct changes to health services which influence processes, policies, and procedures	• financial • analytical technical • problem-solving • change management

Source: HIMSS.org
Attribution: Deanna Howe
License: CC BY-SA 4.0

The professionals noted above and more are found in many healthcare settings and will certainly be a part of any team that introduces new technology or updates existing technology or processes.

- - - - - - - - - - - - - - - - - - - -

First Person Perspective

Nurse S, RN-BC, BSN, has a Master of Science (MSN) in Patient Centered Technologies. She has twenty-five years of experience as a nurse, twelve years certified in nursing informatics, and works with a national physician services group.

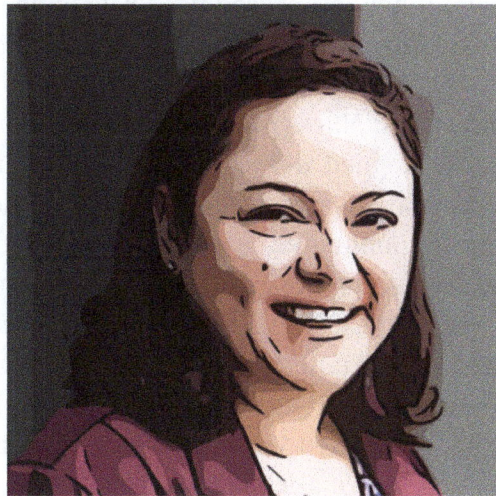

Figure 11.1: First Person Perspective

Source: Original Work
Attribution: Deanna Howe
License: CC BY-SA 4.0

It's an exciting time in healthcare with the introduction of a worldwide pandemic. Technology use, especially telehealth and mobile technology, have pushed my fellow nurses and me to really use our critical thinking skills to deliver innovative, solid, and collaborative work in the interest of increasing patient safety, provider satisfaction and organizational goals. I feel that my nursing foundation, learned during nursing school, has given me the ability to always deliver in an environment that is typically dominated by non-clinicians. The road has been long in blending different perspectives on how technology, as a healthcare tool, should be designed, developed and implemented. Early in my informaticist journey, I identified that my role would be as a mediator and translator of ideas so that any given project would continue to move forward. There is always something new to learn and because of my clinical experience and the valuable critical thinking skills learned along the way, I don't see myself leaving the field. I really enjoy my cohorts (physicians, scientists, tech analysts, legal teams, operators, accountants) and working with them.

As a nurse informaticist, I have grown with health information technology and the needs of healthcare organizations, who in general have come to recognize the importance of having a group of specialists that can support the cognitive interaction between providers, nurses, clinical processes, patients, and the technology delivered by any given healthcare organization. Not all informaticists perform this role specifically. There are many of us who choose to be trainers, educators, builders of software, and who focus on quality improvement, data analysis, system optimization, testers, and more. The opportunities are vast for those of us working in informatics. I don't regret switching from bedside nursing to playing a larger though unrecognized role in healthcare. Satisfaction is gained when our clients are happy, and patients have better outcomes.

For your consideration: Nurse S states that blending perspectives on how healthcare tools should be designed, developed, and implemented has taken a long time. Her nursing foundation has given her the ability to deliver in a high-tech environment that is typically dominated by non-clinicians. Did you know that some nurses specialize in the field of nursing informatics, which combines a clinical and technical language for use in healthcare? Because nurses working in healthcare today are often required to use new technology in reporting patient outcomes, should they or should they not have a voice and be placed on implementation teams? How does Nurse S's clinical experience and feedback benefit a health technology team? How would nursing informatics courses and continuing education help nurses and other health professionals strengthen healthcare organizations?

11.5 ELECTRONIC HEALTH RECORD/ DIGITALIZATION OF HEALTH RECORDS

The **electronic health record (EHR)** is a digital version of a patient's paper medical record and includes **protected or personal health information (PHI)** (HealthIT.gov, 2019a). EHRs promote availability of readily-accessible medical records. This reduces duplicity in orders and prevents unnecessary delays in service. EHRs also makes healthcare providers privy to information pertaining to conditions being monitored and treated by other specialists. The implementation of an EHR system helps create a level of consistency and fluidity regarding patient information. Patients can see various providers without worrying about how to obtain their healthcare records. EHR systems can eradicate the fragmentation of care by improving care coordination. Of note is the EHR's being a real-time tool that is updated upon every use.

The electronic health record (EHR) provides a record of appointments, medications, treatments, procedures, diagnosis, laboratory test results, immunizations, and any other related medication information. Creating a health record in digital format allows for broader access of one's medical information. For example, an individual comes to the emergency room (ER) unconscious with seizure activity and is unable to provide important data regarding vital statistics and medical history. The patient's driver's license is used to conduct a query-based exchange of information to look up the patient's past history in the medical system. The system finds a match as a result of a recent visit to a participating physician. The record shows a history of epilepsy. Consequently, the ER physician is able to quickly identify the current problem and order proper diagnostic tests and treatments based on access to the digital health record. While this scenario exemplifies how the EHR worked well for one patient, this is not always the case in our current healthcare system.

The electronic medical record is a positive tool overall. However, time spent documenting within a system can be extensive. In a four-week study of family physician attendings and residents, covering 982 patient visits, researchers observed specific components of a patient visit to include pre-visit EHR time, face-to-face time with the patient, time working in the EHR during patient visit, time in EHR after visit, and EHR time outside of operating hours (Young et al., 2018). Results showed an average of 18.5 minutes face-to-face time with a patient and 18.6 minutes overall working in the EHR for the same patient. The results demonstrate the large amount of administrative time physicians spend working in an EHR. Other countries have noted similar administrative time. According to Kane et al. (2019), "at least half of physicians in many countries spent between 10 and 24 hours per week on paperwork, on top of the hours spent seeing patients" (slide 9). Table 11.2 notes the amount of time physicians from different countries spent on paperwork. Time-saving measures introduced with the use of artificial intelligence (AI), however, may decrease the administrative time and allow for more concentrated time with direct patient care.

Table 11.2: Physician Hours Per Week Spent on Paperwork and Administrative Tasks

Country	1–9 Hours	10–24 Hours	25+ Hours
United States	26%	56%	18%
United Kingdom	26%	57%	17%
Germany	18%	59%	24%
France	37%	52%	11%
Spain	36%	50%	15%
Brazil	33%	44%	23%
Mexico	33%	42%	25%

Source: Medscape
Attribution: Leslie Kane, MA; Bernardo Schubsky, MD; Tim Locke; Maria Kouimtzi; Veronique Duqueroy; Claudia Gottschling; Mariana Lopez; Leoleli Schwartz
License: Fair Use

11.5.1 Interoperability

Many medical offices today have some sort of electronic system to store your health information. However, many electronic health record (EHR) systems do not "talk" to one another, nor do they allow transmission of data across systems. A lack of interoperability remains a major issue in today's EHR systems and often leads to fragmented bits of information rather than a full, complete accounting on one's health information. To elaborate,

> Interoperability describes the extent to which systems and devices can exchange data and interpret that shared data. For two systems to be interoperable, they must be able to exchange data and subsequently present that data such that it can be understood by a user (HIMSS, 2019, para. 1).

More simply, **interoperability** is the ability for different technology systems to communicate and exchange health information in a meaningful way. The reality is that with all of the breakthroughs in EHRs, there still remains interoperability issues within systems and between systems. Hospitals are not immune from interoperability issues. For example, a patient is transported to the local hospital ER following a motorcycle accident. Upon arrival to the ER, the patient is stabilized and noted to have multiple open, compound fractures of arms and legs requiring surgical repair. The patient is transferred to the operating room (OR). Following a successful operation, the patient is transferred to the musculoskeletal unit for monitoring and recovery. There is nothing remarkable about this scenario, except it is not uncommon for one hospital to operate separate computer systems within the same facility.

In the above scenario, each unit (ER and OR) had to fax a copy of the patient record to the inpatient unit for copy to the EHR because the systems are unable to "communicate" and "share" with one another. This creates the potential for lost records, extra work for the unit administrator personnel, and barriers to a seamless system that communicates and shares the health data of a patient who is seen in all areas. According to HIMSS (2019), there are four levels of interoperability:

- Level 1 (foundational)—establishes inter-connectivity from one system to another; no interpretation needed

- Level 2 (structural)—defines the format of data exchange; more purposeful and information is evident

- Level 3 (semantic)—two or more systems can communicate and share information more readily; the systems do not have to be the same

- Level 4 (organizational)—secure, seamless, timely sharing of data within and between organizations, entities and individuals; includes governance, policy, social, and legal considerations

Interoperability is affected in many ways by the lack of agreement among vendors to share proprietary system information. This means that the multiple vendors of EHR systems have partially created the inability for EHRs to operate according to the highest functional ideal, sharing health information within and throughout all systems. While ensuring there is accessibility and interoperability of medical information within systems, a larger goal is the ability to move health information among different information systems to ensure the highest quality, most accurate data, and timely medical care. According to HealthIT.gov (2019b), there are three types of Health Information Exchanges (HIE): directed, query-based, and consumer-mediated.

An example of a directed exchange is a health provider's sending laboratory results to another physician as part of a referral for specialized care. This type of exchange enables coordination of care between the two providers. An example of query-based exchange is similar to the emergency room scenario above, in which a search for patient health information is conducted to learn more about the patient's history. Consumer-mediated exchange occurs when a patient has access to their own health information and can actively take part in their care. This can be realized through patient portals, which will be discussed later in this chapter. Most HIEs are built, owned, and managed by hospitals or hospital systems. This works well for those patients able to direct all or most care within a specific system (See Figure 11.2). The obvious downfall is when a patient must seek care outside of the HIE system.

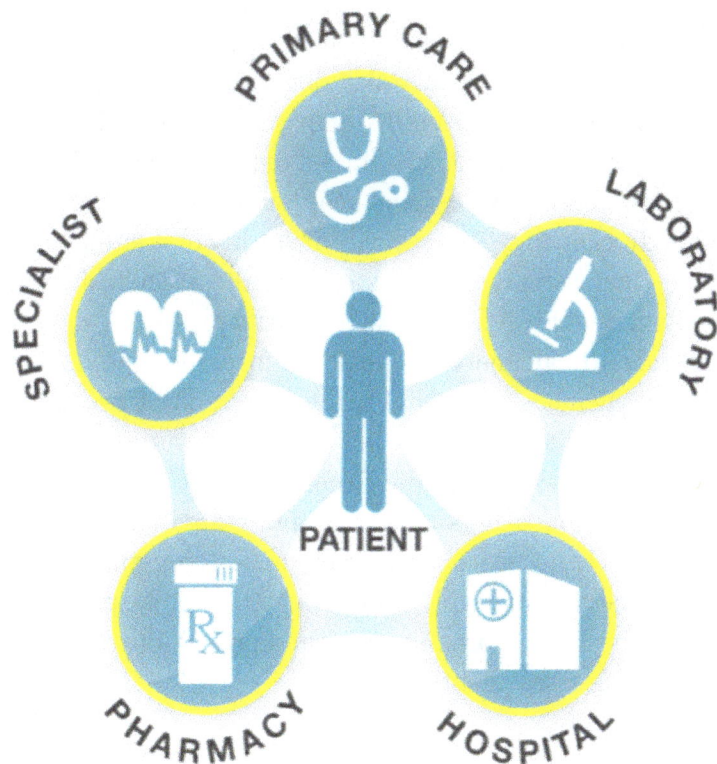

Figure 11.2: Diagram of Health Information Exchange Within One System

11.5.2 HIPAA and Security

As a result of the enhanced use of electronic medical information, the **Health Insurance Portability and Accountability Act (HIPAA)** was introduced in 1996: "The HIPAA Privacy Rule establishes national standards to protect individuals' medical records and other personal health information and applies to health plans, healthcare clearinghouses, and those healthcare providers that conduct certain healthcare transactions electronically" (HHS, 2015, p. 1). HIPAA also requires patient authorization and ensures patients are aware of their rights regarding personal health information. For example, patients visiting a physician office or other healthcare related area that collects personal information, will likely have to read and sign a HIPAA authorization form. This form informs each patient about their rights in regard to personal information collected and allows the patient to authorize sharing of certain information, all information, or no information with others.

With advancements in technology and technology use growing, our health information systems are put at high risk for the possibility of misuse, inappropriate use, or stolen information. Security standards and maintenance of health information systems, such as electronic medical records, is very important. Healthcare facilities face remarkable challenges when it comes to security, privacy, and confidentiality; therefore, both patients and all employees must be educated regarding health information safety. Most healthcare providers are required to complete corporate health information security training annually. Many organizations will require employees to sign documents stating they will not share or discuss private patient information with anyone who is not directly related to the patient's care team without authorization from the patient. Further, providers are not authorized to access any personal health information of persons for whom they do not directly care for. The security form likely includes descriptions of fraudulent actions and penalties for committing these acts. Most organizations terminate employment of those who breach security protocols.

Security extends to safeguarding health information within the computer system. This requires that hospitals, clinics, physician offices, and any other sources that collect, manage, or have access to personal health information, ensures the security of the computer system in which information is stored. Specifically, areas that must have ongoing measures to protect private patient health information includes "unsecured wireless access, inadequate encryption, authentication failures and other access control vulnerabilities" (OIG, 2019, para. 2).

Security tips for healthcare organizations and providers are as follows:
- security risk assessments
- encryption of data
- controlled access to the system
- authentication of users

- providing secure remote access
- adoption of role-based access
- scanning audit log
- backing up data off site
- obtaining business associate agreements (Medical Economics, 2017).

Security tips for healthcare professionals include the following:
- logging out of computer systems before walking away from the computer
- ensuring passwords are complex and not shared with anyone
- shredding documents with PHI before disposal
- not sharing any patient PHI with unauthorized sources
- ensuring corporate emails are from valid sources (HIPAA Journal, 2017).

Security tips for patients include the following:
- never sharing health information online
- password protecting health documents stored on personal computers
- verifying all sources before sharing personal information
- shredding all documents before disposal (HealthIT.gov, 2017a).

It is difficult to know to what extent health information is protected from hackers. Cybersecurity is a growing concern as ransomware attacks are on the rise. Therefore, vigilance by all persons who access healthcare information is essential.

Pause and Reflect

You are visiting a hospital cafeteria to eat lunch with a friend. There are three healthcare workers at the table next to you loudly discussing a patient they had cared for earlier in the morning and sharing identifiable personal health information. You now know this is a violation of HIPAA and hospital policy. Understanding HIPAA, what can you share about this privacy act with others?

11.5.3 HITECH Act and Meaningful Use

The Health Information Technology for Economic and Clinical Health Act (HITECH) is part of a stimulus package (The American Recovery and Reinvestment Act [ARRA] of 2009) which emerged to provide financial incentives to promote the use of electronic health records (EHR) by healthcare providers (HIPAA Journal, 2018). In addition, a major component of the HITECH Act was the "meaningful use" of certified electronic health records. Prior to the HITECH Act, less than 8% of all entities used EHRs. Today, 95% of hospitals have a certified EHR (Parasrampuria & Henry, 2017). Physicians and hospitals who have adopted EHRs must meet meaningful-use criteria to earn incentive payments. Those who do not meet the established criteria will incur reduction in reimbursements from Medicare and Medicaid. HITECH Act also influenced HIPAA by "addressing the development, adoption, and implementation of health information technology (HIT) policies and standards and provided enhanced privacy and security protection for patient information" (Mastrian & McGonigle, 2021, p. 87).

11.6 EMERGING TECHNOLOGIES

Healthcare is experiencing exciting times regarding emerging technology. According to *Managed Healthcare Executive* (2017), healthcare organizations are investing in several types of technology to improve efficiency, support decision making and personalized medicine, empower patients, protect against cyber threats and data breaches, and improve remote health monitoring. Technology discussed in this chapter that is expected to transform healthcare includes artificial intelligence (AI) technologies, telehealth, wearable health monitors, patient portals, medication management software, and clinical decision support systems. Other emerging technologies not discussed include 3D printing, augmented and virtual reality, and next-generation sequencing.

11.6.1 Artificial Intelligence

Artificial Intelligence (AI) is emerging as a significant instrument in healthcare through use with time-saving strategies for administrative tasks, assisting with the analysis of diagnostic tests such as imaging, and through data analysis and the ability to improve diagnostic decision-making. Handing off tedious tasks to a computer decreases costs and increases accuracy associated with, for example, the multi-level, ongoing need to ensure healthcare providers are meeting all requirements for practice. Organizations who utilize computer software to manage the many timelines and paperwork associated with provider licensure, ongoing certifications, and education, will resolve issues, such as lapses in licensure and accreditation, that state boards and national accreditation organizations require (Ferrazzi, 2015).

Automating administrative tasks creates more time for professionals to concentrate on patient care. Physicians, nurses, administrators, human resource managers and countless other professionals have time freed up to focus on patient care initiatives when automation takes care of more common tasks. According to *Healthcare Weekly* (2018), physicians spend less than 27% of their time on direct patient care. Administrative tasks, such as reading paper medical records or filling out forms, can take up a large amount of time. Physicians also note a time-consuming process with phone calls to insurance companies requesting authorization for medications and/or procedures (Medical Economics, 2018). Automating these tasks with simple point-and-click technology could greatly reduce administrative tasks and recapture some much-needed patient time.

AI has the potential to improve detection of abnormalities in radiographs, skin images, and cardiac disease (eye imaging). Scientists are involved in deep learning techniques to "teach" computer systems to recognize abnormalities of diagnostic tests. While this technology is emerging, the prediction is that AI systems will improve the overall rate of detection of diseases, such as breast cancer, as well as improve the potential for individualized treatments (Newman, 2019). Studies are currently underway to discover if AI accuracy in detection of abnormalities through diagnostic imaging surpasses that of human (physician) detection accuracy. In a small study with fifty-eight dermatologists, their completing a 100-image test screening for melanoma had a lower mean for sensitivity and specificity of lesion classification than an AI, known as convolutional neural networks (CNN), created by Google (Haenssle et al., 2018). In simple terms, this means that the artificial intelligent agent detected lesion classification for skin melanomas more accurately than did the humans. While more studies are needed, these promising results indicate the potential of AI in healthcare.

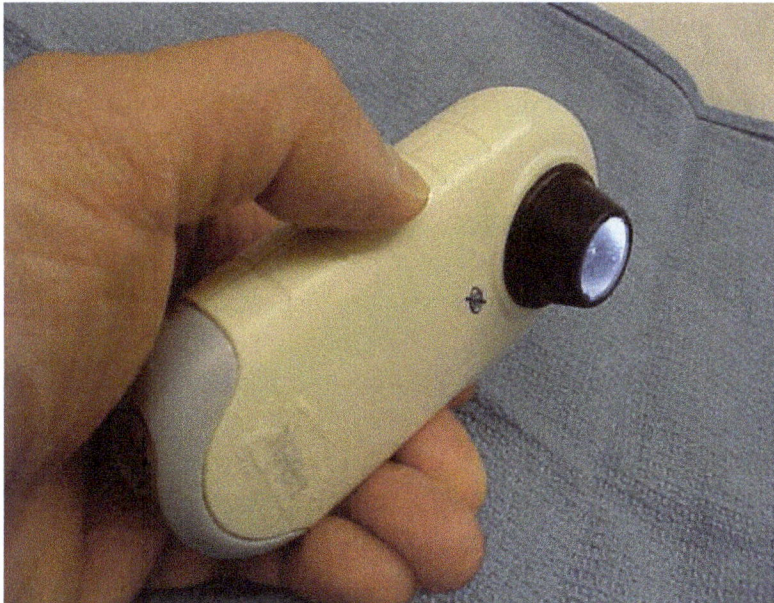

Figure 11.3: A dermatologist uses a dermatoscope, a type of handheld microscope, to look at skin

Source: Wikimedia Commons
Attribution: Northerncedar
License: Public Domain

Speech recognition (SR) software is another form of AI in which deep learning also occurs. SR is most often seen in electronic medical record use in which a physician or other healthcare worker dictates patient clinical notes. Rather than taking time to type directly into the EHR system or having billers and coders decipher notes, SR allows for more accuracy and a seamless upload of clinical notes into electronic medical records. SR systems are "taught" different languages and accents, so reliability is generated. A physician can read several paragraphs of text and the SR software will develop recognition of speech patterns. In a study of 217 clinical notes, SR had an error rate of 7.4%; after a transcriptionist review, the error rate dropped to 0.4%; and after the final version physician review, a drop to 0.3% occurred (Zhou et al., 2018). The initial SR error rate indicates the need for more testing and "learning" by the software but also shows—with the essential human review—that speech recognition software can be a good first step in the documentation process. The use of SR can help increase the speed and accuracy of medical record documentation.

Supply chain management (SCM) technology is emerging as a significant tool. A good workflow is extremely important in healthcare to increase efficiency and facilitate improved patient safety. Technology is an instrument to assist in improving old and creating new workflow processes. Technology is meant not to determine or define healthcare workflow but rather to serve as a complementary addition. According to LaPointe (2016), "healthcare supply chain management is the regulation of the flow of medical goods and services from manufacturer to patient" (para. 1). Tracking inventory helps eliminate waste and increases efficiency in resource allocation. In a survey of 100 healthcare organizations, chief administrators noted SCM as a priority; however, it did not drive investment in the technology. Half of those surveyed still use manual processes to manage supplies (Miliard, 2019).

SCM technology can help reduce workflow procedures in many ways. One example is reduction of time and waste ordering and stocking supplies. SCM technology can reduce costs associated with the management of supply levels by moving from the manual inventory and spreadsheet update method to a format that assesses stock levels through automation. For example, imagine medical supplies needed for a medical-surgical unit in a hospital. Typical items stocked would include intravenous start kits, syringes, urinary catheter start kits, 4X4 gauze, bandage tape, urinals, and bedpans. Prior to technology, a hospital would order large amounts of medical items for storage in a central supply point, and each unit would requisition specific items to desired levels appropriate for that unit. In some cases, supplies are poorly monitored, leading to high stock levels of rarely-used items and low levels of high-use items. For example, a urology unit would use more urinary catheters than a pediatric floor, while a pediatric unit would use more diapers than an operating room. SCM technology for supply management allows for a streamlined workflow process. Barcoding and collection of meaningful-use data will reduce costs associated with manual procedures. Manual processes slow down workflow, and SCM is useful technology for supply management.

Staffing technology can assist by automating the application process; housing employee personnel files; updating employee credentials, such as continuing education credits; and creating an employee portal. It takes tremendous time to onboard (hire and collect documents) new employees. Technology can decrease the human time spent collecting and organizing applicant information, such as background checks, credentials, drug screenings, and payroll information. Consider a human resource department with five employees managing the credentialing documents of a hospital with 600 health professionals. Every year, employees will need to be notified throughout the year about required updates for licensure, special credentials, cardiopulmonary resuscitation (CPR), continuing education credits, flu shots, and other hospital or professional required training. Once a new employee is hired, all specific documents needed must be uploaded into a system, after which, system software will initiate the reminders as needed. Employees can then upload any required documentation into the faculty portal. The use of automated systems reduces the human error associated with manual processes. According to Ferrazzi (2015), "digital onboarding tools can help managers collect leading indicators of success—such as faster ramp to productivity, greater retention rates, and higher employee engagement" (para. 5).

Another advancement is the use of technology to make evidence-based staffing assignments within a healthcare setting. Without doubt, this issue largely affects nurses working within inpatient units. However, any urgent care center, emergency room, or doctor's office can be affected by the ebb and flow of daily patient care. Poorly-managed healthcare environments lead to employee dissatisfaction and patient safety issues. The unpredictability of patient acuity levels (how much care is needed) and patient census (how many patients to be cared for) requires the continuous assessment of staffing. Factors, such as the number of staff available and experience of staff, can also contribute to the complexity of staffing. Too many staff on shift creates financial integrity issues, while too little staff create potential quality and patient safety issues (Mossberger, 2018). Digital applications for upload to a smart phone can allow employees to request time off as well as give administrators real time data to understand staffing needs throughout multiple departments (Healthcare Weekly, 2018). Technological tools that integrate data regarding past shifts, patient acuity, current needs of patients, and existing staff expertise assist administrators to staff units properly, decrease costs, and improve patient outcomes.

11.6.2 Point of Care Technology

Technology that improves patient safety, enables a shorter distance of information exchange, enhances the effectiveness of healthcare delivery, and decreases time spent on patient documentation, is **point of care (PoC)**. PoC technology currently appears in healthcare settings in a variety of ways, including blood glucose meters, such mobile devices as smart phones and iPads, stationary computers located in exam rooms or patient hospital rooms, and mobile computers that can be wheeled to any location. Using PoC technology allows providers to view patient medical records, medication list, and lab results at the bedside using the most up-to-date patient data. PoC also enables healthcare providers to document at the time of examination or diagnostic test, thus eliminating the time between the two activities. This leads to less errors in the documentation process caused from interruptions or memory lapse. Another use of PoC is the scanning of medication barcodes. This technology directly links the patient information, medication administration time, and patient outcomes into the electronic medical record, thereby decreasing errors in manual documentation efforts. The ultimate goal of PoC technology is to improve patient outcomes and enhance administrative processes.

11.6.3 Telehealth

Healthcare reform has created advancement in technology and access to care that includes telehealth. Telehealth is expected to rise to a $36 billion industry in 2020 (AHIP, 2019). According to HRSA (2019), "**telehealth** is defined as the use of electronic information and telecommunications technologies to support long-distance clinical healthcare, patient and professional health-related education, public health, and health administration" (para. 3). The growing number of persons in the U.S. who have chronic illnesses with multiple co-morbidities highlights the need for increased collaboration and continuity of care. Readmission rates within thirty days of hospital discharge for persons with heart disease is a staggering 20% (O'Connor, 2017). This indicates the need for more intensive follow-up care and ongoing education. Telehealth offers improved accessibility to healthcare and decreases in cost; it also enables self-care for patients. The increasing use of telehealth services offers professional care in small rural clinics, hospitals, or a patient's home. Access to ongoing maintenance of health is critical for patients living with chronic conditions, such as diabetes or heart failure. In addition, telehealth services support patients who live remotely, have limited or no access to transportation, or are unable to drive.

During the COVID-19 stay at home order, many healthcare providers have turned to telehealth functions to continue care with patients. According to Henry (2020), COVID-19 has propelled the use of telehealth forward for the American Medical Association (AMA) and physicians working with telehealth, which will likely result in continued wide-spread use. One issue that must be addressed is that many households do not have access to broadband internet and increased efforts to ensure rural communities have access to technology will help telehealth opportunities expand. In recent COVID-19 news, the divide has become evident, with approximately 30% of homes without the basic technology of even a slow broadband connection (Scheiber et al., 2020). The quarantine for safety, while necessary during the COVID-19 virus pandemic, simultaneously puts added stress on those with chronic conditions and who are unable to safely access their doctor's office in person. A proper internet connection and use of a laptop or cellphone could provide much-needed continuation of care through telemedicine.

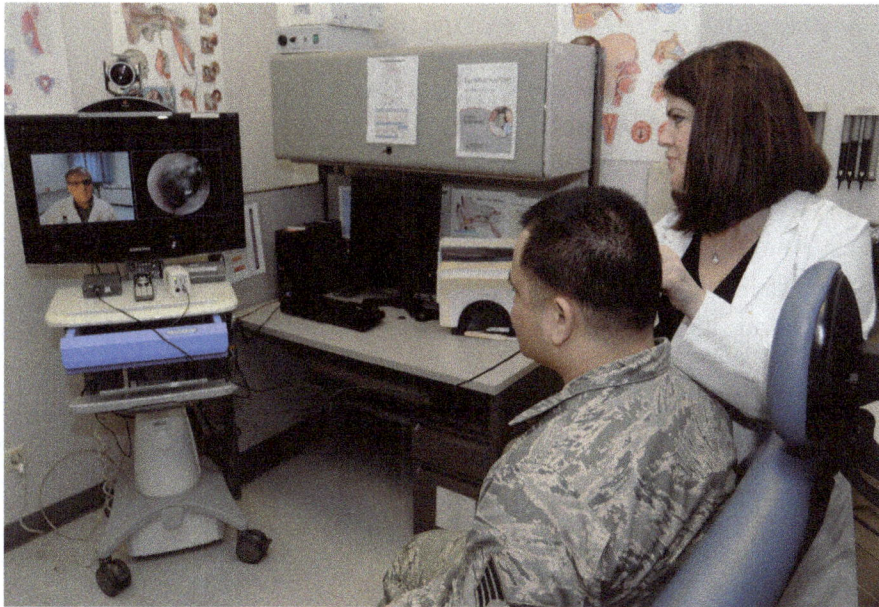

Figure 11.4: Telehealth Makes Possible Long Distance Medical Appointments

Nurse Director for the Telehealth Program at Landstuhl Regional Medical Center, demonstrates using the Telehealth cart otoscope to conduct a real-time tympanic membrane exam. On screen is a Physician Assistant, who from a remote location can see and evaluate the patient and provide an appropriate plan of care.
Source: Flickr
Attribution: Phil Jones
License: CC BY 2.0

Another benefit of telehealth service is the connection with and between healthcare providers. For example, health providers working in remote areas can use telehealth to collaborate with specialists regarding patient diagnosis and management. Finally, insurance companies are using telemedicine remote kiosks to enable employees to connect with healthcare providers for illness and workman's compensation issues. Customer satisfaction ratings are 4.8 out of 5.0 for those using the Blue Cross Blue Shield of Massachusetts (BCBSMA) "Well Connection" telehealth service (AHIP, 2019). This positive satisfaction reveals that patients are finding the technology useful and beneficial. In addition, a healthy workforce decreases costs of healthcare overall. Telehealth thus has the ability to reach many patients who would otherwise be unable to see a healthcare provider because of distance or physical limitations.

Pause and Reflect

Your family member who needs to see a specialist but is unable to make the trip to a larger city is introduced to new technology (telehealth). The family member is concerned about the privacy of this technology and just does not understand it. Based on readings and activities in this chapter, what can you share to alleviate their concerns?

11.6.4 Wearable Health Technology

It would be difficult to miss the number of wearable health technology flooding the market today. Most notable, because worn by millions of people are the watches created by Fitbit, Apple Watch, Garmin, and Nike. The **wearable health technology** that companies have developed allows the average citizen to monitor their heart rate, sleep cycles, daily steps, distance traveled, and much more. The power of this technology is the ability to track our daily, weekly, and monthly activity and fitness. In addition, this technology has expanded to the medical monitoring level with technology that measures vital signs, electrocardiogram (ECG), blood oxygen saturation (SpO2), blood glucose, skin perspiration, and body temperature (Dias & Silva-Cunha, 2018). These technologies allow the patient to perform normal daily functions while recording data, thus increasing the reliability and usefulness of this data. A benefit of wearable health technology is the ability to capture data away from the clinical site so the health provider can make timely diagnosis and informed medical decisions. In addition, wearable health devices improve patient engagement, which can lead to better health outcomes.

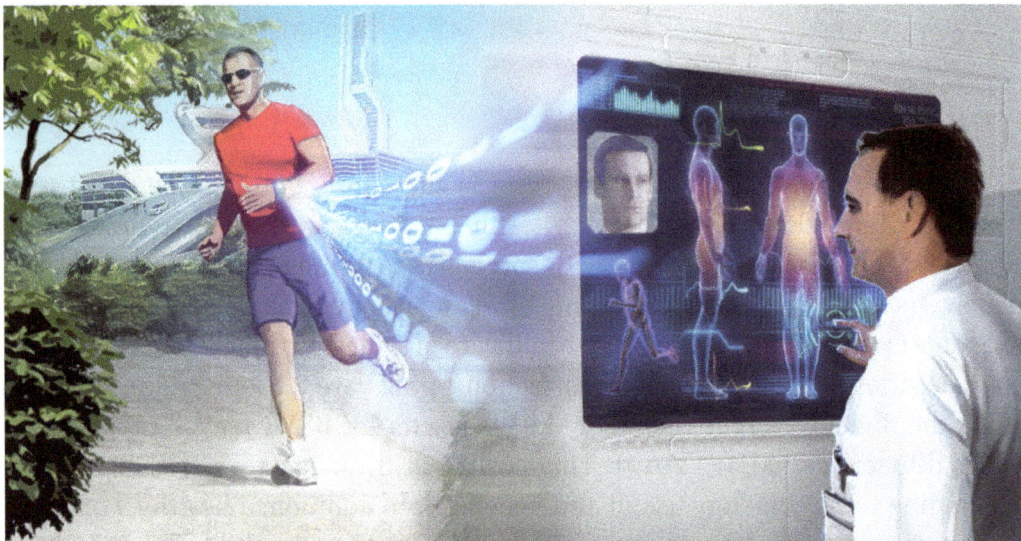

Figure 11.5: Wearable Devices and Smart Watches for Fitness and Hospital Health Tracking

Individuals are taking increased ownership of personal health with use of wearable devices. In the future, we are likely to see health providers monitoring patients' health using data sent from wearable devices in real time.
Source: Flickr
Attribution: Brother UK
License: CC BY 2.0

11.6.5 Patient Portal

The patient portal is an excellent tool for patients to monitor their health. Patients have access to their health records, and most patient portals include a variety of services, such as appointment set up, follow up communication, and education. Portals allow patients to communicate with their doctor or nurse about medical concerns, and a response typically is sent in the same day. Patients can also view results of diagnostic testing as well as track medical history. The **patient portal** is a great feature for patients attempting to manage, and trend data related to, such chronic conditions as diabetes. For example, a patient could review the hemoglobin A1C trends over time to detect if improvement is being made. A visual look at how well an individual is controlling their health is an excellent way to promote healthy living.

The patient portal is a good example of creating communication between provider and patient as well as allowing the patient to participate in self-management. Benefits of patient portals are increased office efficiency through online form completion, updates to insurance information, and offline appointment scheduling. In addition, medical errors are decreased because patients can view and verify their health information, physicians and other providers can include patient education sources, and medications can be screened for drug-to-drug interactions. Further, patients can be provided with billing information and consent forms and scheduled for annual checkups (HealthIT.gov, 2017b).

11.6.6 Medication Management Technology

Without doubt, medication management is an important patient safety initiative. Whether at an individual's home, a doctor's office, or inpatient care, ensuring that the right medication is given to the right person, at the right time is important. According to King and Russell (2019), medication errors are the third leading cause of death in the U.S. Medication management technology covers an array of capabilities, including electronic prescribing, bar-coded medication administration (BCMA) systems, smart infusion pumps for intravenous administration, and medication reconciliation solutions. Many hospitals use medication scanning as a way to improve patient safety with incorporation of health information technology (HIT). Point-of-care barcode scanning decreases medication errors while contributing to patient safety (Patient Safety Network, 2019). Scanning medications is equivalent to a second set of eyes checking what medication is being administered and to whom it is being administered. Alerts are built into the computerized system to alert the nurse or other provider if the medication is correctly dosed for the right patient to be given at the time of scan. Although errors and workarounds do occur, medication errors have been reduced through the use of barcode scanning. Another benefit of most point-of-care barcode scanning technology is the incorporation into the electronic medication record. Once a medication is scanned, the details are updated automatically to the patient's medication record. However, providers should not rely solely on medication technology but rather view it as a supplemental tool for safe practices in medication administration and management.

Pause and Reflect

You have just learned about the benefits of scanning medications for patient administration. Brought to your attention is that sometimes the barcodes do not scan at the point of care. This can lead to frustration from some healthcare professionals who then find workarounds to this technology. This means that some medication is given to a patient without using the proper medication management system. What safety issues might you expect? How does a workaround affect the documentation process?

Computerized physician order entry (CPOE) allows physicians to prescribe and manage patient medication orders within a computerized system. Basic functions of CPOE are the available safeguards, which include drug-drug interaction, drug-disease interaction, and drug-age (Connely & Korvek, 2019). In addition, the software has significantly reduced errors from transcribing written orders. CPOE technology provides clinical decision support through alerts regarding patient allergies and potential medication interactions with food and health conditions. For example, a provider orders a blood thinner medication to a patient with a previously-diagnosed anemia condition. The system would send an alert regarding the medication contraindication in the anemic patient. This alert, then, would help physicians prevent potential drug interactions and improve patient safety.

Pharmacies are also benefitting from medication management software through automating the filling and dispensing of medications. Automated systems reduce manual pill counting thus decreasing errors. In addition, pharmacies are collecting personal health information on customers and creating medication portfolios that include a medical history, medications, immunizations, and education. With large, national pharmacies, such as CVS, Walmart, and Walgreens, patients are able to access their medications from any pharmacy within the chain.

11.7 DATA ANALYTICS

In today's healthcare environments, vast amounts of data are collected on every individual. Many in healthcare are attempting to sort through this data with highly specialized systems that make sense out of the information being collected. There are three types of analytics: descriptive, predictive, and prescriptive. *Descriptive analytics* uses the data to understand what has happened. For example, this could include the number of infection rates on an orthopedic floor in the first quarter, the number of medication errors hospital wide for a year, or how many admissions from flu occurred in the month of October. *Predictive analytics* uses the data to tell what is likely to happen. For example, if a patient is unable to purchase enough insulin to cover an entire month so he or she rations out each day's worth of insulin doses, they will likely end up with higher overall blood glucose levels. Based on the record of higher daily blood glucose levels transmitted via a wearable health device and data collected showing an elevated serum A1C levels in the past three months, the predictive analytics calculates the patient is at risk for crises, such as Diabetic Ketoacidosis (DKA). In *prescriptive analytics*, the data is used to enhance the prediction by giving the provider information on what can be done about the problem.

Each of these data analytic types builds from one another to create pathways from the data that can lead to clinical decision support systems (Bresnick, 2017). **Clinical decision support (CDS)** "provides timely information to help inform decisions about a patient's care and has the ability to significantly impact improvements in quality, safety, efficiency, and effectiveness of healthcare" (eCQI Resource Center, 2019, para 1). One should note, however, that CDS is not a replacement for clinician judgement but a tool to enhance and assist in making high-quality decisions.

11.8 SUMMARY

This chapter described the use of technology in today's current healthcare settings. It explored the types of technology currently in use as well as the emerging technologies. Healthcare costs can be reduced with the use of EHRs through the reduction in waste and redundancy of tests (HealthIT.gov, 2019c). The seamless sharing of health information can decrease additional costs related to duplication of services, such as diagnostic tests. Redesigning and easing workflow assists in reducing healthcare costs and improving operational efficiency. Finally, this chapter reviewed security issues and the protection of individual health information.

11.9 REVIEW QUESTIONS

1. What ways can you protect your private health information (PHI)? What activities put your PHI at risk?

2. What are the benefits of implementing an electronic health record (EHR)?

3. How does the Health Insurance Portability and Accountability Act (HIPAA) address security and improper use by authorized users?

4. What are the benefits of telehealth technology?

5. What are the benefits of interoperability of electronic health record systems?

6. How does wearable health technology benefit both the patient and healthcare provider?

11.10 REFERENCES

AHIP.org. (2019). Telehealth: Connecting consumers to care everywhere. Insurance
      Journal. Retrieved from https://www.ahip.org/telehealth-connecting-consumers-to-

care everywhere/

Bailey, D., Weeks, J., Evans, E., Lowery, J., & McFarland, L. (2017). Technologies for managing virtual data warehouse access and identifying appropriate levels of staffing as CHI Institute for Research and Innovation. Journal of Patient-Centered Research and Reviews, 4(3), 197–198.

Bresnick, J. (2017). The difference between clinical decision support, big data analytics. HealthITAnalytics. Retrieved from https://healthitanalytics.com/news/the-difference-between-clinical-decision-support-big-data-analytics

Connelly, T. P. & Korvek, S. J. (2019). Computer provider order entry (CPOE). NCBI. Retrieved from https://www.ncbi.nlm.nih.gov/books/NBK470273/

Dias, D., & Silva-Cunha, J. P. (2018). Wearable health devices. Vital sign monitoring, systems and technologies. Sensors (Basel), 18(8), 2414. 10.3390/s18082414.

eCQI Resource Center. (2019). CDS-Clinical decision support. Retrieved from https://ecqi.healthit.gov/cds

Edelmann, S. (2019). 6 technologies that will transform health care. Healthcare Transformers. Retrieved from https://health caretransformers.com/6-technologies-that-will-transform-health care/

Ferrazzi, K. (2015). Technology can save onboarding from itself. Harvard Business Review. Retrieved from https://hbr.org/2015/03/technology-can-save-onboarding-from-itself

Haenssle, H. A., Fink, C., Schneiderbauer, R., Toberer, F., Buhl, T., Blum, A., Uhlmann, L. (2018). Man against machine: Diagnostic performance of a deep learning convolutional neural network for dermoscopic melanoma recognition in comparison to 58 dermatologists. Annals of Oncology, 29(8), 1836-–842. https://doi.org/10.1093/annonc/mdy166

Healthcare Weekly. (2018, May 30). 5 ways technology can reduce health care costs. Retrieved from https://health careweekly.com/5-ways-technology-can-reduce-health care-costs/

HealthIT.gov. (2019a). What is an electronic health record (EHR)? Retrieved from https://www.healthit.gov/faq/what-electronic-health-record-ehr

HealthIT.gov. (2019b). What is HIE? Retrieved from https://www.healthit.gov/topic/health-it-and-health-information-exchange-basics/what-hie

HealthIT.gov. (2019c). What are the advantages of electronic health records? Retrieved from https://www.healthit.gov/faq/what-are-advantages-electronic-health-records

HealthIT.gov. (2017a). What you can do to protect your health information. Retrieved from https://www.healthit.gov/topic/privacy-security/what-you-can-do-protect-your-health-information

HealthIT.gov. (2017b). What is a patient portal? Retrieved from https://www.healthit.gov/faq/what-patient-portal

Henry, T. A. (2020, April 29). COVID-19 makes telemedicine mainstream. Will it stay that way? American Medical Association. Retrieved from https://www.ama-assn.org/practice-management/digital/covid-19-makes-telemedicine-mainstream-will-it-stay-way

HIPAA Journal. (2018). What is the HITECH Act? Retrieved from https://www.hipaajournal.com/what-is-the-hitech-act/

HIMSS. (2019). Interoperability in the health ecosystem. Retrieved from https://www.himss.org/what-interoperability

HIPAA Journal. (2017, October 13). How to secure patient information (PHI). Retrieved from https://www.hipaajournal.com/secure-patient-information-phi/

Kane, L., Schubsky, B., Locke, T., Kouimtzi, M., Duqueroy, V., Gottschling., . . . Schwartz, L. (2019). International physician compensation report 2019: Do US physicians have it best? Medscape. Retrieved from https://www.medscape.com/slideshow/2019-international-compensation-report-6011814#9

King, J. & Russell, C. (2019). Transforming medication management. New insights from the HIMSS medication management technology index. HIMSS Media. Retrieved from https://www.himsslearn.org/transforming-medication-management-%E2%80%93-new-insights-himss-medication-management-technology-index

LaPointe, J. (2016). Exploring the role of supply chain management in health care. RevCycleIntelligence.com. Retrieved from https://revcycleintelligence.com/news/exploring-the-role-of-supply-chain-management-in-health care

Managed Health care Executive. (2017, November 22). Top five technology investment areas for health care organizations. Retrieved from https://www.managedhealth careexecutive.com/business-strategy/top-five-technology-investment-areas-health care-organizations

Mastrian, K.G. & McGonigle, D. (2021). Informatics for health professionals. 2nd ed. Jones & Bartlett Learning.

Matthews, K. (2019, November 20). How centralized data improves the health care industry. Retrieved from https://info.cgcompliance.com/blog/how-centralized-data-improves-the-health-care-industry

Medical Economics. (2018). What's ruining medicine for physicians: Paperwork and administrative burdens. Medical Economics, 95(24). Retrieved from https://www.medicaleconomics.com/business/whats-ruining-medicine-physicians-paperwork-and-administrative-burdens

Medical Economics (2017, April 25). 10 ways to improve patient data security. Retrieved from https://www.medicaleconomics.com/e-h-r/10-ways-improve-patient-data-security

Miliard, M. (2019, March 8). Half of hospitals still managing supply chain data manually, if at all. Health careITNews. Retrieved from https://www.health careitnews.com/news/half-hospitals-still-managing-supply-chain-data-manually-if-all

Mossberger, M. (2018). Using technology to address nurse staffing challenges. Health

IT outcomes. Retrieved from https://www.healthitoutcomes.com/doc/using-technology-to-address-nurse-staffing-challenges-0001

Newman, T. (2019, July 16). Could artificial intelligence be the future of cancer diagnosis? Medical News Today. Retrieved from https://www.medicalnewstoday.com/articles/325750.php#1

Nursing Solutions, Inc. (2019). 2019 National health care retention report. Retrieved from www.nsinursingsolutions.com › Files › assets › library › retention-institute

O'Connor, C.M. (2017). High health failure readmission rates. Is it the health system's fault? JACC: Heart Failure, 5(5). DOI: 10.1016/j.jchf.2017.03.011

Office of Inspector General (OIG). (2019). Management issue 9: Integrity and security of health information systems and data. Retrieved from https://oig.hhs.gov/reports-and-publications/top-challenges/2012/issue09.asp

Parasrampuria, S. & Henry, J. (2019, April). Hospitals' use of electronic health records data, 2015-2017. ONC Data Brief, No. 46. Retrieved from https://www.healthit.gov/sites/default/files/page/2019-04/AHAEHRUseDataBrief.pdf

Patient Safety Network. (2019). Medication administration errors. AHRQ.gov. Retrieved from https://psnet.ahrq.gov/primer/medication-administration-errors

Reddy, M. (2019). 9 health technologies every executive should be excited about in 2019. Healthcare Weekly. Retrieved from https://health careweekly.com/health-technologies/

Scheiber, N., Schwartz, N. D., & Hsu, T. (2020, March 28). How the pandemic is magnifying America's class divide. The New York Times. Retrieved from https://www.yahoo.com/news/pandemic-magnifying-americas-class-divide-140718064.html

U.S. Department of Health & Human Services. (2015). Health information privacy. The HIPAA privacy rule. Retrieved from https://www.hhs.gov/hipaa/for-professionals/privacy/index.html

Young, R. A., Burge, S. K., Kumar, K. A., Wilson, J. M., & Ortiz, D. F. (2018). A time-motion study of primary care physicians' work in the electronic health record era. Family Medicine, 50(2), 91–99. 10.22454/FamMed.2018.184803

Zhou, L., Blackley, S. V., Kowalski, L., Doan, R., Acker, W. W., Landman, A. B., . . . Goss, F. R. (2018). Analysis of errors in dictated clinical documents assisted by speech recognition software and professional transcriptionists. JAMA Netw Open, 1(3); e180530. DOI:10.1001/jamanetworkopen.2018.0530

12 National Healthcare Systems

12.1 LEARNING OBJECTIVES

By the end of this chapter, the student will be able to:
- Describe the four types of healthcare systems: Beveridge model, Bismark model, national health insurance model, and out-of-pocket model
- Compare the U.S. healthcare system with systems from countries such as Germany, Canada, and United Kingdom
- Compare the healthcare plans submitted in 116th Congress in 2019
- Describe the pros and cons of a universal or national healthcare system in the U.S.

12.2 KEY TERMS

- Beveridge model
- Bismark model
- Fee-for-Services
- multi-payer
- national health insurance model
- out-of-pocket or entrepreneurial model
- single-payer

12.3 INTRODUCTION

Healthcare is extremely important to the overall health of a nation. This chapter will discuss four basic healthcare models throughout the world, digging deep into how each is used in a select country. It will include a discussion of how the models of Germany, Canada's, and the United Kingdom's healthcare systems work, including funding, benefits, and statistics about each country. As previously discussed, the U.S. healthcare system is complicated and does not serve all members of the population. In today's politics, many are voicing the need for a universal healthcare system, Medicare-for-all, or some sort of blended system which includes a comprehensive health system for all citizens and the use of private health insurance for those that wish to continue with their current health plans. This chapter will include a description of several healthcare bills submitted to the current 116th Congress (2019–2020).

12.3 BASIC MODELS OF HEALTHCARE SYSTEMS

Basically, four different models of healthcare systems are used throughout the 195 countries recognized by the United Nations. Each country has created its own healthcare system to ensure people stay healthy, care for those who are sick, and protect people from medical bills that could place personal finances in jeopardy. Only about forty of the developed, industrialized countries have an established healthcare system (PNHP, 2019). Table 12.1 shows the four types of healthcare models discussed in this chapter, including when each was created, how the health model is financed, which countries use the specific health model, and what parts of the U.S. healthcare system are similar to each model.

Table 12.1: Characteristics of Different Models of Healthcare Systems and Relevance to the U.S. (Chung, 2017)				
Type of Model	Created	Financed by	Countries Using	Relevance to the U.S.
Beveridge model	After World War II in 1948. Named after Sir William Beveridge, a social reformer.	The government through tax payments; Many hospitals owned by the government and some doctors are government employees. No doctor bills; government controls charges.	Great Britain; Hong Kong; most of Scandinavia; Spain	Similar to the Veterans Administration

Bismarck model	Dates back to the late 1800s. Named after Chancellor Otto von Bismarck.	Insurance system (sickness funds) jointly financed by employers and employees' payroll. Everyone must be covered. Insurance companies cannot make a profit. The government controls costs through regulations.	Belgium; Germany; France; Japan; Latin America; Netherlands; Switzerland	Employer-based health plans and some aspects of Medicaid
National health insurance model	Has combined elements of Beveridge and Bismarck	Government insurance program that uses private providers. Every citizen pays into it. No profit or financial motives for programs and is cheaper	Canada; South Korea; Taiwan	Medicare
Out-of-pocket model	Self-pay, just as the name suggests	Favors the rich	Poor countries with no organized healthcare system	Uninsured or underinsured

Source: Chung, 2017
Attribution: Deanna Howe, Adapted from Chung, 2017
License: Fair Use

12.3.1 GERMANY

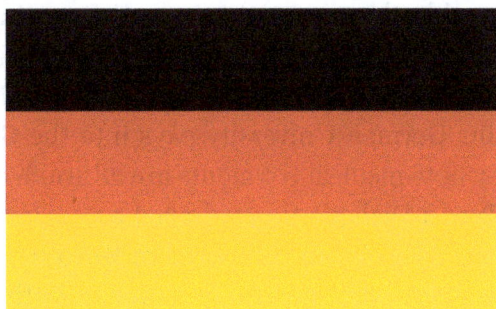

Figure 12.1: German Flag
Source: Wikimedia Commons
Attribution: User "Skopp"
License: Public Domain

The healthcare system in Germany dates back to the late 1800s and offers both private and public health insurance options. The public health system is mandatory for all citizens. In Germany, the health system, known as the **Bismarck model**, is based on the "principle of solidarity," which means that everyone covered through the system has an equal right to medical care and loss of wages while ill (NCBI, 2018). The concept of solidarity emerged in 1883 from the German Chancellor Otto von Bismark, at a time when the first statutory health insurance system was created (Busse et al., 2017). What is significant about the Bismarck model is this system is a shared contribution that all citizens, regardless of health risk, make to a fund that helps all people. The health system is governed by federal authorities and administered by public health insurance companies (GermanyHIS, 2019).

Germany's public health insurance covers the basic preventive services, inpatient care, outpatient care, mental health services, preventative dental care, yearly eye examination, physical therapy, prescription drugs, rehabilitation, and hospice. The public health insurance also provides for sick leave compensation. Mandatory nursing care insurance covers any home care needed. Copayments may be assessed but at much lower ranges than seen in the U.S. Typically, copayments are $10 or less. Children under 18 years of age are exempt from copays. Another advantage of the public health system is Germany has a bilateral agreement with some European Union countries, in a reciprocal plan called European Health Insurance Card (EHIC). This bilateral agreement allows individuals who are covered in their home country to not have to pay for the addition of German statutory health insurance while traveling or working in Germany (GermanyHIS, 2019). In return, Germans with the public healthcare insurance are also covered in participating EHIC countries.

A benefit of those temporarily residing in Germany, such as university students, is the ability to receive health benefits. Germany is obliged to offer affordable coverage for students up to the age of 30. Regardless of student status: language course students, preparatory course students, exchange students, guest scientists, or university students, must obtain mandatory health insurance while studying in Germany (DAAD, n.d.). The low-cost insurance premiums are approximately $130 a month and provide the essential coverage for primary and emergency services. Co-payments for services and prescription drug prices are considerably lower in comparison to the U.S. For example, as noted in an NBC News interview, a U.S. student attending German University pays into the German public health insurance system. They note medical payments are all 100% covered by the health insurance plan. As a Type 1 Diabetic they received a new insulin pump at no cost and the insulin was only $5 a month compared to $100 in the U.S. The student does not have to worry about extra medical fees every month.

As of 2016, the German healthcare system requires each person earning up to €60,750/year ($65,800 U.S. equivalent) or €5,063/month (U.S. $5,483) to pay 14.6% of their gross salary each month (GermanyHIS, 2019). Table 12.2 shows sample income and payment rates into the Germany public health fund. Employers must contribute half of the monthly premium or 7.3% of the total contribution for each individual, thereby decreasing the individual total contribution per month.

Contributions cover dependents and spouses who do not earn an income (Blümel & Busse, 2016). There is no higher fee or rates for households, meaning the premium is capped at the maximum rate of €5,063/month for those earning more than €60,750/year. Approximately 90% of the German population is covered by the public healthcare insurance option (GermanyHIS, 2019). There are some exceptions, such as military, police, and other public sector employees, who are covered under special programs (Blümel & Busse, 2016).

Table 12.2: Sample Income/Payment Rate for Germany's Public Health Fund		
Income per month	Percentage of income	Payment per month into health fund
€1,500/ $1,625	14%	€219 / $237.20
€3,000/ $3,250	14%	€438/ $474.39
€5,063/ $5,483	14%	€739/ $800.40
€12,000/ $12,997	14%	€739/ $800.40
€24,000/ $25,994	14%	€739/ $800.40

NOTE: 1 € (Euro) is equal to approximately $1.08 U.S. dollar (February 15, 2020).
Source: Original Work
Attribution: Deanna Howe
License: CC BY-SA 4.0

German citizens earning more than the maximum income requirements for public insurance can stay in the public system at no higher cost than the maximum premium or opt out and get private health insurance. Similarly, those who are self-employed, working part-time, or earning less than $487 U.S. dollar equivalent per month, can opt for private health insurance. According to Nadash et al. (2018), 8.8 million people in Germany had private health insurance plans in 2015. In addition to health insurance, all citizens by law must have nursing care insurance (Long-term care insurance, LTCI), which is currently set at 3.3% of the individual gross income (with no children). Introduced in 1995, the nursing care insurance covers the cost of long-term services and supports for elder care if these services are necessary (Nadash et al., 2018).

Private healthcare insurance offers more flexibility than the public health plan. In some cases, private health insurance can be a cheaper alternative to public insurance, depending on an individual's health status. Priority for appointments is often given to privately-insured individuals, which could ultimately save time and money. For those with private health insurance, there are no restrictions on doctor availability—meaning a person can choose who they want to see, including specialists.

Medical school in Germany takes six years and up to an additional thirteen years of training, depending on the specialty. The average annual cost of education is approximately $19,900 to $38,200 U.S. equivalent per year for private medical school or $600 per year for public medical school (Kane et al., 2019). Physicians in Germany are not government employees. However, general practitioners and specialists who work in ambulatory care are reimbursed by the statutory health insurance (SHI) system and required by law to serve in regional associations that negotiate contracts with sickness funds (Blümel & Busse, 2016). Approximately 60% of physicians work in a solo private practice and another 25% in group practices. Physicians annually earn approximately $163,000 U.S. dollar equivalent. A gender pay gap exists, with male physicians earning 20% more than female physicians (Kane et al., 2019).

Pause and Reflect

As noted in the example above, Germany's healthcare system has significantly lower prices for prescription drugs, such as insulin. How would a similar price structure in the U.S. impact those with such chronic illnesses as diabetes? Do you think pharmaceutical companies should be able to charge considerably higher prices for medications to U.S. citizens? Is there a relationship between higher prices for service and medications and higher insurance rates?

Basic Statistics of the German Healthcare System and Citizens

- The current population in Germany is 83,763,525 as of June 2, 2020. The median age is 45.7 years, and it ranks 19th in the list of countries by population as of October 21, 2020 (Worldometers, 2020a).

- Ranking 13th in the world, Coronavirus cases: 3,776,721; Deaths: 92,171 as of August 1, 2021 (Worldometers, 2021).

- The public health insurance plan is one of the largest in the world.

- Highest expenditures for healthcare in Europe. In 2017, statistics show EUR376 billion in health expenditures; approximately one billion Euros a day.

- Approximately $4,550 U.S. dollar equivalent is spent annually on healthcare for each resident.

- Germany spends over 11% of the GDP (gross domestic product) for the nation's healthcare.

- The German healthcare system covers more than 80% of pharmaceutical costs of residents.

- The cost of an inpatient hospital stay is $10 per night (public health insurance).

- More than 20% of residents are over 65 years of age, leading to an increase in nursing care expenditures (GermanyHIS, 2019).

- Life expectancy at birth for females is 83.79 years; men is 79.05 (World Population Review, 2020).

- Maternal mortality rate is seven deaths per 100,00 live births (2017 est.) (CIA, 2019).
- Infant mortality rate is three infant deaths per 1,000 live births for 2018 (The World Bank, 2019).

* €1.00 (Euro) equivalent to U.S. $1.08 (February 15, 2020).

12.3.2 Canada

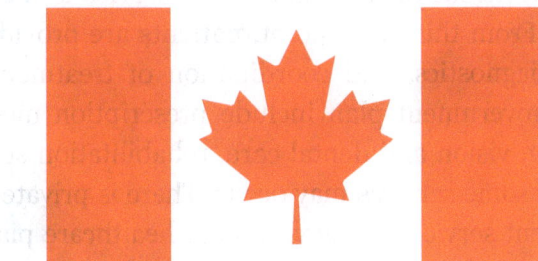

Figure 12.2: Canadian Flag

Source: Wikimedia Commons
Attribution: User"Mzajac"
License: Public Domain

The history of healthcare in Canada shows a country that has overcome many challenges to create a national healthcare system for all. Citizens of Canada call their health plan "Medicare." But one should not confuse Canada's Medicare with what the U.S. calls Medicare. As discussed in previous chapters, the U.S. Medicare program primarily serves elderly persons. Canada's healthcare system is a **national health insurance model**, single-payer system with health services as a right for all citizens and is a point of great pride in Canada.

Publicly-funded healthcare came to the forefront during the Great Depression (1929–1939) when 60% of citizens could not afford the private healthcare that predominated in the country. It took another twenty years for the creation of the Saskatchewan Hospitalization Act (1946), which guaranteed all citizens of Saskatchewan full hospital coverage, paid by the government. This beginning led to tremendous support by the Canadian people, and in 1949, 80% of citizens polled said they would support a government-funded healthcare system that would require an individual contribution. The government passed new legislations in 1957 called the Hospital Insurance and Diagnostic Services Act (HIDS), which led to the government financing 50% of hospital expenses for provincial and territorial hospitals. By 1961, all provinces had HIDS Act programs in place.

In 1962, Saskatchewan again led the country with the first public healthcare program for physician services. This new initiative quickly led to other provinces creating similar plans. The Medical Care Act (Medicare) of 1966 broadened the HIDS Act expense-sharing, and each province and territory (ten provinces and three territories) in Canada began to initiate universal coverage. The healthcare system continued to evolve, and in 1984, the Canada Health Act was created. This new legislation replaced federal hospital and medical insurance acts in addition to setting criteria on portability, accessibility, universality, comprehensiveness, and public administration. The act further prohibited physician extra billing and user fees for already-insured services (Government of Canada, 2019). Although the healthcare system continues to evolve, the overall principle remains: Canada's healthcare system is based on individual need versus an ability to pay for services.

Healthcare services vary depending on the province or territory where one is seeking care. All provinces and territories offer emergency medical services even without a government health card. Primary care service is the first line of care provided in Canada. From this entry point, patients are provided with essential early intervention, diagnostics, and coordination of treatment plans. Services not covered by the government plan include prescription medications outside of the hospital setting, vision and dental care, rehabilitation services, and home care. Cost sharing for some services may occur. There is private health insurance available to supplement services the government healthcare plan does not cover (Luthra, 2017). Provinces and territories provide supplemental assistance to those unable to afford care of uncovered services. According to Allin and Rudoler (2016), approximately two-thirds of Canadians have private health coverage for services not covered by the government plan.

The cost for individual healthcare is difficult to calculate. Canadians will not see a bill nor make any payments for physician or hospital expenses directly. No specific healthcare tax is deducted from individual payroll to fund healthcare. Rather, healthcare is funded through general government revenues. This makes it difficult for individuals to know exactly how much healthcare services cost. Table 12.3 shows the average tax bill based on income, the tax rate percentage and the cost of healthcare insurance. Several government funds contribute to the funding of healthcare: income tax, employment insurance, Canada Pension Plan premiums, property taxes, profit taxes, sales taxes, taxes for alcohol and tobacco consumption, fuel taxes, carbon taxes, motor vehicle license fees, natural resource fees, and import duties (Ren et al., 2017).

Table 12.3: Average Income and Total Tax Bill in Each Decile, 2017

Family Type	Average Cash Income ($)	Average Total Tax Bill ($)	Tax Rate	Healthcare Insurance ($)
Unattached individuals	44,674	19,570	43.8%	4,596
2 parents, 0 children	109,446	52,296	47.8%	12,283
2 parents, 1 child	129,099	52,839	40.9%	12,410
2 parents, 2 children	127,814	51,336	40.2%	12,057
1 parent, 1 child	60,063	19,981	33.3%	4,693
1 parent, 2 children	62,377	17,003	27.3%	3,994

Source: Frasier Institute
Attribution: Feixue Ren, Milagros Palacios, and Bacchus Barua
License: Fair Use

Canada has seventeen medical schools: fourteen in English and five in French. Medical schools in Canada require four years of study and an additional three- to seven-years residency training. Medical training costs are shared by provincial governments, medical schools, and students. The average annual cost of education is $16,798 Canadian dollars per year ($12,676 U.S. equivalent) (AFMC, 2017). Most physicians in Canada are self-employed and paid on a **Fee-for-Service** plan. Provincial and territorial ministries of health negotiate the fee schedule with physician providers (Allin & Rudoler, 2016).

Doctors in Canada earn a comfortable six-figure income. The average income varies depending on province. Alberta province is among the highest earners, with $380,384 annually, compared to Nova Scotia province, which is among the lowest average earners at $259,368 annually (Keith, 2018). Physician specialists can earn significantly higher wages. For example, ophthalmologists are the highest earners, with an average gross salary of $714,000. A gender pay gap exists with male physicians earning more than female physicians. There is little published data regarding gender pay gaps in Canada, and the issue appears to be complex. Women make up about 40% of physicians but, in regard to specialties, predominantly work in pediatrics and obstetrics-gynecology, which has lower average incomes than the male-dominated specialties of general surgery, ophthalmology, and diagnostic radiology (Izenber et al., 2018).

Pause and Reflect

Canadians are very proud of their healthcare system in spite of some needed improvements. Each person pays taxes to ensure all citizens have access to healthcare services. Would U.S. citizens consider higher taxes if all Americans could have better healthcare access? Would you? Why, or why not?

Basic Statistics of the Canadian Healthcare System and Citizens

- The current population in Canada is 37,845,431 as of October 21, 2020. The median age is 41.1 years; and ranks 39th in the list of countries by population as of October 21, 2020 (Worldometers, 2020b).

- Ranking 25th in the world, Coronavirus cases: 1,430,825; Deaths: 26,598 as of August 1, 2021 (Worldometers, 2021).

- Health expenditures for 2019 is 11.6% of the gross domestic product.

- $264.4 billion spent on health, a 3.9% growth, $7,068 per person (CIHI, 2019a).

- 15.3% of spending is on pharmaceuticals, a 1.8% growth, $1,078 per person (CIHI, 2019b).

- Life expectancy at birth for females is 84.45 years; men is 80.56 (World Population Review, 2020).

- The public sector will pay for about 70% of total health expenditures (65.1% from the provincial and territorial governments and 5.3% from other parts of the public sector) (CIHI, 2019c).

- Private-sector spending will account for the other 30% of total health expenditure in 2019. The private sector has three components, the largest of which is out-of-pocket spending (14.4%), followed by private health insurance (12.3%) and non-consumption (2.9%) (CIHI, 2019d).

- Maternal mortality rate is 10 deaths per 100,00 live births (2017 est.) (CIA, 2019).

- Infant mortality rate is four infant deaths per 1,000 live births for 2018 (The World Bank, 2019).

* Can $1.00 (Canadian dollar) equivalent to U.S. $0.75 (February 15, 2020).

12.3.3 United Kingdom

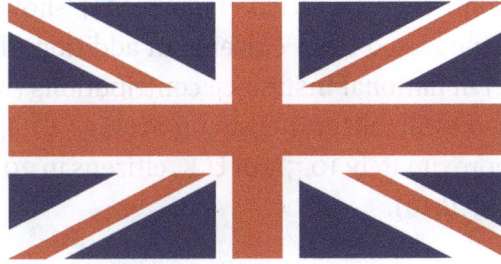

Figure 12.3: United Kingdom Flag

Source: Wikimedia Commons
Attribution: User "Zscout370"
License: Public Domain

Healthcare in the United Kingdom has evolved from the earliest centuries. Prior to the National Health System (NHS), healthcare was primarily different for each social class. During the Victorian Era (1837–1901), the middle and upper classes would help to finance hospitals for the working class. The stigma associated with charitable hospitals meant that most middle and upper-class people who could afford private doctors would avoid hospitals and assume home care for illness.

The U.K. has the largest single-payer healthcare system in the world. The current healthcare system was created by William Beveridge and established in 1948. The **Beveridge model** is a national health, single-payer system funded by general taxation and national insurance which is paid by employers, employees, and self-employed individuals. At just over seventy years old, the NHS is a source of national pride, with two-thirds of citizens considering the establishment of the health system to be Britain's greatest achievement (Duncan & Jowit, 2018).

The U.K. has four major countries: England, Wales, Scotland, and Northern Ireland. The national healthcare system includes the National Health Service (NHS) in England, Department of Health, NHS Wales, NHS Scotland, and Social Services and Public Safety in Northern Ireland. Each country participates in the national health system, but the organization and management vary by country. The founding principle of the NHS is that health services be free at the point of service to all citizens. The NHS provides urgent and emergency care; inpatient hospital; general practitioners; dental (not all are free and shared costs may be required); pharmacy; mental health; sexual health; and optical services (children and adults over 60). NHS has an app, similar to a patient portal, allowing for patients to access medical records, book and manage appointments, refill prescriptions, and check symptoms. Services not included through the NHS include eye exams for working adults,; physiotherapy (there are long wait times so many opt for private care); chiropractic care; podiatry; and tests or scans not ordered by the general physician and some shared cost dental services (Connington, 2018). Private health insurance is available to purchase and used to cover services not supported through the NHS.

Citizens pay into NHS through taxation. The amount of tax contribution depends on the amount one earns. For example, an employee earning £28,000

($36,531 U.S. equivalent) will pay nearly £6,000 ($7,828) in income tax and National Insurance contributions (NIC). Figure 12.4 shows the percentage of national tax from income raised from citizens. In addition, the employer will pay nearly £3000 ($3,912) in national insurance contributions (Miller, 2019). Private health insurance is also available and costs on average £1,435 ($1,872) per year (Woodfield, 2018). Approximately 10.5% of U.K. citizens in 2015 had private health plans (Thorlby & Arora, 2016).

How much tax does the government raise?
Percentage of national income

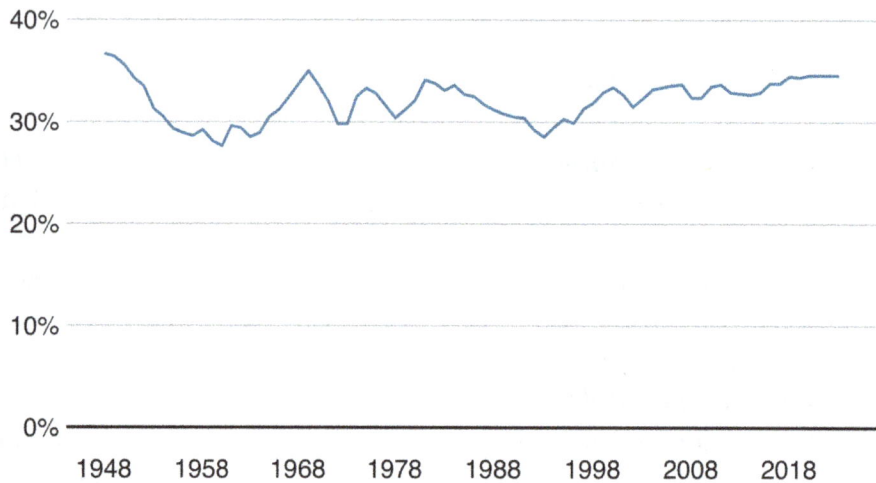

Values for 2019 to 2024 are projected figures

Source: Office for Budget Responsibility   BBC

Figure 12.4: Percentage of National Income the U.K. Government Raises

Source: Office for Budget Responsibility
Attribution: BBC News
License: Fair Use

Medical school in the U.K. takes five-to-six years and up to an additional twelve years of training, depending on specialty. The average annual cost of education is $45,000 U.S. equivalent per year for private medical school or $11,000 per year for public medical school (Kane et al., 2019). Physicians who work in hospitals are salaried employees of the NHS. However, they may also serve in private practice. General practice doctors and other specialists, such as optometrists and dentists, are self-employed and work within the NHS through service contracts. The latter is similar to fee-for-service contracts in the U.S. between physicians and government health programs, such as Medicare and Medicaid. General practitioners in the U.K. earn on average £104,000 ($135,690) and specialists £115,000 ($150,000) annually in 2018 (Locke, 2019). A gender pay gap exists with male physicians earning 26% more than female physicians (Kane et al., 2019).

Basic Statistics of the U.K. Healthcare System and Citizens

- The current population in the United Kingdom is 67,996,758. The median age is 40.5 years; and ranks 21 in the list of countries by population as of October 21, 2020, (Worldometers, 2020c).

- Ranking 6th in the world, Coronavirus cases: 5,856,528; Deaths: 129,654 as of August 1, 2021 (Worldometers, 2021).

- Healthcare spending was 9.769% USD estimated GDP for the year 2018 (OECD, 2018).

- Government-financed healthcare expenditure in 2017 accounted for 79% of total healthcare spending, at £155.6 billion (202.28 billion U.S. equivalent) (Office of National Statistics, 2017).

- Life expectancy at birth for females is 82.05 years; men is 79.71 (World Population Review, 2020).

- There are 12 million people aged 65 and above in the U.K. (AgeUK, 2019).

- Maternal mortality rate is seven deaths per 100,00 live births (2017 est.) (CIA, 2019).

- Infant mortality rate is four infant deaths per 1,000 live births for 2018 (The World Bank, 2019).

* £1 (British Pound Sterling) equivalent to U.S. $1.30 (January 19, 2020).

12.3.4 United States

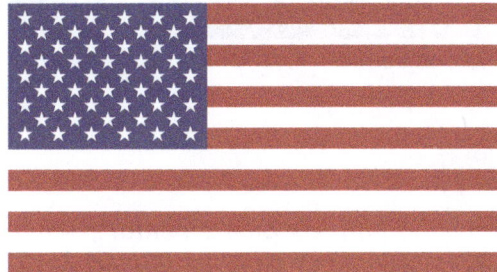

Figure 12.5: United States Flag

As discussed throughout this book, the U.S. has a very complicated healthcare system. There is much room for improvement, and the topic of a national or universal healthcare system that covers all citizens has been debated for many decades. As previously presented, the U.S. healthcare system is a combination of government-run health programs, such as Medicare, Medicaid, Public Health, Veteran's Administration, and multi-payers, which includes many health insurance plans. In addition, the Affordable Care Act (ACA) was signed into law March 23, 2010, by President Barack Obama. ACA is mentioned here because it is the closest the U.S. has come to capturing the many uninsured individuals and providing affordable health insurance. According to Morgan and Abutaleb (2017), approximately 20 million Americans were able to get healthcare coverage under the ACA. Yet, ACA has had issues, and many leaders in the industry believe the country can do better to address healthcare needs for all. Since its creation, the ACA has faced congressional bills to enhance, repeal, or defund it, but for now the ACA still stands.

First Person Perspective

Ms. S. is an early elementary school teacher who lives in Maine.

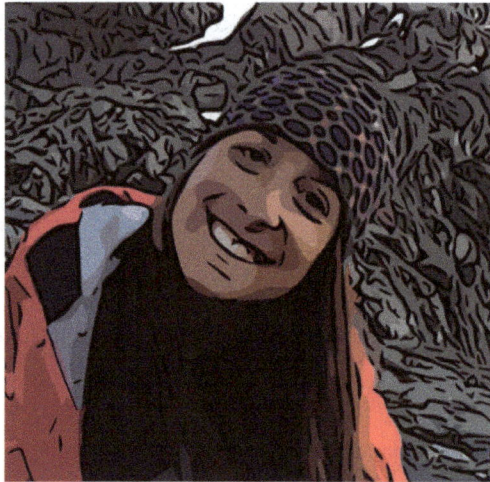

Figure 12.6: First Person Perspective

Source: Original Work
Attribution: Deanna Howe
License: CC BY-SA 4.0

I enrolled in an ACA plan as an elementary school teacher at a small independent school in rural Maine where there no was no employer-based plan on offer. I was making about $32,000 and was paying around $300 per month for my premium. This amount was high but in-line with all the ACA plans on offer and one I thought would work for me, given my health and lack of pre-existing conditions. My out-of-pocket maximum on this plan was around $7500, the same as all the other silver plans through the exchange.

In early December of that year, I was diagnosed with a rare tumor that required immediate medical attention. Unfortunately, given the timing of this, my care was spread out over two calendar years. As a result, I was hit with two out of pocket maximums at once and was on the *hook for $15,000 in medical bills plus my monthly premiums, a medical debt I am still paying off and will be paying off for many years to come. Had this whole ordeal started just a few weeks later, my bill would have been $7500 instead of $15,000.*

Later in that same year, the marketplace raised my income level without me experiencing any change of income. I was still working the same job and making the same amount of money. That change retroactively raised my deductible and I received a new bill for another few thousand dollars. It took months of phone calls to the insurance company and the marketplace to finally get that issue resolved.

My experience with the ACA, I'm afraid, can't be all that uncommon. I had a plan, but I couldn't afford to use it. Even when things went well, I still had to call insurance companies and hospital billing offices repeatedly to verify that things would be covered. Multiple times, new bills came from people who were out of network, even though the hospital I was at was in network. In the middle of the scariest and most traumatic experience of my life, my family and I had to deal with battling insurance companies, confusing bills, and the knowledge that I would come out of this with long-term medical debt, when all we should have been focusing on was my treatment, recovery, and supporting each other.

First person perspective vignette collected and created by D. Howe, 2020.

For your consideration: Ms. S. notes that her elementary school teaching position did not offer a healthcare insurance plan. How does the ACA serve to support those without another option for healthcare insurance coverage? What are the implications for professionals such as Ms. S. whose employment does not offer healthcare insurance? Ms. S. notes the high deductible and now $15,000+ debt she has incurred because of an unexpected health condition. How could the ACA be improved to decrease the debt burden to participants?

12.4 ISSUES SURROUNDING THE U.S. HEALTHCARE SYSTEM

Healthcare system performance rankings of the top eleven wealthiest countries recognized by the Organization for Economic Cooperation and Development (OECD) (2017) finds the U.S. is ranked last or nearly last in four of five categories: care process, access, administrative efficiency, equity, and healthcare outcomes. Compared to other countries, the U.S. spends approximately 50% more on healthcare services but still has the worst health outcomes of all other countries evaluated. According to Tikkanen and Abrams (2020), the Commonwealth Fund analysis of the U.S. in comparison to the other ten wealthiest countries found that the U.S. has the following:

- The lowest life expectancy rate

- The highest suicide rates

- The highest chronic disease burden

- An obesity rate two times higher than the OECD average

- Americans had fewer physician visits than peers in most countries (indicating an access or supply issue)

- Among the highest number of hospitalizations from preventable causes (diabetes and hypertension)

- The highest rate of avoidable deaths (mortality amenable to healthcare)

But in good news, the U.S. outperforms most other countries in preventative health screenings (specifically mammography for breast cancer) and flu vaccinations.

In today's political environment, there is little movement towards implementation of a healthcare system that provides benefits for all. Frankly, Congress is more divided along party lines than ever before. The same can be said for U.S. citizens. In a poll of U.S. voters, the divide in support of a single-payer plan is growing (see Figure 12.7). However, 74% of U.S. citizens overall favor an inclusive healthcare plan (KFF, 2019).

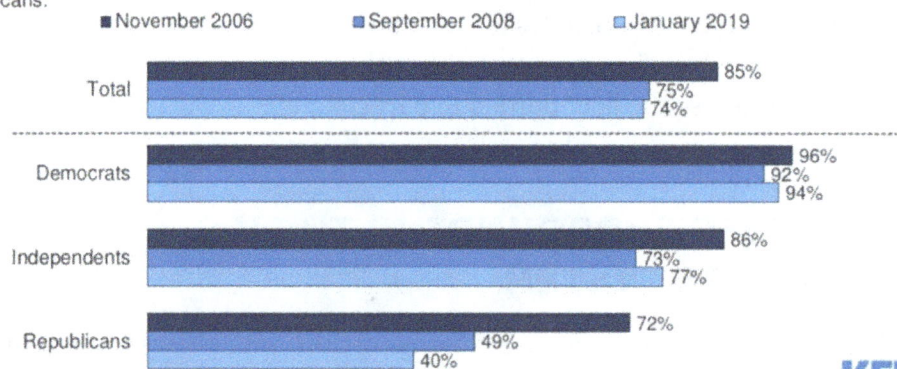

Most Support Federal Government Doing More To Help Provide Health Insurance, But Republican Support Has Declined Over Time

Percent who say they **favor** the federal government doing more to help provide health insurance for more Americans:

■ November 2006   ■ September 2008   ▨ January 2019

	November 2006	September 2008	January 2019
Total	85%	75%	74%
Democrats	96%	92%	94%
Independents	86%	73%	77%
Republicans	72%	49%	40%

SOURCE: KFF Polls. See toplines for full question wording and response options.

KFF

Figure 12.7: Support for Federal Government Providing Health Insurance Along Political Party Lines

Source: Kaiser Family Foundation
Attribution: Kaiser Family Foundation
License: © Kaiser Family Foundation. Used with permission.

Nearly every developed country in the world has some type of universal healthcare system. Yet, the U.S. remains unable or unwilling to ensure all citizens have access to or funding for healthcare. Is healthcare a human right? According to the World Health Organization (2017), "the right to health for all people means that everyone should have access to the health service they need, when and where they need them" (p. 1). It is well known that the burden of healthcare expenses leads to stress on businesses that must assist with funding healthcare for employees. This is especially true for small businesses. In addition, the individual financial burden to meet deductibles, copays, and out-of-pocket expenses, as well as catastrophic health conditions, often leads to a personal bankruptcy. According to Yabroff et al. (2019), in a non-cancer related study by American Cancer Society conducted from 2015 to 2017, researchers found more than 100 million people in the U.S. experienced medical financial hardship. For those without healthcare, the most prevalent hardship is the lack of access to medical care and an inability to pay the high cost of medical bills if care is sought. Unfortunately, persons with no medical insurance are less likely to seek primary preventative healthcare services or seek care for chronic illnesses (Tolbert et al., 2019).

Health insurance in America is primarily obtained as a benefit through employment. Federal programs, such as Medicare and Medicaid, offer health benefits to non-working adults, children, and those earning less than the federal poverty level. The Affordable Care Act (ACA) has done a good job in closing the gap of those who are without healthcare coverage and ineligible for Medicaid. However, there remains millions of uninsured Americans today. A provision of the ACA called for states to adopt Medicaid expansion in which eligibility for Medicaid allowed people with annual incomes below 138% of the federal poverty level, or $17, 236 for an individual, to obtain health insurance coverage (Garfield et al., 2020). Funding for Medicaid expansion is primarily through federal funds, but states must also contribute. The goal was for Medicaid expansion to be nationwide; however, the Supreme Court ruled that state participation was optional. Currently, twelve states do not participate in the Medicaid Expansion program. This creates a gap in coverage for adults with "incomes above Medicaid eligibility limits but below the poverty level, which is the lower limit for Marketplace premium tax credits" (see Figure 12.8) (Garfield et al., 2020, para 2). Interestingly, the twelve states not participating in Medicaid expansion overwhelmingly are southern states which have a disproportionate number of black Americans (Pearson, 2019).

Gap in Coverage for Adults in States that Do Not Expand Medicaid Under the ACA

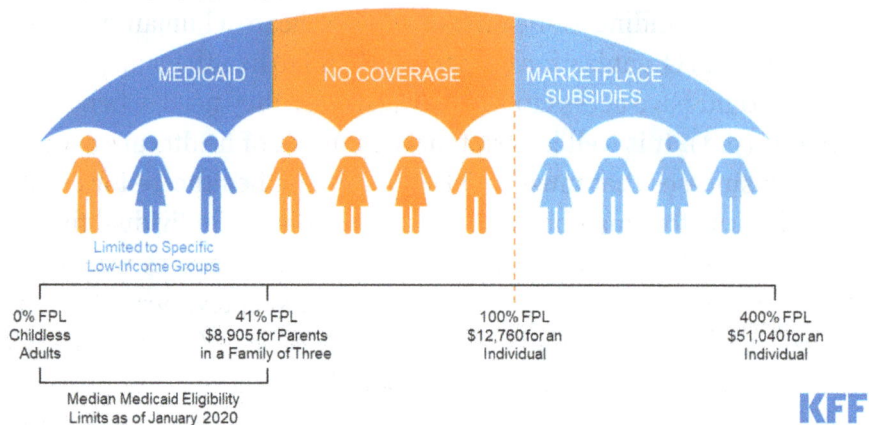

Figure 12.8: Gap in Coverage for Adults in States that Do Not Expand Medicaid Under the ACA, 2020

Source: Kaiser Family Foundation

Attribution: Kaiser Family Foundation

License: © Kaiser Family Foundation. Used with permission.

Who are the uninsured in America? According to Tolbert et al. (2019), individuals who live in low-income households and have at least one worker in the family are the primary uninsured population. Adults are more likely than children to be uninsured because Medicaid primarily covers children's health insurance needs. An individual's race is a factor, with African Americans and Hispanics at higher rates of uninsured than Caucasians. Literature reveals that socioeconomic characteristics of income, employment, citizenship and language are associated with uninsurance in minority populations (Sohn, 2017). The problem has been identified and now a solution is necessary.

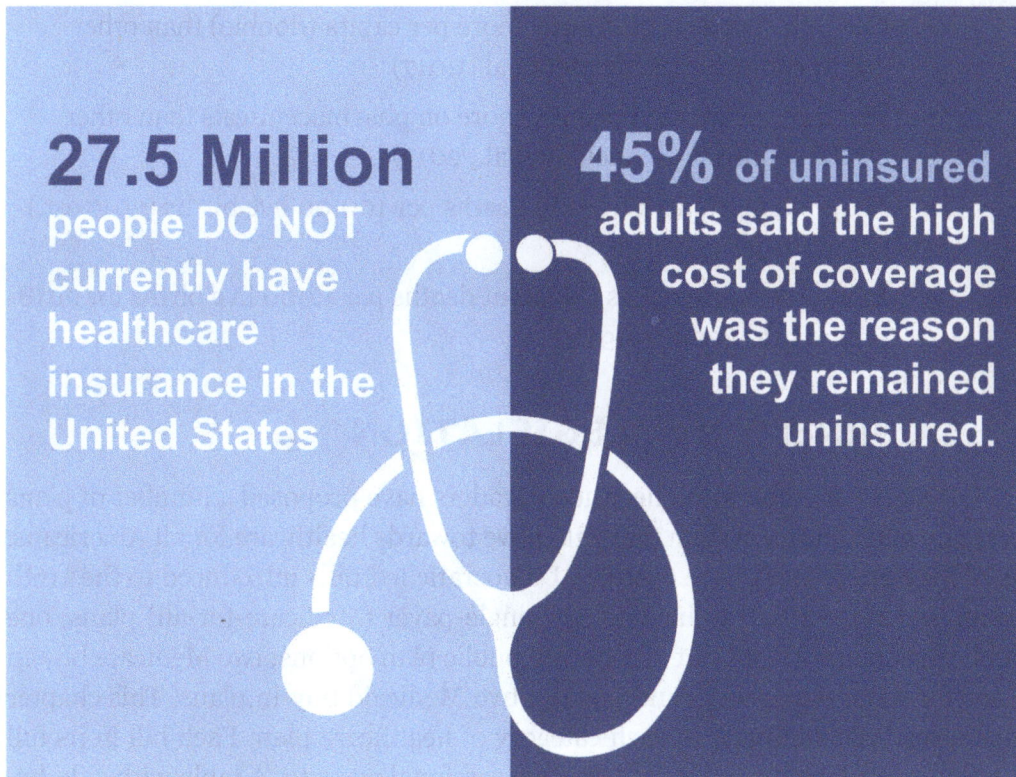

Figure 12.9: Uninsured Americans

Source: Kaiser Family Foundation
Attribution: Corey Parson
License: CC BY-SA 4.0

Basic Statistics of the U.S. Healthcare System

- The current population in the U.S. is 331,605,982 as of October 21, 2020. The median age is 38.3 years; and it ranks number three in the list of countries by population (Worldometers, 2020d).

- Coronavirus cases: 35,745,024; Deaths: 629,315 as of August 1, 2021 (Worldometers, 2021).

- U.S. life expectancy at birth for females is 81.46 years; men is 76.42 (World Population Review, 2020).

- No uniform health system, no universal healthcare coverage; hybrid system

- In 2018, 8.5% or 27.5 million people had no health insurance at any point during the year (Berchick et al., 2019).

- In 2018, 67.3% of the population had private insurance (of which 55.1% was employer based) and 34.4% had public coverage (Berchick et al., 2019).

- Uninsured children under the age of 19 increased to 5.5% in 2018 (Berchick et al., 2019).

- The U.S. spends significantly more per capita (double) than other OECD countries (Schneider et al., 2017).
- The U.S. spends significantly more on pharmaceuticals than other OECD countries (Schneider et al., 2017).
- Maternal mortality rate is 19 deaths per 100,00 live births (2017 est.) (CIA, 2019d).
- Infant mortality rate is six infant deaths per 1,000 live births for 2018 (The World Bank, 2019).

12.5 CURRENT U.S. LEGISLATION

Legislative members and healthcare leaders have proposed a number of plans to create a healthcare system that will move towards healthcare for all Americans. As of May 2019, there were fourteen Democratic led bills introduced to the 116th Congress (2019–2020) to include two single-payer (Medicare-for-all) plans; one public program with opt-out plan; seven public plan options; two Medicare buy-in plans for those between 50 and 64; and two Medicaid buy-in plans. This chapter includes a brief summary of each category of healthcare plan. Each bill in its full version is available through the U.S. congressional website. A table with side-by-side comparison of all plans is included in the supplemental resources.

12.5.1 Medicare for All

Medicare-for-all legislature has been submitted to both the House of Representatives H.R.1384 and the Senate S.1129 in 2019. Both bills are very similar and have the same title. The Medicare for All Act of 2019, submitted by Senator Bernie Sanders, would establish a universal, single-payer health program to ensure healthcare for all residents of the U.S. Main points of the bill include the eligibility, benefits, patient choice, patient costs, cost controls, and timeline for implementation (PNHP, 2019b) (see Table 12.4). The Medicare for All bill would replace all private insurances, Medicaid, Medicare, and CHIP for covered benefits and move to a single-payer system (Congress.gov, 2019a).

Table 12.4: Medicare for All Act of 2019 Program Highlights.	
Eligibility	Covers everyone residing in the U.S.
Benefits	Covers medically-necessary services including primary and preventive care, mental healthcare, reproductive care (bans the Hyde Amendment), vision and dental care, and prescription drugs. Also provides home- and community-based long-term services and supports, which were not covered in the 2017 bill.
Patient Choice	Provides full choice of any participating doctor or hospital. Providers may not dual-practice within and outside the Medicare system.
Patient Costs	Provides first-dollar coverage without premiums, deductibles, or copays for medical services, and prohibits balance billing. Copays for some brand-name prescription drugs.
Cost Controls	Prohibits duplicative coverage. Drug prices negotiated with manufacturers.
Timeline	Provides for a four-year transition. In year one, improves Medicare by adding dental, vision, and hearing benefits and lowering out-of-pocket costs for Parts A & B; also lowers eligibility age to 55 and allows anyone to buy into the Medicare program. In year two, lowers eligibility to 45, and to 35 in year three.

According to berniesanders.com (2020), "all Americans are entitled to go to the doctor when they're sick and not go bankrupt after staying in the hospital" (para. 1). A key point of the Medicare for All plan is comprehensive healthcare coverage, free at the point of service. This includes no networks, premiums, deductibles, or copays. In addition, the plan expands Medicare coverage to include dental, hearing, vision, home and community long-term care, inpatient and outpatient services, mental health and substance abuse treatment, reproductive and maternity care, and prescription drugs (berniesanders.com, 2020). The plan also notes private health insurers and employers may only offer supplemental coverage. Private health insurers and employers are prohibited from coverage that duplicates benefits covered under the Medicare for All plan. According to sanders.senate.gov (2019), financing of the Medicare for All plan would include $26 trillion, or 55%, from the current $47 trillion (tax financed) projections of what the U.S. will spend on healthcare from 2018 to 2027. According to berniesanders.com (2020), funding the Medicare for All plan includes using the $30 trillion expected government expenditures for the next ten years and an additional $17.5 trillion in revenue option. The extra revenue is created through a 4% income-based premium paid for by employees (exempting the first $29,000 in income for a family of four). Employers will pay an additional 7.5% income-based premium (exempting the first $1 million in payroll to protect small businesses (berniesanders.com, 2020). Strategies to increase revenue through taxation primarily targets super-rich citizens by increasing income tax rate, taxing capital gains at the same rates as income from wages and enacting corporate tax reform. The bill plans an incremental roll out with full implementation four years from enactment.

12.5.2 Public Program with Opt-Out

Introduced to the House of Representatives, a bill has been submitted to amend the Social Security Act to establish a Medicare for America Act (H.R.2452) which will provide for comprehensive health coverage to all Americans. The bill provides coverage to uninsured; those who have purchased plans on the open market; and those with Medicare, Medicaid, and CHIP. Employer-sponsored private coverage remains an option in this plan. This plan caps premiums at 8% of individual or household income. The Medicare for America Act includes all of the services currently provided through the government-subsidized programs but also includes prescription drugs, dental, vision, and hearing services. Additional services include long-term services for seniors and those with disabilities. Exemptions are noted for households earning 200% or less than the federal poverty level. The plan blocks undocumented immigrants and Deferred Action for Childhood Arrivals (DACA) from receiving coverage. Medicare for America Act is financed by sunsetting (expiration) of the Republican tax bill, imposing a 5% surtax on adjusted gross income over $500,000, and excise tax on all tobacco products, beer, wine, liquor, and sugar-sweetened drinks (Congress.gov, 2019b).

Pause and Reflect

The Medicare-for-all Act of 2019 plan described above is a drastic change to the current U.S. healthcare system. Considering the benefits, costs, and timeline for this program, do you think this is a good idea for the U.S.? Why, or why not? Do you think Americans would benefit from this plan? In what ways?

12.5.3 Public Plan Option

Seven public plan options, most similar to one another, were introduced in 2019 to both the Senate and House of Representatives (grouped here S.3; S.1261. & H.R.2463; S.981 & H.R.2000; H.R.2085 & S.1033). One of the plans, Medicare-X Choice Act of 2019, was reintroduced leaving the current sources of health insurance in place but adds a new option. A less dramatic change than the Medicare for All plan, Medicare-X Choice Act gives citizens a choice but ensures everyone has access to a government plan. The 2019 version of this bill lowers premiums and increases coverage for Medicare-X consumers and those in the individual market. Its rationale notes that "Despite the success of the Affordable Care Act, too many Americans still live in areas with limited competition and unaffordable healthcare costs. In 2019, 17% of those enrolled on the exchanges lived in an area with just one insurer" (Kaine.senate.gov, 2019, para. 4). Eligibility for this plan includes all citizens currently eligible to participate in the Marketplace and not eligible for

Medicare. Initially, this plan would focus on rural areas with few medical providers and higher costs and expand to the entire country by 2024. The plan would use the current Medicare network of doctors and add affordable prescription drugs. Individual income taxes are capped at 13% for premiums.

12.5.4 Medicare Buy-In for Older Adults

Two bills, similar in nature, are currently submitted to Congress (S.470 & H.R.1346). The Medicare Buy-In and Healthcare Stabilization Act of 2019 provides an option for citizens aged 50 to 64, who are lawful citizens and not eligible for Medicare Parts A and B (Govtrack.us, 2019). There is no employer buy-in option leaving eligible individuals, if they choose, the sole responsibility to purchase coverage in this plan. Benefits include those currently noted in Medicare Parts A, B, and D. Cost sharing remains current in Medicare plans, and there is no annual limit on out-of-pocket cost sharing. Premiums are set to cover 100% of benefits (Govtrack.us, 2019).

12.5.5 Medicaid Buy-In

The Medicaid Buy-In plan (S.489 & H.R.1277) is submitted as the State Public Option Act. In these plans, states will offer a public plan option based on Medicaid. With this plan, the Marketplace is unchanged, and current sources of private and public coverage continue. Those eligible would include residents of states offering the Medicaid Buy-In plan who are eligible for marketplace and not concurrently enrolled in other health coverage (Congress.gov, 2019c). There is no employer provision in this plan. The benefits include a Medicaid alternative plan which includes the ACA 10 essential health benefits. Cost-sharing is set by each state, but annual out-of-pocket limits cannot exceed the ACA limit of $7,900. Premiums are set by each state but cannot be more than 9.5% of annual household income (Congress.gov, 2019c).

12.6 TIME FOR CHANGE

The U.S. has the capacity to strengthen the healthcare system to ensure equitable health services for all Americans. This requires tremendous effort on the part of policy-makers. Based on conclusions from the Commonwealth Fund assessment of other industrialized nations, Tolbert et al. (2019) suggest three areas for focus:

1. Reduction of healthcare costs through better budgeting practices and assuming value-based pricing of new technology
2. Addressing the risk factors and creating better management of chronic diseases
3. Providing incentives for effective care and disincentives for less effective care

Clearly, countries that provide healthcare services to all of their citizens have overall better health outcomes. An effort to untie health insurance benefits from employment and move to a single-payer national system would be difficult. However, all American citizens deserve access to healthcare services so that optimal health can be obtained.

What are the pros and cons of a national or universal healthcare system? It depends on who is answering the question. From a patient's perspective, the positives would include no bills, no co-pays, no deductibles, no exclusions for pre-existing conditions, no bankruptcies because of high medical bills, and no long-lasting effects or death as a result of no healthcare coverage (White, 2020). The negatives might include decreases in flexibility for patients and fewer physicians available as a result of decreased opportunity for higher compensation (White, 2020).

- -

First Person Perspective

Mr. L. is an outdoor educator, guide, and carpenter.

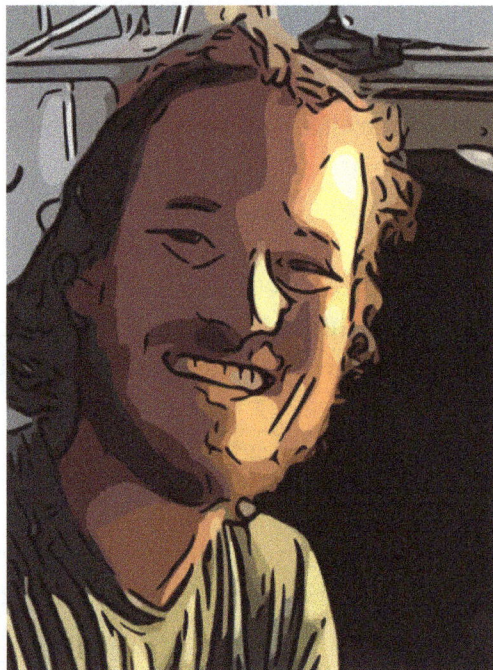

Figure 12.10: First Person Perspective

My ACA experience relates to the past few years while I have been located in a rural mid-coast town in the northwestern region of the U.S. I have experienced continual confusion, questionable bills, difficulty in tracking down answers, a lack of clarity on what a given medical service would *cost me, long waits for responses from insurance companies, and deferred or cancelled medical care as a result of not wanting to pay the high fees associated with my plans. During my years on the ACA plans, I have had multiple income streams from a combination of gig, self-employed, and W-2 without benefit work. As I sit here this year, during a pandemic, after having lost my W-2 job, it is nearly impossible for me to determine my income. If I tell the ACA that I will make $26,000, my deductible is $2,500–3,000 with an out-of-pocket maximum of $6,200. If I tell them I will make $25,600, that deductible drops to $600.*

I have watched the trends on the ACA Marketplace, as my doctors and preferred hospitals appear and disappear and as deductibles and out-of-pocket maximums have sky-rocketed, even as premiums have remained flat or come down. The premium fees are only important if you don't use any care. A few medical visits over the course of the year and the out-of-pocket costs become far more important in terms of the financial burden. The most frustrating part of this, as a young healthy person, is I have one consistent healthcare need, which is the ability to see a mental health provider, and there is virtually no plan available that will cover this before I have exhausted my deductible. This issue isn't simply limited to mental healthcare. Outside of a primary care visit, nearly any medical procedure or specialist office visit on these plans requires you to pay the entire deductible before the plan starts covering a percentage of the service.

Without the ACA, I would surely go bankrupt in that catastrophic scenario; however, the chances of a catastrophe are relatively low. Instead, on a yearly basis, I am offered the opportunity to spend thousands of dollars in premiums for a plan that doesn't cover my most basic health need, which I then have to spend thousands of more dollars in order to cover, effectively removing the chance for me to amass any type of savings. That feels like a slow but continuous catastrophe. If a public plan were available to me, I would take it in a heartbeat.

First person perspective vignette collected and created by D. Howe, 2020.

For your consideration: Mr. L. shares his experience with ACA and the unpredictability of services, payments and fees. Consider if, as a young adult, there was an expectation to pay nearly 20% of your gross income in deductibles and copays to meet your most important health need. How would you manage this expense? Many in Mr. L.'s situation would decide not to seek care. What if the condition were communicable (spread to others)? Would this change your perspective? If the U.S. had a universal healthcare plan, Mr. L. and millions of Americans would not have to worry about basic health needs being met. How might a universal healthcare program funded by the government help to create a healthier population?

12.7 THE IMPACT OF COVID-19 ON THE U.S. HEALTHCARE SYSTEM

At the end of 2019, the COVID-19 virus spread quickly through provinces in China and then to countries throughout the world. COVID-19 hit the shores of the U.S. in early 2020 and quickly spread because of the highly contagious nature of this virus. The COVID-19 virus pandemic has been like no other health threat to our nation since the Spanish flu (1918-1920). Symptoms of individuals affected with COVID-19 vary depending on age and underlying health conditions. Some individuals show no symptoms at all and can easily spread the virus unwittingly, while others suffer with severe symptoms that require hospitalization and potentially cause death.

The numbers of people seeking care for symptoms as a result of COVID-19 has created a tremendous strain on the U.S. healthcare system. In March 2020, federal officials began spreading the word that social distancing was necessary to help slow down the spread of the virus. Hospitals and other health service entities canceled most non-emergency services and worked to create more intensive care space to manage the influx of patients with severe symptoms who would require respirators and other life-saving interventions. Many cities declared a state of emergency, and the hunt for personal protective equipment and ventilators went to the federal level. At the same time, the nation began to shut down, asking citizens to shelter in place and avoid any public gatherings. Businesses began to close and, as a result, millions were suddenly out of work. Panic set in, and the legislative branch met to create emergency funds to assist families with stimulus money to aid in meeting financial obligations. However, healthcare insurance coverage and access has been severely affected. In contrast, citizens of countries highlighted in this chapter—Germany, Canada, and the U.K.—as well as most of the world's wealthiest countries, will not lose health insurance coverage as a result of job loss during the pandemic (Stankiewicz, 2020).

A persistent problem in the U.S. continues to be the lack of healthcare for all citizens, and this has been exacerbated by the COVID-19 virus pandemic. As noted earlier in this chapter, health insurance is largely tied to employment. Millions of Americans have been fired or furloughed, resulting in loss of health insurance for themselves and their family members. Of the approximate 31 million people who filed for unemployment, an estimated 27 million Americans will lose employer-sponsored health insurance coverage (see Figure 12.11) (Garfield et al., 2020). The slight good news is that an estimated half of Americans who became uninsured after job loss (12.7 million) will be eligible for Medicaid, and another 8.4 million will be eligible for ACA health coverage (Garfield et al., 2020). Yet, this still leaves several million without health insurance coverage as a result of the COVID-19 virus pandemic. With no health insurance, people tend to delay care or not seek care due to cost, which could risk the health of countless Americans.

Health Insurance Coverage Before and After Job Loss Among People in a Family Experiencing Job Loss as of May 2, 2020

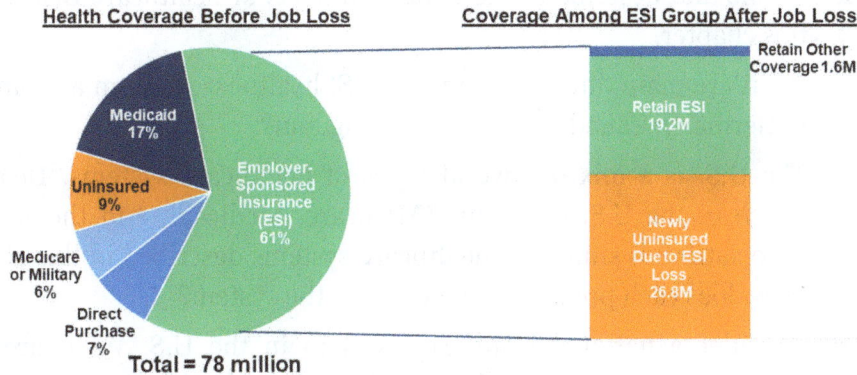

Figure 12.11: Health Insurance Coverage Before and After Job Loss Among People in a Family Experiencing Job Loss, as of May 2, 2020

Source: Kaiser Family Foundation
Attribution: Kaiser Family Foundation
License: © Kaiser Family Foundation. Used with permission.

COVID-19 has forever changed the U.S. healthcare system. According to Facher (2020), the pandemic could upend the tradition of health insurance being tied to employment. Other predictions include the accelerated use of telemedicine, noted in Chapter 11; home health aides in replacement of nursing homes; recognition of racial disparities in our current system; affordability of medications; pandemic preparedness; a larger role of advanced practice providers in healthcare; and changes in the medical fee structure.

12.8 SUMMARY

This chapter described health systems in Germany, Canada, and the United Kingdom, which provide all citizens with healthcare coverage. The description of each country health system includes a short history and notes components of the healthcare system, such as the cost, benefits, and scope. This chapter included legislative proposals submitted to the 116th Congress which expand health services within the U.S. healthcare system or propose a complete overhaul with Medicare for All plans. The U.S. has a healthcare system that includes many government programs (e.g. Medicare, Medicaid) as well as private payer's (insurance companies). Yet, there remains no single plan to address the millions of people without health coverage. Finally, this chapter included a discussion of the COVID-19 virus and its impact on Americans and the health system. The recent COVID-19 virus pandemic shines a light on the inadequacies of the U.S. healthcare system.

12.9 REVIEW QUESTIONS

1. Define and describe the four basic models of healthcare discussed in this chapter.

2. What are main differences in the U.S. healthcare system as compared to Germany, Canada, and United Kingdom?

3. The U.S. is a mix of several types of healthcare systems. Designate which of the U.S. programs (Medicare, Medicaid, and the Veterans Association) is similar to healthcare systems described in this chapter. How does each program's structure fit the system?

4. Consider a national healthcare system in the U.S. What are three advantages and three challenges of a national healthcare system?

5. Describe a Medicare for All in the U.S. healthcare plan. How is it financed?

12.10 REFERENCES

AgeUK. (2019). Later life in the United Kingdom 2019. Retrieved from https://www. ageuk.org.uk/globalassets/afe-uk/documents/reports-andpublications/later_life_ uk_factsheet.pdf

Allin, S. & Rudoler, D. (2016). The Canadian health care system. The Commonwealth Fund. Retrieved from https://international.commonwealthfund.org/countries/ canada/

American Public Media. (APM Research Lab). The color of coronavirus COVID-19 deaths by race and ethnicity in the U.S. Retrieved from https://www.apmresearchlab.org/ covid/deaths-by-race

The Association of Faculties of Medicine of Canada. (2017). How much is tuition at a Canadian medical school? Retrieved from https://afmc.ca/node/247

Berchick, E. R., Barnett, J. C., & Upton, R. D. (2019, November 8). Health insurance coverage in the United States: 2018. United States Census Bureau, P60-267 (RV). Retrieved from https://www.census.gov/library/publications/2019/demo/p60-267. html

Berniesanders.com. (2020). Health care as a human right-Medicare for all. https:// berniesanders.com/issues/medicare-for-all/

Blümel, M. & Busse, R. (2016). The Germany health care system. The Commonwealth Fund. Retrieved from https://international.commonwealthfund.org/countries/ germany/

Booth, S. (2019). Medicare for all: What is it and how will it work? Healthline. https:// www.healthline.com/health/what-medicare-for-all-would-look-like-in-america#1

Busse, R., Blümel, M., Knieps, D., & Bärnighausen, T. (2017). Statutory health insurance in Germany: A health system shaped by 135 years of solidarity, self-governance, and competition. The Lancet, 390(10097), 882–897. https://doi.org/10.1016/S0140-6736(17)31280-1

Canadian Institute for Health Information. (2019a). How much will we spend on health in 2019? National Health Expenditure Database. Ottawa, ON: CIHI, 2019. Retrieved from https://www.cihi.ca/en/how-much-will-we-spend-on-health-in-2019

Canadian Institute for Health Information. (2019b). Where is most of the money being spent in 2019? National Health Expenditure Database. Ottawa, ON: CIHI, 2019. Retrieved from https://www.cihi.ca/en/where-is-most-of-the-money-being-spent-in-2019

Canadian Institute for Health Information. (2019c). Canada continues to lag behind other OECD countries on measures of patient safety. Ottawa, ON: CIHI, 2019. Retrieved fromhttps://www.cihi.ca/en/canada-continues-to-lag-behind-other-oecd-countries-on-measures-of-patient-safety

Canadian Institute for Health Information. (2019d). Who is paying for these services? National Health Expenditure Database. Ottawa, ON: CIHI, 2019. Retrieved from https://www.cihi.ca/en/who-is-paying-for-these-services

Central Intelligence Agency (CIA). (2019). The world factbook. Maternal mortality rate. Retrieved from https://www.cia.gov/library/publications/the-world-factbook/fields/353.html

Chung, M. (2017). National health care reform: Learning from other major health care systems. Princeton Public Health Review. Retrieved from https://pphr.princeton.edu/2017/12/02/unhealthy-health-care-a-cursory-overview-of-major-health-care-systems/

Congress.gov. (2019a). S.1129- Medicare for All Act of 2019. Retrieved from https://www.congress.gov/bill/116th-congress/senate-bill/1129

Congress.gov. (2019b). H.R.2452- Medicare for America Act of 2019. Retrieved from https://www.congress.gov/bill/116th-congress/house-bill/2452

Congress.gov. (2019c). H.R.1277- State Public Option Act. Retrieved from https://www.congress.gov/bill/116th-congress/house-bill/1277?q=%7B%22search%22%3A%5B%22H.R.1277%22%5D%7D&s=1&r=1

Connington, J. (2018). What conditions and treatments aren't covered on the NHS and how much do they cost? The Telegraph. Retrieved from https://www.telegraph.co.uk/money/consumer-affairs/conditions-treatments-arent-covered-nhs-much-do-cost/

Deutscher Akademischer Austauschdienst (DAAD) (n.d.). Health Insurance. https://www.daad.de/en/study-and-research-in-germany/plan-your-studies/health-insurance/

Duncan, P. & Jowit, J. (2018, July 2). Is the NHS the world's best health care system? The Guardian. Retrieved from https://www.theguardian.com/society/2018/jul/02/is-the-nhs-the-worlds-best-health care-system

Facher, L. (2020, May 19). 9 ways COVID-19 may forever upend the U.S. health care industry. STAT. Retrieved from https://www.statnews.com/2020/05/19/9-ways-covid-19-forever-upend-health-care/

Garfield, R. & Orgera, K, & Damico, A. (2020, January 14). The coverage gap: Uninsured poor adults in states that do not expand Medicaid. Kaiser Family Foundation. Retrieved from https://www.kff.org/medicaid/issue-brief/the-coverage-gap-uninsured-poor-adults-in-states-that-do-not-expand-medicaid/

Garfield, R., Claxton, G., Damico, A., & Levitt, L. (2020, May 13). Eligibility for ACA health coverage following job loss. Kaiser Family Foundation. Retrieved from https://www.kff.org/coronavirus-covid-19/issue-brief/eligibility-for-aca-health-coverage-following-job-loss/

Germany Health Insurance System. (2019). German health care system guide. Retrieved from https://www.germanyhis.com/

Government of Canada. (2019). Canada's health care system. Retrieved from https://www.canada.ca/en/health-canada/services/health-care-system/reports-publications/health-care-system/canada.html

Govtrack.us. (2019). H.R. 1346: Medicare Buy-In and Health Care Stabilization Act of 2019. Retrieved from https://www.govtrack.us/congress/bills/116/hr1346

Izenberg, D., Oriuwa, C., & Taylor, M. (2018). Why is there a gender wage gap in Canadian medicine? Healthydebate. Retrieved from https://healthydebate.ca/2018/10/topic/gender-wage-gap-medicine

Kaine.senate.gov. (2019). Bennet, Kaine reintroduce Medicare-X to provide low-cost, high-quality insurance to every American. Retrieved from https://www.kaine.senate.gov/press-releases/bennet-kaine-reintroduce-medicare-x-to-provide-low-cost-high-quality-insurance-to-every-american

Kaiser Family Foundation (KFF). (2019). Public opinion on single-payer, national health plans, and expanding access to Medicare coverage. Retrieved from https://www.kff.org/slideshow/public-opinion-on-single-payer-national-health-plans-and-expanding-access-to-medicare-coverage/

Kane, L., Schubsky, B., Locke, T., Kouimtzi, M., Duqueroy, V., Gottschling, C., Lopez, M. & Schwartz, L. (2019, September 19). International physician compensation report 2019: Do US physicians have it best? Medscape. Retrieved from https://www.medscape.com/slideshow/2019-international-compensation-report-6011814

Keith, E. (2018). Here's how much a doctor is getting paid per year by province in Canada. Narcity. https://www.narcity.com/life/heres-how-much-a-doctor-is-getting-paid-per-year-by-province-in-canda

Locke, T. (2019). UK Doctors' salary and satisfaction report 2019. Medscape. Retrieved from https://www.medscape.com/slideshow/2019-uk-doctors-salary-report-6011623#2

Luthra, S. (2017). Canada's single-payer health system: What is true? What is false? 2019

Kaiser Family Foundation. Retrieved from https://khn.org/news/canadas-single-payer-health-system-what-is-true-what-is-false/

Miller, H. (2019, November 19). General election 2019: How much tax do British people pay? BBC News. Retrieved from https://www.bbc.com/news/business-48988052

Morgan, D. & Abutaleb, Y. (2017). U.S. House passes republican health bill, a step toward Obamacare repeal. Scientific American. Retrieved from https://www.scientificamerican.com/article/u-s-house-passes-republican-health-bill-a-step-toward-obamacare-repeal/

Nadish, P., Doty, P., & von Schwanenflügel. (2018). The German long-term care insurance program: Evolution and recent developments. The Gerontologist, 58(3), 558–597. https://doi.org/10.1093/geront/gnx018

National Center for Biotechnology Information, U.S. National Library of Medicine. (2018). Health care in Germany: The German health care system. Retrieved from https://www.ncbi.nlm.nih.gov/books/NBK298834/

Office of National Statistics. (2017). Health care expenditure, UK health accounts: 2017. Retrieved from https://www.ons.gov.uk/peoplepopulationandcommunity/healthandsocialcare/healthcaresystem/bulletins/ukhealthaccounts/2017

Organisation for Economic Co-operation and Development. (2019). OECD Data. Health spending (indicator). 10.1787/8643de7e-en https://data.oecd.org/healthres/health-spending.htm

Pearson, C. (2019, April 3). Protecting and expanding Medicaid means confronting racism baked into the program. National Women's Health Network. Retrieved from https://www.nwhn.org/protecting-and-expanding-medicaid-means-confronting-racism-baked-into-the-program/

Physicians for a National Health Program (PHNP). (2019a). Health care systems-Four basic models. Retrieved from https://pnhp.org/resource/health-care-systems-four-basic-models/

Physicians for a National Health Program (PHNP). (2019b). Understanding the Medicare for All Act of 2019. Retrieved from https://pnhp.org/what-is-single-payer/senate-bill/

Ren, F., Palacios, M., & Barua, B. (2017). The price of public health care insurance 2017. Fraser Research Bulletin. Retrieved from https://www.fraserinstitute.org/sites/default/files/price-of-public-health-care-insurance-2017.pdf

Sanders.senate.gov. (2019). Financing Medicare for all. Retrieved fromhttps://www.sanders.senate.gov/download/medicare-for-all-2019-financing

Schneider, E. C., Sarnak, D. O., Squires, D., Shah, A., & Doty, M. M. (2017). Mirror, mirror 2017: International comparison reflects flaws and opportunities for better U.S. health care. The Commonwealth Fund. Retrieved from https://www.commonwealthfund.org/publications/fund-reports/2017/jul/mirror-mirror-2017-international-comparison-reflects-flaws-and

Sohn, H. (2017). Racial and ethnic disparities in health insurance coverage: Dynamics of gaining and losing coverage over the life-course. Population Research and Policy Review, 36(2): 181–201. doi: 10.1007/s11113-016-9416-y

Stankiewicz, M. (2020). Millions lose health insurance during a pandemic. Only in America. Public Citizen. https://www.citizen.org/article/millions-lose-health-insurance-during-a-pandemic-only-in-america/

Thorlby, R. & Arora, S. (2016). The English health care system. The Commonwealth Fund. Retrieved from https://international.commonwealthfund.org/countries/england/

Tikkanen, R., & Abrams, M. K. (2020). U.S. health care from a global perspective, 2019:Higher spending, worse outcomes? The Commonwealth Fund. Retrieved from https://www.commonwealthfund.org/publications/issue-briefs/2020/jan/us-health-care-global-perspective-2019#:~:text=In%202018%2C%20the%20U.S.%20spent,%2C%20Switzerland%2C%20spent%2012.2%20percent

Tolbert, J., Orgera, K., Singer, N., & Damico, A. (2019, December 13). Key facts about the uninsured population. Kaiser Family Foundation. Retrieved from https://www.kff.org/uninsured/issue-brief/key-facts-about-the-uninsured-population/

Woodfield, D. (2018). What does private health insurance cost? Bought by Many. Retrieved fromhttps://boughtbymany.com/news/article/private-health-insurance-cost-uk/

The World Bank. (2019). Mortality rate, infant (per 1,000 live births). Retrieved from https://data.worldbank.org/indicator/SP.DYN.IMRT.IN

World Health Organization (WHO). (2017). Health is a fundamental human right. Human rights day 2017. Retrieved from https://www.who.int/mediacentre/news/statements/fundamental-human-right/en/

Worldometers (2020a). Germany population (Live). https://www.worldometers.info/world-population/germany-population/

Worldometers (2020b). Canada population (Live). https://www.worldometers.info/world-population/canada-population/

Worldometers (2020c). U.K. population (Live). https://www.worldometers.info/world-population/uk-population/

Worldometers (2020d). United States population (Live). https://www.worldometers.info/world-population/us-population/

Worldometers (2021). Coronavirus Cases. https://www.worldometers.info/coronavirus/#countries

World Population Review. (2020). Life expectancy by Country 2020. Retrieved from http://worldpopulationreview.com/countries/life-expectancy-by-country/

Yabroff, K. R. Zhao, J., Han, X., & Zheng, Z. (2019). Prevalence and correlates of medical financial hardship in the USA. Journal of General Internal Medicine, 2019. DOI: 10.1007/s11606-019-05002-w

Glossary

access: the timely use of personal health services to achieve the best possible health outcomes

accreditation: occurs when an entity's processes are reviewed by an impartial organization to ensure the entity is measuring up to national standards

acute: short-term episodes of symptoms or illness

adult disability: the law defines disability as the inability to engage in any substantial gainful activity (SGA) by reason of any medically-determinable physical or mental impairments which can be expected to result in death or which has lasted or can be expected to last for a continuous period of not less than twelve months

Advanced Alternative Payment Models (APMs): an option of the Quality Payment Program that rewards healthcare providers for providing high-quality, more affordable care

advanced practice provider (APP): a group of non-physician medical professional providers that who have graduated from accredited programs, passed national licensure examinations, and are licensed in the state they practice. APPs include physician assistants and advanced practice registered nurses

allied health professionals: a broad group of health professionals made up of specialty trained individuals who are typically licensed or certified to perform specific duties

ambulatory care center: a free-standing center or part of a hospital where same-day surgical services or procedures are performed

American Indian and Alaskan Native: refers to a person having origins in any of the original peoples of North or South America (including Central America) and who maintains tribal affiliation or community attachment (as defined by OMB)

Americans with Disabilities Act (ADA): a federal legislation passed in 1990 that prohibits discrimination against people with disabilities. The law made it illegal to discriminate against a disabled person in terms of employment opportunities as well as access to transportation, public accommodations, communications, and government activities. The law prohibits private employers, state and local governments, employment agencies, and labor unions from discriminating against the disabled. Employers are required to make reasonable accommodations in order for a disabled person to perform their job function.

artificial intelligence (AI): the use of complex algorithms and software to emulate human cognition in the analysis of complicated medical data

assisted living facilities: facilities often associated with nursing homes. In assisted living facilities, housing is provided, meals are usually provided, and medications are often provided. The resident is able to provide other activities of daily living.

Basic Health Program: a program created by the ACA granting states an option to expand Medicaid coverage to individuals in the 138th to 200th percent of the federal poverty guidelines

Beveridge model: healthcare is provided and financed by the government through tax payments

Bismarck model: an insurance system in which insurers, called "sickness funds", is financed jointly by employers and employees through payroll deduction. This system provides health insurance plans to cover everyone.

Centers for Medicare and Medicaid Services (CMS): a federal agency within the U.S. government's Health and Human Services department (HHS). CMS administers and operates the Medicare program. Medicaid, although administered by individual states, also receives oversight by CMS.

childhood disability: a child under age 18 will be considered disabled if they have a medically-determinable physical or mental impairment or combination of impairments that causes marked and severe functional limitations and can be expected to cause death or that has lasted or can be expected to last for a continuous period of not less than 12 months

Children's Health Insurance Program (CHIP): a program created to provide healthcare to children whose family income exceeds the guidelines set forth by Medicaid yet are not able to purchase private coverage

Choosing Wisely Campaign: a campaign designed to encourage collaboration between healthcare providers to provide the most cost effective, necessary care to patients

chronic disease: a condition that lasts one year or more and requires ongoing medical attention or a limitation of activities of daily living or both

civilian: noninstitutionalized person

clinical decision support (CDS): are computer-based programs that analyze data to provide prompts and reminders to assist healthcare providers in implementing evidence-based clinical guidelines at the point of care

complementary and alternative medicine (CAM) providers: medical products and practices that are not part of standard medical care, such as chiropractors and

Chinese medicine practitioners

correctional health: the medical specialty in which healthcare providers care for people in prisons and jails. Alternate terms include *jail health* or *prison health.*

data analytics: the process of analyzing raw data to find trends and answer questions

deductible: a cost the consumer is required to prepay to receive the benefits indicated in the health insurance policy. See *high deductible.*

defensive medicine: the manner in which healthcare providers offer care in attempts to eliminate chances of litigation

dentist: a doctor who specializes in the prevention and treatment of oral disease, including the teeth, gums, and mouth

disability: an impairment of a body part or function, an activity limitation, or a restriction preventing participation in life situations

elderly: persons aged 65 and older

electronic health record (EHR)- a digital record of patient health information generated by encounters in any care delivery setting

epidemiology: the study of diseases and illnesses and the factors that determine their presence in a population

equitable care: care provided that is the same for all people with improved health outcomes and reduced healthcare costs

Fee-for-Service- a system of health insurance payment in which a doctor or other healthcare provider is paid a fee for each particular service rendered

Flexner Report: a report developed in 1910 that helped established the educational preparation of physicians

gender pay inequality: differences in annual pay between what men and women earn for the same job or responsibilities

gross domestic product: the comprehensive value of goods and services generated in a country

health: a state of complete physical, social and mental well-being, and not merely the absence of disease or infirmity

healthcare disparities: differences in health and healthcare between population groups

healthcare system: within the context of this book, an interconnecting network which provides multi-layers of components to manage the health of U.S. citizens

healthcare quality: the extent to which health services provided to individuals and patient populations improve desired health outcomes

health determinant: factors that interact to create the health of each individual

health disparities: preventable differences in the burden of disease, injury, violence, or opportunities to achieve optimal health that are experienced by socially-disadvantaged populations

Health Insurance Marketplace: a healthcare coverage option for individuals who are employed yet do not have healthcare coverage with their employer

Health Insurance Portability and Accountability Act (HIPPA): a U.S. law designed to provide privacy standards to protect patients' medical records and other personal health information

health literacy: overall encompassing of what is needed for healthcare services to be accessed and utilized by an individual

Health Maintenance Organization (HMO): a type of managed care coverage that requires enrollees to have a primary care provider and preferred approval before services are rendered

health-seeking behaviors: seeking healthcare services when needed

health status: a description and/or measurement of the health of an individual or population at a particular point in time against identifiable standards, usually by reference to health indicators

high deductible: a plan with lower monthly premiums but where the beneficiary pays a large sum of money for healthcare costs before the insurance company pays for any of the healthcare costs. For 2020, the IRS defines a high deductible health plan as any plan with a deductible of at least $1400 for an individual or $2800 for a family.

home health: services provided in the patient's home and the patient is considered homebound. Often, skilled services are provided by nursing or other professionals.

hospice: service where the patient is seen in their home for healthcare. The patient has been given a limited time to survive, usually six months.

incarcerated: the act of confining someone in a prison

incidence: the rate at which individuals develop a condition or disease

infant mortality: the ratio of infant deaths to live births in a given year

inpatient: services are provided in hospitals where patients are usually admitted for an *acute* illness or a scheduled surgery and spend one or more nights

interoperability- the ability of different information systems to access, exchange, and integrate data across systems

length of stay: how long a person stays in the hospital; it is an indicator of hospital efficiency

life expectancy: how long, on average, a person can expect to live

long-term care facility: a non-acute facility that provides around-the-clock nursing services to patients, usually for rehab or recuperation after a hospitalization, or as a permanent residence when loved ones can no longer care for the aged or disabled person

managed care: care that consists of contractual agreements between medical facilities and healthcare providers to render healthcare at lower consumer costs.

Medicaid: a government-sponsored healthcare program that offers coverage to lower-income individuals

medical underwriting: the process that enabled insurance market companies to decide the costs of premiums and whether to accept or deny individuals' healthcare coverage based on pre-existing conditions

Medicare: a U.S. healthcare program that provides healthcare coverage to those individuals 65 or older, those diagnosed with end-stage renal disease, or those under 65 years old receiving Social Security Disability Insurance

Medicare Advantage: Also known as Part C, Medicare Advantage is the counterpart to *Original Medicare*. With Medicare Advantage, *Part A* (hospitalization), *Part B* (outpatient services), and usually *Part D* (medications) are bundled. Medicare Advantage is provided by private insurance companies. Individuals with Medicare Advantage must choose healthcare providers and hospitals within a specific network; using outside providers will result in additional costs.

Medicare Part A: part of *Original Medicare* and covers hospitalizations, skilled nursing homes, some skilled nursing home health services after hospitalization, and hospice. Monthly premiums are not required but deductibles are.

Medicare Part B: covers physician's office visits, outpatient care, home health visits without prior hospitalization, medical supplies, and preventive services

Medicare Part D: provides coverage for prescription drugs. This is a separate plan and beneficiaries pay a monthly premium.

Medigap supplemental insurance: an optional insurance bought from private companies for persons with *Original Medicare Part A* and *Part B*. Medigap supplemental insurance may pay for some of the costs not covered by Original Medicare.

military veteran: Title 38 of the Code of Federal Regulations defines a veteran as "a person who served in the active military, naval, or air service and who was discharged or released under conditions other than dishonorable"

morbidity: a term used to describe illness within a population

multi-payer system: allows multiple entities (e.g., insurance companies) to collect and pay for healthcare services

National Health Expenditure Accounts (NHEA): provides an estimated total cost of U.S. healthcare

national health insurance model: a system of health insurance that insures a national population against the costs of healthcare. May be administered by public sector, private sector, or both.

network (healthcare): a network includes hospitals, physicians, and possibly insurers and community agencies who are linked together to provide a broad range of services for the community

optometrist: a practitioner who provides primary eye and vision care and also performs eye examinations to detect defects in vision, signs of injury, ocular diseases, or abnormalities

Original Medicare: provided directly through Medicare and includes *Part A* and *Part B*

out-of-pocket: in the health insurance industry, portion of the bill that the insurance company doesn't cover and that the individual must pay on their own. Includes deductibles, copays, and coinsurance.

outpatient: services are provided at a facility the patient enters to receive healthcare and then they return to their home after the service or procedure

overutilization: practice that occurs when patients undergo unnecessary healthcare exams and procedures

patient portal: a secure online website that gives patients access to personal health information

Patient Protection and Affordable Care Act: provides healthcare coverage to individuals who may not otherwise receive healthcare coverage for reasons such as pre-existing conditions and gender-related issues. Also known as the Affordable Care Act (ACA) or Obamacare.

personal or protected health information (PHI): all individually-identifiable health information, including demographic data, medical history, test results, and other information used to identify a patient

pharmacist: a professional licensed to engage in pharmacy with duties including dispensing medications, monitoring drug interactions, administering vaccines, and counseling patients regarding the effects and proper use of drugs and dietary supplements

physician: a person who is educated, clinically experienced, and licensed to practice medicine

point of care technology: the devices and systems that support healthcare professionals in daily activities of monitoring patients, caring for them, and documenting their health progress; mostly often used at the bedside

Point of Service plan (POS): a type of managed care plan that allows a client to choose a provider outside of the network with a referral from their primary healthcare provider, thereby allowing the cost of services to be covered by the medical insurance

Preferred Provider Organization (PPO): a type of managed care program that allows enrollees to have a choice to use providers and hospitals within the network or not

prevalence: the number of actual cases of an illness or disease or disability

private insurance: Healthcare coverage not sponsored by the government

provider networks: a conglomerate of healthcare providers who work with healthcare entities to provide the most efficient, cost-effective care for consumers

psychologist: a person who specializes in the study of the mind, its behavior, and in the treatment of mental, emotional, and behavioral disorders

quality improvement: a process investigating patient care, its effectiveness, and how processes can be improved

Quality Payment Program: program that provides incentives for healthcare providers offering value-based care

registered nurse: a nurse who has graduated from a college's nursing program or from a school of nursing, has passed a national licensing examination, and holds a license in the state in which they practice. Includes Licensed Practical/Vocational Nurses.

service price and intensity: refers to the price and complexity of healthcare services

service utilization: refers to the types of services used to healthcare which prevent and cure disease, promote health, and provide information about health status

single-payer system: a single entity (government) is responsible for collecting the funds that pay for healthcare services on behalf of an entire population

skilled: indicates a higher level of care that is provided by professionals, such as sterile dressings by registered nurses or speech, physical, and occupational therapy services

Social Security Act of 1935: an act passed that provided coverage for underprivileged, jobless, aging Americans

Sustainable Growth Rate Formula: formula that helped determine how Medicare would pay physicians

system: a multihospital arrangement or a single-hospital system that also owns other services, such as a long-term care facility, an outpatient ambulatory surgical center, or ambulatory healthcare clinic

telemedicine: the use of telecommunication technology to support and promote long-distance clinical healthcare, such as healthcare provided through phone or video. Also called *telehealth*.

usual place of healthcare: Having an easily-accessible location with appropriate services provided, where rapport has been developed with the caregivers, and where the individual goes for healthcare needs regularly

wearable health technology: electronic devices that consumers can wear to collect data of their personal health and exercise

workers compensation insurance: provides medical expenses, lost wages, and rehabilitation costs to employees who are injured or become ill during the course of their work.

DEANNA HOWE BIOGRAPHY

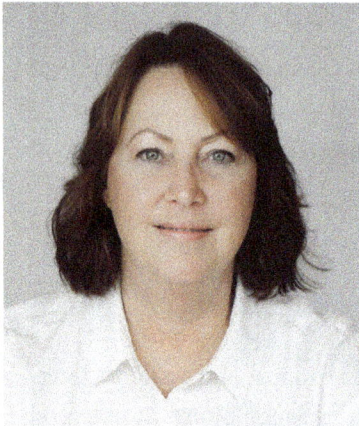

Dr. Deanna Howe has worked in healthcare since 1985 when she first entered the field as a medical technician in the Air Force. After active duty she began nursing school and initially graduated with an Associate of Science in Nursing degree. She continued with education while working in the field as a registered nurse and earned a BSN, MSN, and Ph.D. in nursing. Dr. Howe has worked in community health, public health, medical-surgical nursing, operating room and the last 16 years teaching nurses of the future. She teaches post-licensure and graduate courses from a distance as a full-time professor with Albany State University. Her research focus and writing to date has been on faculty experiences and satisfaction teaching online. She has lived and visited several countries, working with many different cultural groups, has been exposed to numerous unique health practices and experienced eastern and western health systems. Through these diverse experiences, she has developed a global point of view regarding healthcare. Dr. Howe currently lives in Germany with her husband and two dogs (Lucy and Beau) and has two grown children.

ANDREA DOZIER BIOGRAPHY

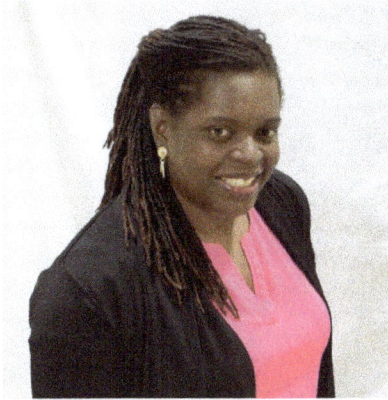

Dr. Andrea Lovett Dozier received her Associate of Science in Nursing degree from Darton State College, Bachelor of Science in Nursing from Georgia Southwestern State University, Master of Science in Nursing from Albany State University, and Doctorate in Curriculum and Instruction from Valdosta State University. She also received her Online Teaching Certification from Valdosta State University. Dr. Dozier has over 25 years of nursing experience and has been providing instruction in higher education for over 18 years. She is currently employed as an associate professor of nursing and currently serves at the Associate of Science in Nursing Programs Director at Albany State University. Her research interests include teacher efficacy, instructional methodologies, and course design in nursing education.

SHEREE DICKENSON BIOGRAPHY

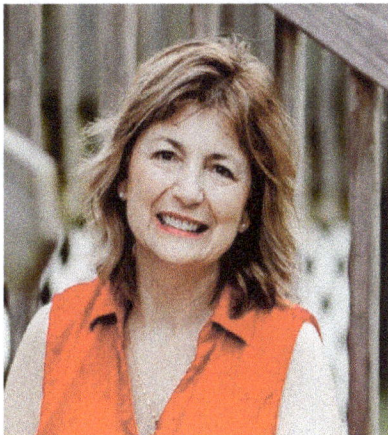

Dr. Sheree Dickenson received her undergraduate A.S.N. and B.S.N. degrees from Georgia Southwestern University, A M.S.N degree in Adult Health/Nursing Education from Valdosta State University, and an Ed.D. for nurse educators from The University of Alabama. She has recently accepted an adjunct nursing teaching position after over 40 years in nursing with the last more than 15 of those years teaching undergraduate nursing students. She has served on various boards and committees within the school, hospital, and community. Her research interests are clinical judgement of nursing students and the care and teaching of patients with diabetes mellitus.

www.ingramcontent.com/pod-product-compliance
Lightning Source LLC
Chambersburg PA
CBHW080231270326
41926CB00020B/4208